TEXBOOK *of* NATUROPATHIC

Family Medicine & Integrative Primary Care

TEXTBOOK *of* NATUROPATHIC

Family Medicine & Integrative Primary Care

SHEHAB EL-HASHEMY, MBCHB, ND

with
Martin Downorowicz, ND
Philip Rouchotas, MSc, ND
Jared Skowron, ND
Lorinda Sorenson, ND
Zeynep Uraz, ND
Alan Vu, ND

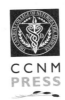

CCNM
PRESS

Dedication: This book is dedicated to my mentors and teachers at the Canadian College of Naturopathic Medicine, the many naturopathic physicians from whom I continue to learn, the dedicated cadre of primary care instructors of CLE 303 – and to my students for their feedback and critical thinking that undoubtedly shaped the evolution of this book.

Acknowledgments: The author would like to thank Dr Nick De Groot, BSc, ND, Dean of The Canadian College of Naturopathic Medicine (CCNM), for his ongoing support to this project; Dr Aubrey Rickford, BA, ND, former Associate Professor of Asian Medicine & Clinic Faculty at CCNM, for his valuable input in the Hypertension module; Dr Philip Rouchotas MSc, ND, Associate Professor of Clinical Nutrition at CCNM, for contributing to the Dyslipidemia module; Dr Martin Downorowicz, BSc, ND, for contributing to the Ophthalmology module; Dr Jared Skowron ND, Associate Professor of Pediatrics at the University of Bridgeport College of Naturopathic Medicine, for contributing to the Pediatrics module; Dr Lorinda Sorenson, ND, Associate Professor of Naturopathic Medicine at the National University of Health Sciences, for contributing to the Geriatrics module; Dr Zeynep Uraz, ND, Assistant Professor of Women's Health & Clinic Faculty at CCNM, for contributing to the Gynecology module; Dr Alan Vu, ND, for contributing to the Gynecology module; Dr Maria Shapoval, ND, for verifying references; and Bob Hilderley, Executive Director of CCNM Press, for his unwavering attention to detail in editing this manuscript.

Disclaimer: The medical and health information presented in this book is based on the research, training, and professional experience of the authors, and is true and complete to the best of their knowledge. However, this book is intended only as an informative guide for those wishing to know more about medicine and healthcare; it is not intended to replace or countermand the advice given by the reader's personal healthcare provider. The publisher and the authors are not responsible for any adverse effects of consequences from the use of information in this book. It is the responsibility of the reader to consult a qualified healthcare professional regarding personal care.

The author of this book has taken every effort to ensure that all information contained is accurate and complies with NABNE, AMA, and CMA guidelines and accepted standards at the time of publication. Due to the constantly changing nature of all medical sciences and the possibility of human error, the reader is encouraged to exercise clinical judgment and incorporate new information that becomes available with continuing research. In particular, the reader is advised to check the manufacturer's published monographs of all prescription and non-prescription agents (pharmacological, botanical, nutritional, and homeopathic) before administration.

ISBN-10:   1-897025-43-2
ISBN-13:   978-1-897025-43-7

Edited by Bob Hilderley.
Designed and typeset by Sari Naworynski.

Printed and bound in Canada.

Published by CCNM Press Inc., 1255 Sheppard Avenue East, Toronto, Ontario, Canada M2K 1E2 www.ccnmpress.com

CONTENTS

Acronyms & Abbreviations

Examination Boards & Licensing Bodies

MCCQE	Medical Council of Canada Qualifying Examination
MCC	Medical Council of Canada
NABNE	North American Board of Naturopathic Examiners
NBME	National Board of Medical Examiners
NPLEX	Naturopathic Physicians Licensing Examination
USMLE	United States Medical Licensing Examination

Regulatory & Professional Associations

AAFP	American Academy of Family Physicians
AAN	American Academy of Neurology
AANP	American Association of Naturopathic Physicians
AAO	American Academy of Ophthalmology
AAP	American Academy of Pediatrics
ACS	American Cancer Society
AHA	American Heart Association
AMA	American Medical Association
ATS	American Thoracic Society
BDDT-N	Board of Directors of Drugless Therapy - Naturopathy
BGS	British Geriatrics Society
BSAC	British Society for Antimicrobial Chemotherapy
CDA	Canadian Diabetes Association
CDC	Center for Disease Control and Prevention
CAND	Canadian Association of Naturopathic Doctors
CMA	Canadian Medical Association
CTFPHC	Canadian Task Force on Preventive Health Care
NKF	National Kidney Foundation
OAND	Ontario Association of Naturopathic Doctors
RCPSC	Royal College of Physicians and Surgeons of Canada
USPTSF	United States Preventive Services Task Force

Health Assessment

#	fracture
AAL	anterior axillary line
ABC	airway breathing circulation
Abx, Abc	antibiotics
ADLs	activities of daily living
AP	anteroposterior (imaging)
A&O x 4	alert & oriented to person, place, time, and date
A/O, A&O	alert and oriented
A&P	auscultation & percussion
Asx, ASX	asymptomatic
Ausc, auscul	auscultation
A&W	alive and well (in family Hx)
BP	blood pressure
CA	chronological age
CAD	coronary artery disease
C&A	conscious and alert
C&S	culture and sensitivity
CC, c/o	chief complaint, complains of
CKD	chronic kidney disease (previously termed CRF)
DOB, D/B	date of birth
DU	diagnosis undetermined
Dx, diag	diagnosis
DDX	differential diagnosis
Ex	examination
F	female
FH, FHx	family history
FOD	free of disease (in family Hx)
F/U, FU	follow up
FUO, FWS	fever of unknown source, fever without identifiable source
h/o	history of
H&P	history and physical
Ht, h	height
Hx, H	history
IADL	instrumental activities of daily living
IBW	ideal body weight
IPPA	inspection, palpation, percussion, auscultation
LRT	lower respiratory tract
LMP	last menstrual period
LMN	lower motor neuron
LWD	living with disease
M	male
MA	mental age
MCI	mild cognitive impairment
MHx, MH	medical history
MMSE	mini mental state examination
NAD	no apparent distress/disease, no acute distress, nothing abnormal detected
N/C, NC	no complaints
NED	no evidence of disease
NKA	no known allergies
NKDA	no known drug allergies
norm	normal
NVS	neurological vital signs
P	pulse
P&A, P/A	percussion and auscultation
palp	palpation
PE, PEx, PX	physical examination
PERRLA	pupils - equal, round, react to light & accommodation
PH	poor health
PMH, PMHx	past medical history
PMI	past medical illness, point of maximal impulse (cardio Ex)
PPHx	previous psychiatric history
Px, prog	prognosis
Pt	patient
R, RR	respiration, respiration rate
R/O, RO	rule out
ROS	review of systems
Rx	prescription
SOAP	subjective, objective assessment, plan
SONP	soft organs non palpable
S/S	signs & symptoms
Sx	symptoms
UT, UTI	urinary tract, urinary tract infection
T	temperature
TPR	temperature, pulse & respiration
Tx, tr, treat	treatment
UCD, UCHD	usual childhood diseases
U/O, UO	under observation
URT, URTI	upper respiratory tract, upper respiratory tract infection
UT, UTI	urinary tract, urinary tract infection (commonly refers to lower UTI)
VS, v/s	vital signs
WDWN	well developed well nourished, well dressed well nourished
WNL	within normal limits
Wt	weight
X&D	examination and diagnosis
y, yr	year
y/o	years old

The principle objective of this textbook is to provide senior medical students, new practitioners, and retraining medical professionals with an introduction to the discipline of naturopathic primary care in a family practice setting. Naturopathic primary care is a developing field of study and discipline of practice now in the process of establishing best practice standards and guidelines based on random controlled trials and empirical evidence.

As a discipline of family medicine, primary care is sanctioned by almost all naturopathic regulatory boards and thoroughly examined in the Naturopathic Physician Licensing Examination Step Two (NPLEx II). This book can be used to prepare for these board examinations; in fact, each module in the book is designed to answer a series of questions derived not only from NPLEx II, but also from the United States Medical Licensing Exam II (USMLE II) and the Medical Council of Canada Qualifying Examination (MCCQE) board exams, thus integrating naturopathic standards of practice with conventional medical and surgical guidelines.

By providing a bridge between conventional and alternative medicine, naturopathic doctors are carving a niche for themselves as healthcare professionals capable of integrating these medical traditions. That is why a considerable effort has been made to present naturopathic primary care standards in conjunction with those of the American Medical Association and the Canadian Medical Association.

Primary care and family medicine are best taught using practice-based learning techniques in the clinic with real patients, but clinical reasoning and problem-solving skills can be taught effectively in the classroom using didactic, Socratic, and case-based questions. Problem solving involves looking for many possible solutions under the circumstances and empowering the patient to choose the best of several options. This book is designed to expand these problem-solving skills beyond symptom recognition and differential diagnosis to arrive at a reasoned assessment and case management plan. Each module is, in fact, structured in imitation of SOAP charting standards so that this pattern of reasoning is reinforced. Socratic and case-based questions provide the opportunity to test clinical reasoning skills before being applied in the clinic.

There is no pretense here of being comprehensive; instead, the book is selective, a primer focusing on the most common conditions seen in day-to-day family practice. The book is an educational tool, designed to teach clinical reasoning, not a complete reference, to be memorized. The book is also dynamic, not final. New research will demand new standards of practice and clinical guidelines, in turn requiring revision of this text even as it is being read. We welcome your participation in this ongoing project. Please contact us at the publisher's website (www.ccnmpress.com).

STANDARDS AND GUIDELINES

Evidence-Based Medicine

Clinical Standards of Practice

Charting Guidelines

Standard Diagnostic Tests

Evidence Quality and Test Validity

The philosophy of naturopathy can be traced to the era of Hippocrates (460-377 BCE). However, the concept of curing illness via natural means was developed further as a result of newfound interest during the 18th and 19th centuries when practitioners such as Vinzenz Priessnitz (1799-1851) and Sebastian Kneipp (1821-1897) established comprehensive hydrotherapeutic interventions to cure many health conditions. The principles and practice of this *Naturheilkunde* (German) were subsequently introduced to the United States by Kniepp's protégé, Benedict Lust (1870-1945), who coined the term naturopathy.

Naturopathic medicine embraces the belief that health is influenced by each individual's inherent healing ability (*vis medicatrix naturae*). In this paradigm, disease is viewed empirically as a direct result of ignoring or violating the general principles of health. Historically, these principles have been defined as comprising internal and external environments. Traditional naturopathic practitioners thus aimed to correct and stabilize these environments as primary interventions to ward off disease.

From a technical perspective, modern naturopathy or *Naturheilverfahren* can be defined as an eclectic system of healthcare, which integrates elements of alternative and conventional medicine to support and enhance self-healing processes. The different therapeutic interventions and modalities vary according to the jurisdiction of practice, but generally include the historical crafts of herbal or botanical medicine, hydrotherapy, dietetics, exercise, and meditation. In some jurisdictions, the practice also includes clinical nutrition, homeopathy, spinal manipulation, iridology, acupuncture, pharmacotherapy, minor surgery, life-style counseling, and traditional Chinese medicine.

Naturopathic medicine has been described as a science and an art. Proponents of evidence-based practices argue that in cases where unbiased evidence exists, science should prevail. Clinical practice is also an art, attending to characteristics of individual human beings. Naturopathic medicine takes into account individual attributes in the context of available evidence.

To a large extent, contemporary naturopathic practitioners have shored-up traditional naturopathic empiricism with the principles of evidence-based medicine to diagnose and manage health conditions. Evidence-based medicine (EBM) can be contextually defined as "an approach to practicing medicine in which the clinician is aware of the evidence in support of clinical practice and the strength of that evidence."

> To a large extent, contemporary naturopathic practitioners have shored-up traditional naturopathic empiricism with the principles of evidence-based medicine to diagnose and manage health conditions.

Evidence-based care combines (1) the best available external evidence, (2) the naturopathic doctor's clinical expertise, and (3) the patient's preferences when making decisions about their healthcare.

1. EXTERNAL EVIDENCE

EBM practices translate into adopting the habit of making selective, efficient, patient-centered "searches" for evidence and then incorporating quality findings into everyday practice.

In the not so distant past, decision making at the level of the primary-care physician was based on recalling a memorized algorithm or part of a didactic lecture. One simply practiced the way one was taught. Views regarding disease processes, diagnostic beliefs, and treatment expectations took generations to evolve. However, in our era of rapid global information exchange, the revision of traditional practices and expectations is occurring at an accelerated pace.

- Should I prescribe *Hypericum perforatum* for severe depression?
- What about S-Adenosyl-Methionine with bipolar II disorder?
- Can hypertensive patients safely stop their medications if they modify their lifestyle?
- Can dietary measures outperform pharmacological agents as primary interventions for hypercholesterolemia? What about diabetes?
- What could an abnormal laboratory test result mean?
- What is a relevant and complete physical examination of a case of frequent sore throats?
- What type of diet induces remission in an IBD flare up?
- Should I recommend vitamin E for patients with atherosclerosis?
- Am I obligated to report infectious diseases to public health? What about adverse reactions?
- Should I stop prescribing L-Arginine for peripheral vascular insufficiency?
- What is the side effect profile of natural hormone replacement?
- Can the calcium and vitamin D supplements I prescribed increase my patient's risk of heart attack?
- Would any of the above issues affect the way I obtain informed consent in my practice?

Standards and guidelines that once answered such questions change, ever so quickly. At any given time, there are approximately 44,000 clinical trials being conducted, which fuel the generation of some 700 monthly systematic reviews in peer reviewed journals that ultimately affect current practices in conventional, complementary, and alternative medicine. To complicate matters further, many reputable organizations, regulatory bodies, professional societies, advisory panels, and government-appointed task forces issue evidence-based guidelines for the practice of family medicine and primary care.

External evidence includes research from the basic sciences and, in particular, patient-centered clinical research into the accuracy of diagnostic tests (including the clinical examination), the markers used for making prognoses, and the effectiveness and safety of treatments, whether for therapy, prevention, or rehabilitation. This external clinical evidence may invalidate previously accepted practices and replace them with new ones that are safer and more effective, with better outcomes.

External evidence is based on verified research information on specific cohorts of patients. Selection criteria for entry into these research studies are often rigid. By design, these clinical trials can only analyze a fraction of a problem or situation that may exist in clinical practice. Conclusions relating to trial cohorts are assumed to hold true for other cohorts that appear to be similar. For example, a particular patient in your practice may exhibit multiple pathologies that render her unlike any other patient in published studies. Is the available "evidence" valid for that particular patient? There is no means to know the answer for certain, only a means of deducing one empirically.

2. CLINICAL EXPERTISE

External clinical evidence can inform but never replace clinical expertise. This expertise even decides whether the external evidence is relevant to the patient at all. To illustrate this point, consider that only 20% to 37% of conventional medical practices are indeed evidence based (Imrie, 2002). The balance of accepted medical practices are based on empiricism. This is the process of learning from daily observation and experimentation rather than theory (for example, give aspirin and observe effect on reported headache) via inductive philosophy (conclude that aspirin relieves headaches). Such empirical knowledge passes from one generation of physician educators to the next. Through this process, the knowledge is upheld, refined, or altogether rejected by the next generation. The traditional Chinese medical doctrine is an example of the empiricist school of thought.

Rather than embarking on the impossible task of reading every report on every medical advance, the doctor interested in EBM learns to be more focused. EBM practices translate into adopting the habit of making selective, efficient, patient-centered "searches" for evidence and then incorporating quality findings into everyday practice.

The clinician also needs to be conscious of the limitations and possible dangers of following external evidence slavishly. For example, the use of intravenous diuretics in acute pulmonary edema has evolved without any formal randomized controlled trial evidence because the application of a trial comparing such intervention with a placebo would be considered unethical. In this case, ignoring clearly successful interventions because of lack of randomized controlled trial (RCT) evidence would simply be illogical. In addition, collating evidence for uncommon conditions (or side effects) is difficult and may not allow for adequate analysis (think Cox II inhibitors). Though EBM-friendly evidence is important, the limitations of adopting austere approaches must be recognized.

Many naturopathic or complementary and alternative medicine (CAM) interventions are difficult to blind or have no satisfactory placebos because they rely on "complex effects" that are a crucial part of the healing process (Kleijnen, 1994). Ted Kaptchuk, author of *The Web that Has No Weaver* and research fellow at Harvard's Center for Alternative Medicine Research, suggests that the most important role for CAM could be to bring these effects into the forefront of medicine. Randomized controlled trials attempt to cancel out variable factors, such as the therapeutic setting, the personality of the therapist, the amount of time given to patients, and even the very words spoken to them. Instead of being hidden within the placebo arm, these should be disentangled and systematically studied so that their therapeutic benefits can be harnessed by all involved in the provision of health care. It follows that the art of both conventional and complementary medicine and the "complexity of caring" is difficult but not impossible to study.

3. PATIENT'S PREFERENCES

> Naturopathic best practices can be defined as a merger between a rich body of empirical knowledge, clinician expertise, good quality external evidence, and preferences of patients to arrive consistently at appropriate management plans.

Patient preference is paramount to the concept of patient-centered care and yields to individualized management plans that foster compliance. For example, your expertise may lead you to believe that acupuncture will most likely relieve a particular patient's sub-acute low back pain. If this patient is afraid of needles or simply does not prefer this approach, he will likely not comply with the treatment plan. In practice, patients may not volunteer their preference – and the therapeutic relationship may ultimately suffer. Where comparable options (this applies to evaluation and treatment) exist, it is imperative to incorporate your patient's unique preferences to inspire compliance and collaborative responsibility.

It follows that naturopathic best practices can be defined as a merger between a rich body of empirical knowledge, clinician expertise, good quality external evidence, and preferences of patients to arrive consistently at appropriate management plans.

PROBLEM-BASED LEARNING

Evidence-based medicine is an active process that enhances the physician's expertise. This process involves five steps:

1. Identifying a clinical question or need for inquiry.
2. Efficiently tracking down the best evidence with which to answer the question.
3. Critically appraising the evidence for validity and ability to withstand scrutiny.
4. Applying the results in clinical practice.
5. Evaluating performance of the evidence in clinical applications.

EVOLVING STANDARDS AND GUIDELINES

From this nexus of external evidence, clinical expertise, and patient preference, standards and guidelines for best practices of naturopathic medicine have been established. The strength of naturopathic medicine has been in chronic care management and longer-term solutions, but increasingly the naturopathic physician is taking on the role of primary care giver in a family medicine setting. Although naturopathic family medicine lacks such publications as *Current Practice Guidelines in Primary Care*, and naturopathic standards are not fully catalogued in the National Guidelines Clearing House, a body of standards has grown within the profession. In many cases, diagnostic test procedures and screening guidelines are shared with other healthcare professionals. These shared guidelines are featured in Part 1 of this book. Where naturopathic medicine shines is in case management, offering more options to the patient than conventional medical and surgical solutions. These case management guidelines are featured in Part 2 of this book.

Standard Bearers

A growing number of licensing bodies, regulatory and professional associations, refereed journals and accredited data bases are involved in disseminating information on naturopathic medical standards of practice. The principal standard bearers are three licensing boards: the Naturopathic Physicians Licensing Examination (NPLEX), the United States Medical Licensing Examination (USMLE), and the Medical Council of Canada Qualifying Examination (MCCQE). Also involved are guideline-generating international and national medical associations, such as the World Health Organization, Center for Disease Control, US Preventive Health Services Task Force, Canadian Diabetes Association, as well as evidence-based trials, literature reviews, and expert opinion.

RECOMMENDED EBM SOURCES OF NATUROPATHIC STANDARDS OF PRACTICE

Examination Boards & Licensing Bodies

MCCQE	Medical Council of Canada Qualifying Examination
MCC	Medical Council of Canada
NABNE	North American Board of Naturopathic Examiners
NBME	National Board of Medical Examiners
NPLEX	Naturopathic Physicians Licensing Examination
USMLE	United States Medical Licensing Examination

Regulatory & Professional Associations

AAFP	American Academy of Family Physicians
AAN	American Academy of Neurology

AANP	American Association of Naturopathic Physicians
AAO	American Academy of Ophthalmology
AAP	American Academy of Pediatrics
ACS	American Cancer Society
AHA	American Heart Association
AMA	American Medical Association
ATS	American Thoracic Society
BDDT-N	Board of Directors of Drugless Therapy - Naturopathy
BGS	British Geriatrics Society
BSAC	British Society for Antimicrobial Chemotherapy
CDA	Canadian Diabetes Association
CDC	Center for Disease Control and Prevention
CAND	Canadian Association of Naturopathic Doctors
CMA	Canadian Medical Association
CTFPHC	Canadian Task Force on Preventive Health Care
NKF	National Kidney Foundation
OAND	Ontario Association of Naturopathic Doctors
RCPSC	Royal College of Physicians and Surgeons of Canada
USPTSF	United States Preventive Services Task Force

REFEREED JOURNALS AND DATA BASES

ACUBRIEFS

http://www.acubriefs.com

Acubriefs was established and is supported by a grant from the Medical Acupuncture Research Foundation (MARF). Its purpose is to make the most comprehensive database of English language references on acupuncture available online. Access to the database is free.

AMED: Allied and Complementary Medicine Database

http://www.bl.uk/reshelp/findhelpsubject/scitectenv/medicine-healthamed/amed.html

Compiled by the British Library, AMED is a literature database, in the English language, in the field of allied and alternative medicine. It offers information from different countries, especially from Europe. The database contains bibliographic data, keywords, and abstracts since 1985. Subjects covered: Acupuncture, homeopathy, hypnosis, chiropractic, osteopathy, rehabilitation, herbalism, holistic treatments, Chinese medicine, occupational therapy, physiotherapy, podiatry.

Agency for Healthcare Research and Quality (AHRQ)
http://www.ahrq.gov
The Agency for Healthcare Research and Quality (AHRQ) produces a range of publications and electronic information products that are available to users through different channels and a variety of formats. This is a well-sourced database of Clinical Information, Evidence-based Practice, Outcomes & Effectiveness, Technology Assessment, Preventive Services, and Clinical Practice Guidelines.

American Indian Ethnobotany Database
http://herb.umd.umich.edu/
Subjects covered: Foods, drugs, dyes and fibers of native North American peoples.

ARCAM and CAMPAIN
http://www.umm.edu/altmed/
The Center for Integrative Medicine at the University of Maryland has developed, and regularly updates, two bibliographic databases: The Arthritis and Complementary Medicine Database (ARCAM) and the Complementary and Alternative Medicine and Pain Database (CAMPAIN). These databases are compiled from regular comprehensive electronic and hand searches of scientific literature sources world-wide. The Cochrane CM register is searchable here as well. Access is free.

Biomed Central
http://www.biomedcentral.com/
Over 100 OPEN ACESS journals covering all areas of biology as well as conventional and complementary medicine (free).

CABI - CAB ABSTRACTS
http://www.cabi.org/

AbstractDatabases.asp?SubjectArea=&PID=125
Subjects covered: Human health and nutrition, animal sciences and veterinary medicine, plant and agricultural sciences, and the management and conservation of natural resources. More than 9,000 serial journals in more than 50 languages are scanned, as well as books, reports, and other publications.

CAMLINE
www.camline.org/
Canadian website on evidence-based CAM.

CAM on PubMed
www.nih.gov/nccam/camonpubmed.html
The National Centre for Complementary and Alternative Medicine (NCCAM) and the National Library of Medicine (NLM) have partnered to create CAM on PubMed, a subset of NLM's PubMed.

Chalmers Research Group
http://www.chalmersresearch.com/epi6188/CAMdbs.pdf
Databases with CAM content from the Chalmers Research Group, Children's Hospital of Eastern Ontario Research Institute.

CINAHL
http://www.cinahl.com/
CINAHL contains references to journal articles, healthcare books, nursing dissertations, selected conference proceedings, standards of professional practice, educational software and audiovisual materials in nursing. Subjects covered: Nursing and allied health.

Cochrane Library – including Cochrane Collaboration CM Field
http://www.cochrane.org
http://www.compmed.umm.edu/Cochrane/
The Cochrane Library consists of a regularly updated collection of evidence-based medicine databases, including The Cochrane Database of Systematic Reviews. The systematic reviews provide high quality information to people providing and receiving healthcare, and those responsible for research, teaching, funding and administration at all levels.

FreeMedicalJournals.com
http://www.freemedicaljournals.com/
The Free Medical Journals Site was created to promote the availability of full text medical journals on the Internet.

Global Health
http://www.cabdirect.org/
CAB HEALTH brings together the resources of the Public Health and Tropical Medicine (PHTM) database and the human health and diseases information extracted from CAB ABSTRACTS since 1973. It contains foreign language journals, books, research reports, patents and standards, dissertations, conference proceedings, annual reports, public health, developing country information, and other difficult to obtain material. Subjects covered: communicable diseases (including HIV/AIDS), tropical diseases, parasitic diseases and parasitology, human nutrition, community and public health, and medicinal and poisonous plants.

HerbMed
http://www.herbmed.org
HerbMed, produced by the nonprofit Alternative Medicine Foundation, is a categorized, evidence-based resource for herbal information. It includes

hyperlinks to clinical and scientific publications and dynamic links for automatic updating.

Herb Research Foundation
http://www.herbs.org/index.html
HRF provides a search service from their specialty research library containing more than 300,000 scientific articles on thousands of herbs.

Hom-Inform
http://www.hom.inform.soutron.net/Catalogues/Search.aspx
Hom-Inform is a database of literature references to homoeopathy, with key terms and some abstracts, provided by the British Homeopathic Library.

IBIDS
http://ods.od.nih.gov/Health_Information/IBIDS.aspx
International Bibliographic Information on Dietary Supplements (IBIDS) is produced by the Office of Dietary Supplements at the National Institutes of Health. It is a database of published, international, scientific literature on dietary supplements, including vitamins, minerals, and botanicals.

MANTIS
http://www.healthindex.com
Manual, Alternative and Natural Therapy is a database for healthcare disciplines not covered by major biomedical databases. The MANTIS Database is a sizable source of osteopathic, chiropractic, and manual medical literature.

Natural Standard
http://www.naturalstandard.com
Natural Standard is a database founded by clinicians and researchers to provide high quality, evidence-based information about complementary and alternative therapies. It is primarily oriented to clinicians and pharmacists. Subjects covered: Alternative and complementary medicine.

Phytobase
http://www.gamed.or.at/archiv/bm/informationsdienste/phyto.htm
Phytobase is a database of literature on toxicology, pharmacology (pharmacodynamics, pharmacokinetics), therapeutic uses for natural compounds, and isolation of natural compounds from plant material. Phytobase indexes 140 scientific journals published worldwide and currently includes approximately 20,000 records from 7,800 publications. The language of the database is German.

PsycINFO
http://www.apa.org/pubs/databases/psycinfo/index.aspx
PsycINFO includes journal articles, books, book chapters, dissertations, and government reports in professional and academic literature in psychology and related disciplines. Subjects covered: medicine, psychiatry, nursing, sociology, education, pharmacology, physiology, linguistics and other areas.

PubMed
http://www.pubmed.org
National Library of Medicine's search interface to access the 10 million citations in MEDLINE, Pre-MEDLINE, and other related databases.

The Chinese Medicine Database
http://www.cm-db.com/
Offers translation of classical chinese medicine texts as well as a searchable database of single herb monographs and herbal formulas.

The Richard and Hinda Rosenthal Center for Complementary and Alternative Medicine
http://www.rosenthal.hs.columbia.edu
Founded in 1993, this center builds bridges between diverse therapeutic traditions and modern medicine.

The Research Council for Complementary Medicine
http://www.rccm.org.uk/static/Links_CAM_databases.aspx?m=11

Tropical Plant Database
http://rain-tree.com/plants.htm
Each plant file contains taxonomy data, phytochemical and ethnobotanical data, uses in traditional medicine, and clinical research from Raintree Nutrition, Inc, Austin, Texas.

SCOPE OF PRACTICE

Various naturopathic medical regulatory boards have defined primary care practice by distinguishing its scope from co-treatment and consulting treatment. For example, the regulatory board of naturopathic medicine in Ontario (BDDTN, 2004) defines these three practices provided by naturopathic physicians as follows:

- **Primary Care Management:** The "provision of patient's overall healthcare management including the monitoring of all treatments in progress with other providers as appropriate."
- **Co-treatment:** The "treatment of a patient in concert with the doctor providing primary care management of the patient."
- **Consulting Treatment:** The provision of "a second opinion or ancillary care for a patient whose primary care management is being provided by another doctor."

Among these three scopes of practice, naturopathic physicians have traditionally concentrated on co-treatment and consulting treatment, often foregoing primary care management either due to lack of familiarity with the legal requisites of primary care practice or failure to receive adequate academic training and clinical mentorship. This book addresses these issues, helping naturopathic medical students and practitioners to add requisite primary care competencies to their repertoire of services.

BASIC AND CASE-SPECIFIC SOPS

Naturopathic doctors in most regulated jurisdictions are expected to adhere to published standards of practice (SOPs) that outline aspects of care delivery and service to the patient and community.

These standards of practice serve two major functions: they identify the responsibilities and scope of practice of naturopathic doctors, and they are used in disciplinary and judicial functions to evaluate the actions of naturopathic doctors. The two types of standards that apply to licensed naturopathic doctors are either Basic or Case Specific SOPs.

Basic Standards of Practice

Regardless of the scope of practice of the naturopathic doctor (primary care, co-treatment, or consulting treatment), the following standards are considered basic:

The naturopathic doctor will …

Naturopathic doctors must comply with local and regional laws in the conduct of their practice.

1. Have knowledge of and comply with the laws and regulations governing the practice of naturopathic medicine in the jurisdiction of practice.
2. Provide a level of care consistent with each patient's individual condition.
3. Actively consult and/or refer as appropriate to other health professionals when the patient condition so warrants.
4. Treat each patient with respect and human dignity regardless of the individual's health condition, personal attribute, national origin, handicap, age, sex, race, religion, socioeconomic status, or sexual preference.
5. Respect the patient's right to privacy by protecting all confidential information.
6. Deal honestly with all patients, colleagues, public institutions, and legal bodies, and refrain from giving any false, incomplete, or misleading information.
7. Report any healthcare provider whose character or competences are deficient or who is grossly negligent or reckless.
8. Maintain clear and adequate patient-care and billing records for at least 7 years after the patient's last visit.
9. Formulate an assessment/diagnosis to a level consistent with the patient based on knowledge, training, and expertise of the naturopathic doctor and the technology and tools available to the profession.
10. Advise the patient regarding significant side effects from the treatment plan.
11. Monitor each patient at a level consistent with the degree of management being exercised.
12. Refrain from providing primary care management for any patient where the relationship with the patient (such as family member, close personal friend) would serve to interfere with the doctor's objective judgment.

Case Specific Standards of Practice

The following case-specific standards are considered a guide for the development of standards for particular incidents or presentations:

1. The scope of the doctor's practice (primary care management, co-treatment, consulting treatment, or expert testimony) shall be identified.
2. The scope of the problem (complaint, specific naturopathic medical modality) and all other pertinent data, such as history and diagnosis shall be identified.

3. The body of knowledge to be used in assessing the problem shall be identified.
4. All management plans should address the entirety of the presenting condition.
5. Diagnosis should be derived from an appropriate body of knowledge that is applicable to the problem, with no possibility of conclusions being drawn out of context.
   - Sources of information used to derive management decisions must be generally accepted by the naturopathic profession.
   - Universally acceptable sources of information include textbooks, journals, information taught in naturopathic medical schools, and recognized expert opinions in the naturopathic community or in the specialty area in question.
   - As with other all other healthcare professions, reliable information sources, expert opinions, and testimony from outside the naturopathic profession are also acceptable.
6. When required, regulatory bodies shall render disciplinary and/or judicial decisions to ensure:
   - Protection of the public and the public interest from risks of physical or mental harm, misrepresentation, inappropriate billing not consistent with fair and accepted practices, full disclosure of treatment and its effects, appropriateness of referral, etc.
   - Compliance with all applicable laws.

UNIFYING IDEALS OF PRIMARY CARE PROFESSIONALS

In addition to these standards, almost all healthcare professionals engaged in rendering primary care services (medical doctors, naturopathic doctors, nurse practitioners, and extended care nurses) agree on the following guiding principles of conduct:

1. Will be committed to wellness and the prevention of disease.
2. Will acquire and apply good knowledge of local community services.
3. Will collaborate with other health providers for the benefit of their community.
4. Will advocate for public policy to promote health.
5. Will promote continuity of patient care and respect patient-physician relationships.

They also agree upon a basic level of competency for primary care practitioners:

1. Will be able to recognize importance of diagnosis of serious life-threatening illnesses.
2. Will be able to diagnose and manage diseases common to their community.

WHEN SHOULD NATUROPATHIC DOCTORS REFRAIN FROM PROVIDING PRIMARY CARE SERVICES?

The following standards of practice were adopted by the Ontario regulatory body of naturopathic medicine in 2004. Although these guidelines are considered universal by most practitioners, the reader is advised to review local or regional standards of practice for clarification.

The naturopathic doctor will refer and/or seek consultation when …

1. A life-threatening situation occurs or is suspected.
2. Diagnosis or treatment is not within the scope of naturopathic practice.
3. Diagnosis is required but cannot be confirmed with the training and technology available to the naturopathic doctor.
4. Treatment requires expertise or technology not available to the naturopathic doctor.
5. Response to treatment is not adequate or the patient's condition deteriorates.
6. Second opinion is desired.

REFERRALS AND CONSULTATIONS IN PRIMARY CARE

Primary care practitioners will commonly refer their patients to or seek advice from other healthcare providers.

Common reasons for consultations and referrals
- Advice (on diagnosis or treatment, for medicolegal purposes)
- Specialized evaluation skill (specialized laboratory tests, specialist scope of practice, mental health evaluation)
- Specialized treatment skill (specialized treatment, failed treatment approach, mental health counseling)
- Patient or third-party request (regulatory body standards, insurance guidelines)

Referrals

A referral is request that another healthcare provider accept the ongoing treatment of a patient. It implies that the accepting provider will be independently and continuously managing at least one significant health problem a patient may exhibit.

Consultations

In contrast, a consultation is a request for management guidance from another healthcare provider. It implies that the primary care provider will receive advice on diagnosis and management, but will retain decision-making and con-

> Primary care practitioners will commonly refer their patients to or seek advice from other healthcare providers.

tinuity of care obligations. Consultations may be informal (a.k.a. curbside consultations) or formal where patients are sent to other providers for in-depth evaluation.

Formal Consultation Requests

In order to respond to a presenting question, the consultant should be supplied with adequate, relevant, and succinct patient information. A good formal consultation request is based on the following criteria:

- Name and age
- Summary of current concern
- Related health history
- List of medications
- Summary of pertinent family and social history
- Summary of related physical findings
- Results of any diagnostic tests
- Results of previous consultations with clear specifications of the:
  1. Question that you need answered; or
  2. Problem that you wish to have evaluated; or
  3. Aspect that you want to be treated.
- Urgency of response
- Any patient's preferences or values that may affect the response.

> The consultant should be supplied with adequate, relevant, and succinct patient information.

Formal Consultant's Reports

Ideally, consultant or specialist reports should include:

- Purpose of consultation as understood by the consultant
- Findings of the consultant's history and physical exam
- Results of any diagnostic tests
- Any treatment provided
- Patient's response to any treatment
- Consultant's assessment or opinion regarding the topic of consultation
- Further treatment recommended
- Further consultations recommended
- Urgency of recommendations
- Summary of instructions given to the patient
- Concluding statement regarding whether consultation is considered complete or consultant's desire to see the patient in the future

Coordination of Care

During consultations or referrals to specialists, the primary care provider must coordinate the patient's care to avoid delays in treatment (falling through the cracks), iatrogenic morbidity, duplication of effort, waste of financial resources, needless tests, and risk of litigation. When several providers are involved in a specific patient's care, someone has to be clearly in charge of coordination (usually the primary care provider). This coordinator must document and follow up on all communications with consultants and secondary care providers.

STRUCTURE OF ENCOUNTERS IN PRIMARY CARE SETTINGS

In primary care settings, the chief task of the physician is to establish a management plan promptly that is appropriate for the resolution of the present complaint (that is, figure out what is going on then acting accordingly). The structure of the encounter is a systematic task list that enables the physician to obtain a story that ultimately leads to proper assessment, treatment, and follow-up.

Many students and perhaps a few practitioners express concern that time constraints of daily practice are not conducive for gathering a "complete" history, ordering a "complete" battery of laboratory evaluations, and performing "head-to toe" physical examinations before implementing a treatment plan. Indeed, part of succeeding in a primary care practice depends on your ability to work within operational constraints, such as reasonable visit durations and cost. In other words, if someone comes to you concerned about bloody diarrhea, you must be able to formulate an effective management plan by the end of the patient's encounter. Below we shall discuss strategies that will enable you to become comfortable with diagnostic uncertainty and provide such time-sensitive, cost-effective, safe, and effective treatment plans within typical and realistic practice parameters.

In private practice, you will rarely have more than 30-40 minutes to do a history and physical. Thus, every question or item on your physical exam has to count. The true clinical challenge for the naturopathic doctor is to ask those questions and do those items on a physical examination that will most directly and effectively sort out likely hypotheses, and screen for impairment in related organs or systems that might reasonably be involved. During follow-up visits, a complete understanding of the patient's story can be obtained.

Acute versus Chronic Presentations

In acute presentations, a more focused approach is required since one is often faced with time sensitive decisions that have to be made (for example, starting rehydration therapy, prescribing provisional treatments, ordering diagnostic tests, consulting with specialists, or sending the patient to the emergency department). Once this complaint-oriented approach is completed, the physician adopts an efficient management plan and can proceed into obtaining a more complete historical database, filling-in the gaps, addressing secondary concerns, and engaging in preventive healthcare, which, in turn, will lead to better patient care.

In primary care settings, the chief task of the physician is promptly to establish a management plan that is appropriate for the resolution of the present complaint.

Data Gathering Methods

At the student level, the following time-honored sequential data-gathering format represents the launching pad for problem solving:

Biographical data → Source and reliability → Reason for seeking care → Present health or history of present illness → Past health history → Family history → Review of systems → Functional assessment → Physical examination

Experienced problem solvers, however, collect required information in a fluid and efficient conversational format that varies considerably depending on the patient's chief concerns. They tend to focus on specific problems, recognize patterns, synthesize provisional impressions, ask questions with high sensitivity (to exclude suspicions) and specificity (to support suspicions), and gather relevant data. In this fashion, the diagnostic reasoning process dictates the format of the doctor-patient interaction. In other words, knowledge of disease processes, clinical reasoning, and evidence-based management guidelines allow problem solvers to identify quickly the underlying cause of illness within the time constrains of daily practice.

Data Gathering Forms

A number of data gathering forms are used routinely in primary care practice, including the following:
* Basic and Advanced Health Assessment
* Physical Exam Checklist
* Functional Assessment
* Past Medical History (PMH)
* Family History (FH)
* Social History (SH)
* Review of Systems (ROS)
* Cognitive Status Examination
* Depression Questionnaire
* CAGE Questionnaire

TASK LIST

Regardless of your choice of data-gathering or data-recording format, the level of competency required of primary-care physicians with regards to episodic interactions can be defined as follows:

1. Identify important cues in the patient's story (Basic Health Assessment):
* Demographic information (gender, age, occupation, residence)
* Symptom analysis

- Functional assessment
- Patient's belief or understanding of their symptoms (and impact on their daily life, family members, and lifestyle)
- Routine vital signs (temperature, pulse, heart rate, blood pressure, weight, height, last menses, smoking status, and recreational drug use)

2. Understand and perform Advanced Health Assessment techniques:
This process focuses on constructing management plans based on "best evidence" that will leave little doubt in the problem-solver's mind:
- Determine what additional questions need to be asked.
- Ask complaint-specific questions to assess patient's risk for certain differential diagnoses.
- Determine what needs to be examined.
- Perform physical examination maneuvers that are suggested by the chief complaint.
- Perform physical examinations appropriately.
- Make selective observation of fine detail during physical examination.
- Selectively requisition high yield (or gold standard) diagnostic/laboratory work-ups.

3. Apply clinical reasoning to test differential or competing diagnoses:
- Identify presenting patterns in light of the doctor's knowledge of known presentations.
- Identify absence of findings that are "sensitive" markers of certain conditions (use a "rule-out" strategy).
- Identify presence of findings that are "specific" markers for certain conditions.
- Recognize your own diagnostic limitations if any, and involve other practitioners in the evaluation plan when indicated.

4. Manage the presentation:
- Discuss diagnostic impression and available treatment options with the patient in order to empower them to choose an effective and practical treatment option.
- Design follow-up plans to ensure resolution of condition and compliance of patient with treatment plan.
- Revise diagnostic hypotheses based on patient's response to initial treatment (no matter how confident you are in your diagnosis, no theory is beyond the threat of disproof).
- Coordinate care and disseminate of information among healthcare providers within the patient's circle-of-care.

The use of data-gathering forms, electronic and printed, is on the rise. However, no form can capture the skill of an experienced primary care provider.

Initial Visit Plan

The duration of a visit varies according to the physician's practice style and level of experience, but similar topics need to be covered. Adjust these time-lines to fit your visitation style.

Time	Duration	Topics
9:00-9:05	5 minutes	Agenda setting, rapport building. Identify patient's goals and motivations, state your goals
9:05-9:35	30 minutes	Interacting time: HPI, focused history, function inquiry, critical ROS, P/E that cannot wait till future visits
9:35 - 9:45	10 minutes	Assembling information and consultation with clinical supervisor
9:45-9:50	5 minutes	Management planning, scheduling next meeting, and closing
9:50 - 10:00	10 minutes	Tidy room if needed, finalize chart, gather equipment and belongings, put away linens, capture last thoughts on patient visit, "self-care", and prep for next patient

Conduct of a First Visit

Now that the objectives of the visit are clear, it helps to place them in the pragmatic context of daily practice. Visits that end well require planning and time-management. From this practical perspective, a primary care outpatient visit with an ND can be described as:

1. Conversation with a purpose (establish trust + gather information + offer information)
2. Action with a purpose (objective evaluation + therapeutic management)
3. Encounter of a predetermined duration

Goals for the Visit

The goals and agendas of the patient, the physician, the institution, and the attending supervisor need to be acknowledged by all bodies to ensure clear communication and no cross-purposes.

- **Patient-centered goals:** seeking relief from suffering, asking for a medical opinion, looking for answers to questions, just wanting to talk
- **Physician-centered goals:** charting history, completing questionnaires, asking particular questions, performing scheduled P/E, requesting labs, explaining your "way of doing things"
- **Institution-centered goals:** completing particular intake forms, signing of consent forms, opening files, or completing patient-centered forms such as Measure Your Medical Outcome Profile (MYMOPs)
- **Attending supervisor-centered goals:** monitoring standing practices and guidelines and the institution's "way of doing things"

Time Management

To provide effective, efficient and humane primary care in a naturopathic setting, physicians must be conscious of the time constraints of a typical office visit and work within these limitations. Running over time may be good for the patient currently in your examination room but not for your patient still in the waiting room. Patients and doctors are left feeling rushed, dissatisfied, or even frustrated at closing. Patients may have obligations and events scheduled after the visit and doctors. Interns may have visits booked back to back.

Failed Visit

Not all visits end well. Here are the most commonly cited reasons associated with a difficult or undesirable ending of an initial primary care visit along with some suggestions for improving the outcome.

1. Patient has many concerns, issues, or questions. You may want to capture these at the outset where possible, acknowledge that you will not be able to address all issues in one office visit, and table less critical issues for future visits.
2. Patient is enjoying talking to you and doesn't want interaction time to end. This is a good thing but has to be managed for the sake of the next patient.
3. The end of the interview approaches abruptly. Give the patient notice that the end of the visit is approaching.
4. Not enough time is budgeted for unpredicted counseling and sensitive issues that the patient has not dealt with for some time. Acknowledge the concerns and allocate time for discussion in future visits.
5. The patient does not understand the plan you have developed or does not draw the connection between the plan and their expected outcomes. Budget time to explain and address these issues.
6. The patient brings up issues during the last few minutes "oh by the way. . ." Use the "Is there anything else" technique early in the visit, triage and table non-critical issue for a future visit.
7. The physician "loses" time while preparing an exam room, acquiring needed supplies and equipment. Where possible, budget time for room set up and preparation.
8. The physician has not had a chance to go to the washroom, eat, wash hands, or get grounded before the next patient visit. Allocate time for these personal things at the outset.

GUIDELINES FOR A SUCCESSFUL PRIMARY CARE VISIT

1. Build rapport with patients and establish a foundation for an effective, long-term, doctor-patient relationship
2. Meet your own performance expectations and prevent feeling rushed, unorganized, or frustrated at closing
3. Be sure patients feel satisfied that the closing plan promises to address their reason for seeking care
4. Be sure patients do not feel rushed or frustrated at the end of the visit and feels motivated to follow-through with your management plan

INTENTIONAL INTERVIEWING

Interpersonal Skills

Honesty and sincerity are the best traits a naturopathic physician can display to inspire cooperation and compliance (heart speaks to heart). If you are a student doctor, introduce yourself as such and tell the patient that you will be sharing your findings with an attending physician. You may also mention that you are working as part of a clinical team with the mandate to provide the best care possible. As a gesture of your respect to the patient, you may also ask them how they wish to be addressed. Your behavior should be calm and confident even when time is limited. Surveys indicate that patients find cleanliness, conservative dresss, and a name tag reassuring.

Interviewing Skill

Open-ended Questions

The effectiveness of your questioning technique relies heavily on how you use open-ended questions (*Tell me about your abdominal pain?*), empathy (*It sounds like you are experiencing a lot of pain*), verbal cueing (*Uh-huh or I see*), encouragers (*Stitching pain!*), summarizing (*So this pain started yesterday night, you feel this stitching abdominal pain every few hours, it wakes you up at night and does not seem to be getting any better – is this correct?*).

Close-ended Questions

When the open-ended strategies are exhausted, you may use more direct close-ended questions, which allow you to test your provisional hypothesis (*Does the pain improve after a bowel movement?*). However, avoid leading (*Is it stitching or stabbing in character?*), multiple, or judgmental questions and comments.

Confidentiality

If the patients report sensitive information of psychosocial, sexual, or emotional nature, they need to be assured of their confidentiality, though you should be aware of the situations where confidentiality would not be upheld, such as your legal obligation to not harm others ("duty to warn"). These requirements may vary by jurisdiction of practice, but generally include situations of suspected child abuse, communicable diseases, disclosure of credible intent to harm someone, or when ordered by a court.

Listening Attentively

Listening without interruption is another interviewing skill that will convey to your patients the feeling that they are attended to. Silence, when used deliberately, may also allow your patients to gather their thoughts and formulate a meaningful answer to your question.

Summarizing

After each major line of questioning, you should again summarize your findings and check with the patient to ensure that no important information was missed. You should also verify information that you think is relevant to the patient's presentation by asking for rationale (*How did you come to know that you are allergic to echinacea?*) or documentation (*Can I take a look at your prescription to check dosages?* or *What were the results of the stress test? Can I obtain a copy?*).

Medical Jargon and Acronyms

It is wise to use language that the patient can easily relate to. If your patients have a medical background, it is unlikely that they will misunderstand you. Otherwise, if you have to use medical terms, then explain them in a manner that is appropriate to the patient's level of education and background.

Transitions

It helps when doctors explain to their patients what information they seek and why. If patients appreciate the necessity and relevance of the information you need, they will likely cooperate and may even expand on certain aspects that were not mentioned before. For example, you may transition between the history of present illness to past medical history by saying, *Now that I have a good description of your concerns, I am going to ask you a few questions about your past health history and family history, because this information will help me identify if there are health risks that may be related to your symptoms.*

Delivering Information and Counseling

Again, the information you provide to your patients should be clear, concise, and appropriate to the patient's level of education and background. Because there may be a power differential, the patient should feel that you are non-judgmental and sincere. Be aware of your body language, for example, when your patients tell you that they consume nothing but doughnuts, coffee, burgers and cola! If you want to suggest a change in lifestyle, an alternative to judgmental behavior is to check with patients if they are ready to receive such advice.

Professional Behavior

Thus far, you have been direct, thorough, sensitive, and honest with your patients. Of equal importance for fostering mutually respectful doctor-patient relationships is not to give premature diagnoses or false reassurances. If the presentation challenges you (if no provisional diagnosis can readily be identified), you should tell your patients that you are not sure of the diagnosis and that you will do your best to figure it out.

In most jurisdictions, naturopathic physicians are required to provide this information explicitly to their patients. For example, the Province of Ontario regulatory board (BDDT-N) requires that naturopathic physicians share their

> The information you provide to your patients should be clear, concise, and appropriate to the patient's level of education and background.

diagnostic impression, evaluation strategy, and follow-up plans with their patients. This is considered to be a requirement of obtaining informed consent.

Doctor as a Teacher

Your ability to educate your patients effectively relies on their understanding and processing of the information they already have. For example, you may ask your patients to explain to you what they consider to be safe sex practices, and then proceed to affirm their practices and address any misunderstandings. To know what it is you need to teach, you may pose hypothetical situations, ask if the patient has additional questions, or ask for a demonstration of particular technique (for example, stretching exercises or use of a peak flow meter).

Closure

At the end of the encounter, you should clearly explain your management plan to the patient:

1. What are you going to do? Schedule diagnostic tests, for example, or make referrals, prescribe provisional treatment, etc.
2. What do you want the patient to do? Make lifestyle changes, for example, or avoid strenuous exercise, go to an occupational therapist, go to the hospital if the situation gets worse, etc.
3. Provide a method for dealing with realistic concerns. For example, "If you have questions about your treatment plan, leave a message at this number," or "If your chest pain is not better after resting for 15 minutes, don't hesitate to seek emergency care."
4. Schedule the time of your next appointment.

FOCUSED HEALTH HISTORY IN PRIMARY CARE

Initially, your attention should be directed towards the patient's reason for seeking care. An efficient approach is to start with open-ended questions and employ facilitative verbal and/or non-verbal communication skills.

Information gathered regarding the History of Present Illness (HPI) should include onset, duration, frequency, character, setting, intensity, aggravating & ameliorating factors, associated symptoms, and the patient's belief or perception regarding their symptoms (why?).

Include relevant Past Medical History (PMH), Family History (FH), Social History (SH), allergies, habits (for example, use of alcohol or drugs), and sexual history (if appropriate to presentation).

REVIEW OF SYSTEMS (ROS)

Go through a complaint-oriented Review of Systems (ROS) as indicated by the presenting symptom. For example, if the chief complaint is abdominal pain, then GI, pulmonary, genitourinary, musculoskeletal, and psychosocial ROS should be explored during your initial encounter.

REVIEW OF SYSTEMS

System	Details
❏ *General Health Status:* Weight gain or loss, weakness, fever, chills, sweats, or night sweats.	
❏ *Cardiovascular:* Retrosternal pain, palpitations, cyanosis, dyspnea on exertion, orthopnea, nocturnal dyspnea, nocturia, edema, known murmurs, hypertension, coronary artery disease, anemia, last ECG or other heart tests.	
❏ *Respiratory:* History of asthma, emphysema, bronchitis, pneumonia, tuberculosis; shortness of breath, chest pain, wheezing, cough, sputum (color/ amount); hemoptysis, toxin or pollution exposure.	
❏ *Gastrointestinal:* Appetite, food sensitivity, dysphagia, heartburn, indigestion, abdominal pain, discomfort, sour eructation, nausea, vomiting, hematemesis, history of abdominal disease, flatulence, recent change in bowel movements, stool characteristics, constipation, diarrhea, black or gray stools, rectal bleeding, rectal itching, hemorrhoids, fistula, use of antacids or laxatives.	
❏ *Skin:* History of eczema, psoriasis, hives; pigment or color change, change in a mole, excessive dryness or moisture, pruritus, bruising, rash or lesion, amount of sun exposure, use of sun tan lotion.	
❏ *Hair:* Recent change in texture or loss.	
❏ *Nails:* Recent change in shape, color, or brittleness.	
❏ *Head:* Frequent or severe headaches, head injury, dizziness, syncope, or vertigo.	
❏ *Eyes:* Change in vision, blurring, blind spots, eye pain, diplopia, redness, swelling, watering, discharge, glaucoma, cataracts, date of last vision test or glaucoma test.	
❏ *Ears:* Earache, infections, discharge, tinnitus or vertigo, hearing loss, hearing aid use, exposure to noise, and method of cleaning ears.	
❏ *Mouth and Throat:* Mouth pain, frequent sore throat, bleeding gums, toothache, lesion in mouth or tongue, dysphagia, change in voice, hoarseness, tonsillectomy, use of chewing tobacco, smoking, change in taste, daily dental care, last dental checkup.	
❏ *Neurologic:* History of seizures, stroke, fainting, blurring of vision, black outs; recent weakness, tic, tremor, coordination problems or paralysis; recent numbness, tingling, memory problems, nervousness, mood change, depression; history of mental illness or hallucinations.	

System	Details
❏ *Neck:* Pain, limitation of movement, lumps, swelling, enlarged and tender nodes, goiter.	
❏ *Breast:* Pain, lump, nipple discharge, rash, history of breast disease; axillary tenderness, lumps or swelling; breast self-examination, last mammogram and results.	
❏ *Peripheral Vascular:* Limb coldness, numbness, or tingling; swelling of legs; discoloration of hands or feet, varicose veins, intermittent claudications, thrombophlebitis, ulcers, long term-sitting or standing, crossing of legs at knees, wearing support socks.	
❏ *Urinary:* Recent changes, frequency, hesitancy, straining, urgency, nocturia, dysuria, polyuria, oliguria, narrowed stream, cloudy urine, dark urine, hematuria, incontinence, flank pain, groin pain, suprapubic pain, low back pain, last DRE or PSA; history or urologic disease, kidney stones, UTI, or BPH; measures to avoid UTIs, use of Kegel exercises after childbirth.	
❏ *Male Genital:* Penile or testicular pain, sores, lesions, penile discharge, lumps, hernia, testicular self-examination.	
❏ *Female Genital:* Age at menarche, last menstrual period, cycle and duration; amenorrhea, menorrhagia, premenstrual pain, dysmenorrhea (primary or secondary), intermenstrual spotting; vaginal itching, discharge, age at menopause, menopausal symptoms, post-menopausal bleeding.	
❏ *Sexual Health:* Presently in a relation involving intercourse? Aspects of sex satisfactory to you and partner? Recent changes or concerns, dyspareunia (for female), changes in erection or ejaculation (for male), use of contraceptives, contact or history or STDs (gonorrhea, herpes, Chlamydia, venereal warts, HIV or syphilis).	
❏ *Endocrine:* History of diabetes, polyuria, polydipsia or polyphagia; thyroid disease, intolerance to heat or cold, change in skin pigmentation or texture, excessive sweating, changes in appetite and weight, abnormal hair distribution, nervousness, tremors, history of hormone therapy.	
❏ *Musculoskeletal:* History of arthritis, gout, joint pain, stiffness, swelling, deformity, limitation of movement, noise with joint movement; recent muscle pain, cramps, weakness, gait instability, incoordination; low back pain, disc disease; physical exercise pattern.	
❏ *Hematologic:* Bleeding tendency, bruising, lymph node swelling, history of blood transfusion; exposure to toxic agents or radiation.	

In some efficiency driven practices, medical practitioners may resort to pre-printed intake forms to collect a patient's entire history (HPI, PMH, FH, and ROS). However, Paul Cutler, author of *Problem Solving in Clinical Medicine* (1998), strongly discourages healthcare practitioners from relying on printed intake forms or computer intake procedures. A primary reason for doctors to take the history is to build rapport and get to know their patients. Experienced physicians are interested in the patient's body language, verbal tone, mood, facial expression, and peculiar reactions in addition to answers to their questions. No machine or printed form can possibly capture such content, which often significantly changes the problem solving focus or the direction of the entire doctor-patient encounter.

Conducting the Physician-Led ROS

Explain to your patient that you will be asking some questions that will help you with your assessment. Remember to use language that is appropriate to the patient's education and background. Record details of positive and relevant negative answers in your chart. A time-saving strategy is to tell your patient that you will "rhyme-off whole sections", and then ask them if they identify with anything that you mentioned. This memory aid for review of systems may be helpful.

FUNCTIONAL ASSESSMENT

There are a number of functional assessments that can be deployed.

Activities of Daily Living (ADL)

This is the capacity of the patient to eat, bathe, go to the toilet, dress, groom, move about the house, transfer from bed, transfer from toilet, and control bowel and bladder. Assess as independent or dependent.

Instrumental Activities of Daily Living (IADL)

These are instrumental capacities, such as cooking, cleaning, using telephone, writing, shopping, doing laundry, taking medications/supplements, using public transit, walking outdoors without getting lost, managing money, independent travel out of town, and driving. Assess as independent or dependent.

Nutritional State

This includes body weight, recent weight gain or loss, 24-hour diet recall, BMI or waist-to-hip-ratio, alcohol/ cigarette/ marijuana/ cocaine/ amphetamines/ heroin/ barbiturates/ caffeine/tea/cola use, and any perceived substance dependency.

Self-Concept and Esteem

This includes personal beliefs regarding education, financial state, appearance, belief system, and methods of self-care.

> Experienced physicians are interested in the patient's body language, verbal tone, mood, facial expression, and peculiar reactions in addition to answers to their questions.

Activity and Exercise
This includes pattern of typical day, exercise regime (type, amount, warm-up, type of stretching, monitoring of body's response to exercise), and leisure activities.

Coping and Stress Management
You may ask patients to describe the stresses in their life, including recent changes, and their methods to relieve stress.

Environmental Concerns
Safety of residential area, adequate heat and utilities, access to transportation, involvement in community services, perceived hazards at home or workplace (asbestos, inhalants, lead paint, chemicals, repetitive motion), use of seatbelts, and travel/residence in other country.

Perception of Own Health
You may ask the patient to define good health, their view of their current health, health concerns, and health goals, as well as their expectations in seeing you.

Depression
If depression is suspected, you should inquire and record your observations regarding the following:
- Does the patient admit to suicidal or homicidal ideation?
- Does patient have a plan?
- Has patient ever acted on this plan?
- Is there any inappropriate blame or guilt?
- Is there any psychomotor retardation or agitation?
- Is there blunted or labile affect? What about diurnal mood variation?
- What about sleep pattern? Any difficulty falling asleep, mid-sleep-cycle awakening, or early morning awakening?
- Is there loss of appetite? What about recent weight gain or loss?
- Does the patient experience loss of mental concentration ability?
- Is the patient able to temporarily forget the depression? Which activities alleviate poor mood?
- Has the patient abandoned social contact?
- Is there any loss of pleasure in previously pleasurable activities?
- Does the patient have hope for the future?
- What are the patient's current or recent stressors?
- Does patient feel able to influence the external environment?

COGNITIVE STATUS EXAMINATION
If there is a need to assess a patient's cognitive status, the standard Mini-Mental State offers a complete and easily conducted cognitive function evaluation.

Chart total Mini-Mental State score along with level of consciousness: alert, drowsy, stupor, or coma.

Abstract Reasoning Assessment

If you need to test abstract (higher-function) reasoning ability you may use proverbs and ask the patient to explain them to you. For example, if you ask a patient to explain the proverb *Don't put all your eggs in one basket*, you may get a concrete answer, such as "If you put a lot of eggs in one basket, they will break," or an abstract one, such as "To reduce risk, one should distribute his investments in more than one project."

PHYSICAL EXAMINATION IN PRIMARY CARE

After taking a good history and generating the differential diagnosis list, you should develop an appreciation of what may be causing the presentation. You may then choose from various physical examination procedures.

- Hypothesis-driven physical examinations: These are aimed at narrowing down your list of possibilities or confirming your clinical impression.
- Complete head-to-toe physical examinations: These may need to be used if the history is complex or vague and you are left without a workable list of differential diagnoses.

> If a hypothesis-driven physical examination is employed in the initial encounter, a complete physical examination should still be completed in subsequent encounters to elaborate possible complications.

Notwithstanding, if a hypothesis-driven physical examination is employed in the initial encounter, a complete physical examination should still be completed in subsequent encounters to elaborate possible complications of the patient's primary problem or to screen for unrelated coexisting problems.

Physical Examination Tips

1. Wash or sanitize your hands before touching the patient. Better yet, do it in front of the patient.
2. Never examine the patient through clothing, such as socks, t-shirts, bras, or undergarments.
3. Determine a logical sequence for your intended PE; then follow this sequence in an organized manner.
4. Explain to your patient what it is you are about to do and why before commencing with the examination. For example you may say, *Your lower abdominal pain may be caused by problems in your digestive, urinary, or genital tract. To figure it out, I'll need to examine your chest, abdomen, genitals, and rectum. Is that all right?*
5. When you disrobe the patient, use serial exposure to preserve the patient's modesty.

Cognitive Status Examination

Function	Instructions	Score
Orientation		
1. What is the date today (year, season, date, month)?	Ask specifically for omitted parts.	(/5)
2. Where are we (country, city, clinic, floor)?	One point for each correct answer.	(/5)
Registration		
Ask patient to repeat a series of three objects after you.	The first repetition determines the score.	(/3)
Name three objects (e.g., lemon, coin, chair), take one second to pronounce each object, then ask the patient to repeat the series.	One point for each correct answer.	
Attention and Calculation		
Serial 7s. Ask patient to begin with 100 and count backwards by 7. Stop after five subtractions (93, 86, 79, 72, 65) OR Ask patient to spell "world" backwards (dlrow =5, while dlorw=3).	Score the total number of correct answers.	(/5)
Recall		
Ask patient if they can recall the three objects you previously mentioned.	Score 0-3	(/3)
Language		
1. Show patient 2 objects (necktie, pen) and ask them what they are?	Score 0-2	
2. Ask patient to repeat one sentence after you "no ifs, ands or buts."	Score 0-1	
3. Give patient a piece of paper and tell them to "take paper in your right hand, fold in half, and put it on the floor."	Score 0-3	
4. Give patient a piece of paper with the following sentence written on it: "Close your eyes." Ask patient to read and do what it says.	Score 1 point if patient closes their eyes.	
5. Ask patient to write any sentence for you on a piece of paper. See if sentence is sensible and contains subject and verb.and punctuation.	Score 0-1 disregard grammar and punctuation	(/9)
6. Ask patient to copy a design of intersecting pentagons (each side should be about 1 inch)	Score 0-1 disregard rotation or tremor.	
	Total Score	(/30)

6. If you feel it is important to perform breast, genital, or rectal examinations, explain the reasoning to your patients and obtain their consent.
7. Prepare your environment so that all necessary tools for your intended examination are readily available – clean and ready medical instruments, charged batteries, specula, thermometer/lens covers, gown, table paper, tongue depressors, cotton swabs, gloves, lubricants, and tissues.
8. If you ask the patient to change positions, offer to assist because this may be difficult for some patients.
9. If your patient expresses acute distress or pain during the PE, acknowledge this and strive to make the patient more comfortable.

PRINCIPLES OF PROBLEM SOLVING IN PRIMARY CARE

The history of knowledge is filled with intellectual milestones, which, to some extent, influence the way we currently think, argue, and express our ideas. The following prominent thinkers undoubtedly have affected the way we reason in contemporary naturopathic and medical circles: Fu Hsi, Shen Nung, Thales, Democritus, Empedocles, Hippocrates, Pythagorus, Plato, Aristotle, Diocles, Herophilus, Erasistratus, Celsus, Galen, Avicenna, Paracelsus, Aquinas, Bacon, Copernicus, Vesalius, Harvey, Descartes, Galileo, Kepler, Gilbert, Newton, Bacon, Hume, Thomson, Hahnemann, Darwin, Einstein, Lindlahr, and Lust (and the legacy continues). Indeed, most contemporary problem-solving strategies bear close resemblance to Frances Bacon's (1561–1626) quest to "Rid the mind of all preconceptions," the experimental method of Galileo Gallilei (1564-1642), and Isaac Newton's (1643–1727) rules of reasoning.

Problem Solving Strategy

1. Acquire information from patient's history and physical examination.
2. Evaluate and group derived information into a well-defined list of problems.
3. Generate a list of hypotheses (based on probability, decision trees, independent research, or database searches).
4. Test your hypotheses systematically (further questioning, examination, testing, following a hunch, consultation or referral),
5. Assume hypotheses that cannot be disproved are true until other more accurate ones displace it. That is, no theory is considered above the threat of disproof.

Although this problem solving strategy may appear to be time consuming, it is indeed required to resolve complex presentations that do not point toward a single key clue. Furthermore, this is the logic we need to apply in order to solve clinical puzzles, consistently and reliably, especially ones that are either new to the primary care provider or peculiar and unanticipated.

The Personal Health Information Protection Act (PHIPA, 01 November 2004) is the privacy legislation that governs the manner in which personal health information may be collected, used, and disclosed within the healthcare system in Canada. For further information on PHIPA beyond the scope of this document, please visit the web-site of the Information Privacy Commissioner at www.ipc.on.ca.

In the United States, you should consult the documentation guidelines for evaluation and management (E&M) developed by the American Medical Association (AMA) and Health Care Financing Administration (HCFA) at www.hcfa.gov.

SOAP CHARTING

As a self-regulating profession, naturopathic doctors are expected to follow accepted professional standards for recording notes in patient files. SOAP charting is one of these standards. SOAP is an acronym for subjective (S), objective (O), assessment (A), and plan (P).

Standard SOAP charting is important for legal purposes. In most jurisdictions, SOAP charting is a cornerstone of many of the Quality Assurance (QA) programs that are required of regulated professions.

Standardized charting is also necessary for effective communication among healthcare professionals. Upon reviewing a patient file, another healthcare professional (ND, MD, RN, RN-EC, NP, DC) should be able to understand easily what has taken place with regard to patient care. SOAP charting is a flexible tool that can be adapted for use in most styles of practice, including those focusing on traditional Chinese medicine (TCM) or homeopathy.

Good charting will provide the practitioner with a tool to guide assessment, goal setting, treatment planning, progress tracking, and treatment plan modification. It reminds the practitioner what has been done and guides what should be done next.

Charting Guidelines
Style

All chart entries must be dated and signed by the physician. All chart entries must be made in black or blue ink. Chart entries must be neat and concise while representing a summarized reiteration of what took place with regards to patient care. All charting corrections or changes should be performed as follows:

> Good charting will provide the practitioner with a tool to guide assessment, goal setting, treatment planning, progress tracking, and treatment plan modification.

- Draw one line through the entry to be changed. The corrected entry should still be legible.
- Write the new entry beside the old entry.
- Initial the change.

Content

Each chart should have the following components: a subjective (S) history, objective (O) physical examination, assessment (A) and diagnosis, management plan (P), and future plan (FP). Note that within the SOAP format, there are variable styles of presenting this required information.

SOAP CONTENT

S: Subjective History: Information you have been given before seeing the patient if relevant + history of presenting complaint(s) + past medical history + family history + relevant ROS + social history.

O: Objective Physical Examination: Data that you inspect, palpate, measure, auscultate, or observe. Indicate only pertinent positive and negative findings relative to the patient's presentation.

A: Assessment or Clinical Reasoning: Problem list → DDx list → Ruled-out list → Likely or Presumptive Diagnosis:

- **Problem List (Assessment):** Different definitions of patient problems in the outpatient setting and their use in patient assessment and management have been described since this convention began in the 1960s. At our clinic, we recently adopted the system designed for use in family practice described by Rakel in *Essentials of Family Practice* (1998;96-97). Rakel defines a problem as "anything that requires diagnosis or management or that interferes with quality of life as perceived by the patient. It is any physiologic, pathologic, psychological, or social item of concern to either the patient or the physician."

  These "problems" can be anything of concern either to you or to the patient, be it anatomic (hernia), physiologic (undiagnosed jaundice), a previous diagnosis, a sign (central edema), a symptom (dysuria), economic concern (financial stress), social problem (family discord), psychiatric condition, physical handicap, abnormal lab or imaging finding, or risk factor (smoking). The criteria are far more inclusive than those of a "diagnosis."
- **Diagnosis (Assessment):** This is where you summarize your clinical reasoning based on the preceding steps. This aspect of assessment is perhaps the most important part of the chart. It may be as simple as stating a particular diagnosis when you are fairly certain about it. When a doctor considers

the diagnoses likely but not certain, a "working" or "presumptive" diagnosis should be used. Diagnostic rational should be included in situations where it would not be easily inferred. Remember that every stated differential diagnosis (DDx) requires a corresponding action in the plan. This is true even when the action is to watch and wait.

P: Plan: All actions recommended or prescribed during the patient's visit should be noted. Remember that the plan must contain an action corresponding to your assessment (again, even if the action is to do nothing).
- Include instructions for diet or lifestyle modification or intervention; any medication (herbal/botanical, homeopathic, nutraceutical, or prescription).
- Where possible, charted prescriptions should include dosages in terms of metric measurement (mg/grams) as well as posology "3 caps t.i.d."
- Important side effects that patients were informed about and what they were instructed to do if they occur.
- Therapeutic application or self-treatment.
- Laboratory testing or imaging.
- Therapeutic order and naturopathic principles that have guided the plan.

FP: Future Plan: This section should include your intended management plan, including follow-up frequency, phone consults, consultations, referrals, and other aspects of coordination of care.

Sample Patient Intake Chart

Patient's Name: _D.V._   **Doctor's Name & #**: _Jane Dow # 885621_
Supervisor: _Dr Adams ND_   **Date**: _____

S: History: Information you have been given before seeing the patient if relevant + History of presenting complaint(s) + Past medical history + Family history + relevant ROS + Social history.

The patient is 40-yr-old male who comes in with a complaint of upper chest "discomfort" for the last 3 months. The discomfort is primarily brought on by exertion and is worse if the weather is cold. Occasionally, he feels similar discomfort when walking or doing heavy work. It has occurred twice when he was upset. He describes the "discomfort" as a steady pressure. It is not affected by breathing or position. It is alleviated by stopping his exertion. He currently gets the "discomfort" 2-3 X/wk. He came in today because three days ago, he awoke at 1 AM with a similar pain but it was severe and radiated to his neck. He sat up for a few minutes and it went away. Since the event, he has not had sex with his wife for fear of pain and wife discovering his "problem."

PMH - He has been told that he has "borderline" hypertension 5 years ago but never addressed it. A routine ECG was normal a year ago.
FH - Father died of cancer at age 72, but also had coronary artery disease.
ROS - He does not report shortness of breath at rest, dizziness or light headedness. He does not know his cholesterol, does not watch his diet, and does not exercise.
Diet - Mainly fast food, doughnuts and coffee.
SH - Has smoked 1ppd X 20 years. He does not consider his job particularly stressful.

O: Physical Examination: Data that you inspect, palpate, measure, auscultate, or observe. Indicate only pertinent positive and negative findings related to patient's presentation.

On PE, Pt is well dressed, well nourished, and is in no acute distress. He does not display much emotion.
BP 140/90
Neck - no venous distension.
Heart - regular rhythm, no murmurs.
Lungs - clear to percussion and auscultation.
Chest wall - no tenderness over rib cage or costochondral joints.
Abd - no tenderness, bowel sounds present, no hepatomegaly or splenomegaly.
Extremities - no peripheral edema, peripheral pulses +2 equal bilat.

A: Assessment or Clinical Reasoning: Problem list → DDx list → Ruled-out list → Likely or Presumptive Diagnosis

Problem List: Complete list of significant concerns include HPI, Meds, FH, ROS, diet, P/E, labs	**DDx List:** Include all possible causes of current presentation	**Ruling out criteria:** Rule out unlikely DDx based on your intake, P/E, problem list and DDx list
HPI Chest Pain - progressive anginal pain with exertion and emotional upset; 3 months, SOB on exercise, Nocturnal dypnea, orthopnea	Acute myocardial infarction	Unlikely from remitting Hx
	Aortic dissection	Unlikely from history and P/E
	Coronary artery insufficiency/ stable angina	Likely need stress ECG to confirm
	Pulmonary embolus	Unlikely from history and P/E
	Pneumothorax	Unlikely from history and P/E
FH - Cancer and CAD - Father	Congenital coronary anomalies	Unlikely from age of onset
	Coronary artery spasm	Maybe, stress ECG is needed to rule out
ROS - does not watch his diet No exercise, smoker, does not know cholesterol level	Myocarditis	No fever, murmur, or friction rub
	Aortic stensis	Unlikely since Radial pulses not diminished
Diet - Poor diet - fast food & Doughnuts	Mitral regurgitation or prolapse	No murmurs
	Dysrhythmia	No tachycardia or irregularity
SH - Sedentary lifestyle Limited stress	Psychogenic origin	No hx of stressful events
	Precordial catch syndrome	Unlikely from age of onset
	Non-coronary chest pain	Maybe, consider if cardiac stress test is negative for CAD
P/E: Bp 140/90	Increased risk of CAD	Yes
	Sedentary lifestyle	Yes
	Poor dietary habits	Yes
	stage 1 hypertension	Yes

Diagnosis: In order of likelihood. Write no more than five likely or provisional Dx.

1. Coronary artery insufficiency with fixed stenosis and angina
2. Coronary artery spasm
3. Stage 1 Hypertension
4. Non-coronary chest pain - GI or MS
5. Lifestyle factors - smoking, Poor diet, sedentary lifestyle, no exercise

P: Management Plan: In order of importance, include immediate plan and, diagnostic workup (required and cost-effective). Write no more than five entries.

1. *Cardiac stress test + Echocardiography*
2. *CBC*
3. *Lipid profile*
4. *Encourage smoking cessation*
5. *Lifestyle counseling*

Follow-up:

_____
_____
_____
_____
_____
_____
_____
_____
_____
_____
_____
_____
_____
_____
_____
_____
_____
_____
_____
_____
_____
_____
_____
_____
_____

Comprehensive Health Assessment Form

Date of Visit: _____

Chart Record #:_____

Telephone: (home) _____ (business) _____

Provider: _____

Language _____ Interpreter present: ☐ Yes ☐ No

Patient Name: _____

Address: _____

Date of Birth: _____ Age: _____ Gender: ☐ Male ☐ Female

Informant/Relationship: _____

Reliability: ☐ Adequate ☐ Inadequate

History of Present Illness

_____

_____

_____

_____

_____

_____

_____

_____

_____

_____

_____

_____

_____

_____

_____

_____

_____

_____

_____

_____

_____

_____

_____

_____

_____

_____

_____

_____

_____

_____

Past surgical History/Trauma/Hospitalization

☐ T & A: ☐ Appendectomy: ☐ Cholecystectomy:
☐ Hernia repair: ☐ Hysterectomy: ☐ Laparotomy:
☐ Cesarean section: ☐ Biopsy:

Other/Details:

Allergies

☐ Drugs   ☐ Environmental   ☐ Foods   ☐ Latex   ☐ IV Contrast
Details:

Reproductive History

Menstrual: _____ Age at menarche _____ LMP _____ Interval _____ Duration _____ Flow _____
☐ Regular ☐ Irregular ☐ Cramping ☐ Intermenstrual Bleeding ☐ PMS
Obstetrical: G _____ T _____ P _____ A _____ L _____ Complications: _____
Menopause: Age _____ Abnl Bleeding: _____ Symptoms: _____
Hormones: ☐ ERT ☐ HRT ☐ topical _____ *Contraceptives:* _____
Sexual Activity: ☐ same sex ☐ opposite sex ☐ abstinent ☐ single partner ☐ multiple partners ☐ > 4 lifetime partners
STD hx: _____

Concerns:

Past Medical History

☐ HTN ☐ Asthma/COPD ☐ Seizure Disorder ☐ Breast Disease ☐ DM ☐ GERD ☐ Renal Disease ☐ Anemia
☐ CVD/CAD ☐ Hepatitis ☐ Thyroid Disorder ☐ Transfusions ☐ CVA ☐ Osteoporosis ☐ Bleeding Disorder
☐ Psychiatric ☐ CA ☐ Arthritis ☐ Infectious Disease ☐ Childhood Illnesses
Other/Details of Above:

Medications

☐ OTC ☐ Vitamins ☐ Supplements/Herbals ☐ Prescriptions

Social History

Marital Status: ☐ Single ☐ Married ☐ Domestic Partner ☐ Divorced ☐ Widowed
Cohabitants: _____   *Children:* _____
Education: _____   *Occupation:* _____
Interests/Activities: _____   *Exercise:* ☐ Aerobic ☐ Weights _____
Diet: ☐ Balanced ☐ Calcium _____   *Sleep/Rest:* _____
Caffeine: ☐ No ☐ Yes cups/day _____   *Tobacco:* ☐ No ☐ Yes PPD ___ # Years _____ Quit Year _____
Smoking in home: ☐ Yes ☐ No _____   *ETOH:* ☐ Yes ☐ No ☐ Daily ☐ Weekly ☐ Monthly # drinks ___
Recreational Drugs: _____   *Support Systems/Coping Skills:* ☐ Adequate ☐ Inadequate

Family History

☐ *Family History Unknown*
Father: _____   *Mother:* _____
Siblings _____   *MGF:* _____
MGM: _____   *PGF* _____
PGM: _____   *Other:* _____
Cultural/Religious Influences: _____

Health Maintenance History

Exam	Last Date	Results	N/A	Refused	Exam	Last Date	Results	N/A	Refused
Pap Test					Dental				
Mammogram					Vision				
SBE/TSE					Hearing				
Stool guaiac					Lipid Profile				
Flex Sig/ Colonoscopy					FBS				
CXR					PSA				
ECG					PPD				

Immunizations (dates):					Safety:
Td	MMR/titers	Hep B	Polio		☐ Seatbelt Use ☐ Cycling Helmet ☐ Sunscreen
Varicella vaccine/chickenpox					☐ Occupational ☐ Smoke Detectors ☐ Housing
Influenza	Pneumovax				☐ Domestic Violence ☐ Firearms

Review of Systems

☐ *General:* ☐ fever ☐ chills ☐ night sweats ☐ fatigue ☐ unexplained weight loss ☐ weight gain

☐ *Skin:* ☐ pruritis ☐ rash ☐ hair loss ☐ worrisome lesion ☐ pigment change ☐ moles ☐ sweating ☐ dry skin ☐ nail change

☐ *HEENT:* ☐ headache ☐ dizziness ☐ earache ☐ hearing loss ☐ tinnitus ☐ vision change ☐ eye pain/sensitivity
☐ excessive tearing ☐ eyeglasses/contact use ☐ glaucoma ☐ rhinorrhea ☐ nasal congestion ☐ post nasal drip ☐ sinus pain
☐ nosebleeds ☐ hay fever ☐ sore throat ☐ mouth sores ☐ hoarseness ☐ toothache ☐ bleeding gums ☐ dentures

☐ *Breast:* ☐ pain ☐ lumps ☐ discharge ☐ history of breast disease ☐ implants

☐ *Pulmonary:* ☐ cough ☐ sputum ☐ hemoptysis ☐ SOB ☐ pain with respiration ☐ wheezing ☐ cyanosis

☐ *CV:* ☐ chest pain ☐ palpitations ☐ DOE ☐ orthopnea ☐ PND ☐ diaphoresis ☐ syncope ☐ heart murmur ☐ leg edema

☐ *PVD:* ☐ claudication ☐ varicose veins ☐ phlebitis ☐ coldness of hands/feet ☐ leg ulcers

☐ *GI:* ☐ dysphagia ☐ heartburn ☐ change in appetite ☐ food intol ☐ nausea ☐ vomiting ☐ hematemesis ☐ abdominal pain
☐ bloating ☐ flatulence ☐ diarrhea ☐ constipation ☐ melena ☐ jaundice ☐ dark urine ☐ BRBPR ☐ change in BM
☐ hemorrhoids ☐ hernia

☐ *GU:* ☐ dysuria ☐ urgency ☐ frequency ☐ hematuria ☐ nocturia ☐ polyuria ☐ suprapubic pain ☐ flank pain
☐ incontinence ☐ lesions
♂ ☐ hesitancy ☐ dribbling ☐ decreased force stream ☐ testicular pain ☐ testicular mass/swelling ☐ penile discharge
☐ erectile dysfunction
♀ ☐ vaginal itch ☐ abnl vaginal discharge ☐ vaginal dryness ☐ dyspareunia ☐ sexual dysfunction ☐ abnl vaginal bleeding

☐ *Endocrine:* ☐ polyuria ☐ polydipsia ☐ polyphagia ☐ heat/cold intol ☐ tremor ☐ lump in throat ☐ unexplained wt change
☐ hair changes

☐ *Heme:* ☐ anemia ☐ easy bruising ☐ swollen glands ☐ bleeding of skin/mucous membranes ☐ freq infections ☐ allergies
☐ delayed healing

☐ *MSK:* ☐ joint pain (location _____) ☐ stiffness ☐ restriction of motion ☐ swelling
☐ erythema ☐ bony deformity ☐ myalgia ☐ muscle cramps ☐ weakness ☐ antalgic gait ☐ back pain

☐ *Neuro:* ☐ focal weakness ☐ paralysis ☐ numbness ☐ tremor ☐ seizure ☐ syncope ☐ gait disturbance ☐ memory loss
☐ aphasia

☐ *Psych:* ☐ anxiety ☐ panic attacks ☐ depression ☐ mood changes ☐ irritability ☐ nervousness ☐ decreased libido
☐ eating disorder ☐ sleep disturbance ☐ suicidal thoughts ☐ impaired judgment ☐ hallucinations ☐ confusion

Comments/Details:

Physical Exam

Vitals

Ht _____ Wt _____ Temp _____ Resp _____ Pulse _____ BP (upright) _____ (supine) _____

Visual Acuity

Right   /   Left   /   Corrective lenses: ☐ yes ☐ no

N = Normal A = Abnormal (Check appropriate box)	N	A
1. **General Appearance**: age • LOC • nutrition • development • mobility • affect • speech • hygiene		
2. **Skin**: hydration • color • texture • hair • nails • lesions		
3. **Head**: shape • size • symmetry • scalp • TMJ • lesions		
4. **Eyes**: lids • conjunctiva • sclera		
Extraocular muscles		
Visual fields		
Pupils: size, reaction to light and accommodation		
Fundi		
5. **Ears**: pinna • canals • TMs • hearing		
6. **Nose**: patency • nares • sinuses • nasal mucosa • septum • turbinates		
7. **Mouth**: lips • gums • teeth • mucosa • palate • tongue		
8. **Throat**: pharynx • tonsils • uvula		
9. **Neck**: ROM • symmetry • palpation • thyroid • trachea • carotids • jugular veins • lymph nodes		
10. **Breasts**: size • symmetry • skin • nipples • palpation • nodes		
11. **Chest/Lungs**: excursion • palpation • percussion • auscultation		
12. **Cardiac**: PMI • palpation • rate • rhythm • S1 • S2 • murmurs • gallops • bruits • extra sounds		
13. **Abdomen**: appearance • bowel sounds • bruits • percussion • palpation • liver • spleen • flank • suprapubic • hernia		
14. **Anorectal**:		
Perianal		
Digital rectal		
Stool guaiac		
Prostate exam		
15. **Female Genitalia**: perineum • labia • urethral meatus • introitus		
Internal: vaginal mucosal • cervix		
Bimanual: vagina • cervix • uterus • adnexa		
16. **Male Genitalia**: penis • scrotum • testes • hernia		
17. **Lymph Nodes**: cervical •subclavian •axillary •inguinal •other		
18. **MSK**:		
Back/Spine: ROM • palpation		
Upper Extremity: ROM • strength • palpation		
Lower Extremity: ROM • strength • palpation		
19. **Peripheral Vascular**:		
Upper extremity: pulses • appearance • temp		
Lower extremity: pulses • appearance • temp		
20. **Neurologic**: cranial nerves • motor • sensory • cerebellar • reflexes • gait • mental status		

Document Abnormals (by number)/Comments

_____
_____
_____
_____
_____
_____
_____
_____
_____
_____
_____
_____
_____
_____

Lab/Studies

_____
_____
_____
_____
_____
_____
_____
_____

Assessment and Plan

_____
_____
_____
_____
_____
_____
_____
_____
_____
_____
_____
_____
_____
_____

Periodic Heath Screening Plan

Exam	Performed	Scheduled	N/A	Refused
Breast Exam				
Mammogram				
Pap Test				
Prostate exam				
Testicular exam				
Digital rectal with guaiac				
Sigmoid/Colonoscopy				
Bone Density				
PPD				

Health Counseling

(Check if discussed; describe any intervention)

☐ Smoking cessation _____
☐ Alcohol / Drug use _____
☐ Diet / Weight _____
☐ Vitamins / Calcium _____
☐ Periodic Dental / Vision care _____
☐ Exercise / Sleep _____
☐ Sun exposure _____
☐ Seatbelts / Helmets _____
☐ Stress / Family issues _____
☐ Safety: Weapons / Domestic Violence _____
☐ Sexual issues / risks _____
☐ Contraception _____
☐ Living will / Power of attorney _____

Other

Lab/Studies Ordered

☐ CXR   ☐ Lipids   ☐ Creat/BUN   ☐ HbA$_1$C   ☐ ECG   ☐ CBC/diff   ☐ LFTs   ☐ TSH
☐ Electrolytes   ☐ FBS   ☐ UA/UC
☐ Other:

_____   _____
Provider's Signature   Date

Sample Clinical Reasoning Chart

Problem List	DDx List	Ruling out criteria
HPI	Acute bronchitis	Unlikely by history & PE
CC1 Chronic cough	Pneumonia	Unlikely by PE (chest is clear to
CC2 High blood pressure		P&A) + no fever or hyperventilation
	Congestive heart failure	Class III CHF unlikely by history
Med History:		and physical exam. Maybe class II
Vasotec 10 mg bid		CHF consider echo
	TB	Possible - Rule out by CXR &
Family History:		Mantoux if persistent
Diabetes, Hypertension	COPD	Unlikely by PE & Spirometry
	Cough due to Med S/E	Likely (onset with a recent dose
Diet & Lifestyle:		increase of Enalapril)
Poor diet, sedentary lifestyle	Essential hypertension	Likely
	Secondary hypertension	Unlikely by ECG and chem panel
ROS:	Stage 2/Moderate HTN	Yes
Fatigue, heartburn, weak	Malabsorption syndrome	Explore by trial ttt
and vertically-ridged nails;	Malnutrition	Likely due to poor diet
SOB with moderate exercise;	Increased risk for DM II	Yes
two-pillow orthopnia	Increased risk for CAD	Yes
	TCM - Yin & Yang	Likely Zang fu presentation &
P/E:	imbalance	pulse
Transient wheeze; BP 160/190	TCM - Liver fire	Unlikely by presentation & pulse
Screening Labs:	No anemia, infection, or hematological dz	
CBC WNL	No dyslipidemia	
Lipid panel WNL		

Sample Diagnosis

1. Cough due to Med S/E - ACEI Enalapril
2. Stage 2 Moderate (Essential) Hypertension
3. Malnutrition
4. Yin & Yang imbalance
5. Risk factor Assessment: Increased for type 2 DM + CAD
?? stage II CHF; TB

Primary Care Performance Assessment

This performance standard reflects the expected level of competency required of primary care naturopathic physicians in clinical practice.

Practitioner: _____ Date: _____ Evaluator: _____

Competency Index			
Not Competent	Below Average	Average	Above average
1	2	3	4

Evaluation Criteria	Competency Index 1- 4	Total Points
1. Identify important cues in the patient's story (Basic Health Assessment):		
1.1 Demographic information (gender, age, occupation, residence)		
1.2 Symptom analysis		
1.3 Functional assessment		
1.4 Patient's belief or understanding of their symptoms (and impact on daily life, family members and lifestyle)		
1.5 Routine vital signs (temperature, pulse, heart rate, blood pressure, weight, height, last menses, smoking status, and recreational drug use)		
Section Total (out of 20)		
2. Understand and perform Advanced Health Assessment techniques:		
2.1 Determine what questions need to be asked. Asking complaint-specific questions to assess patient's risk for certain differential diagnoses.		
2.2 Determine what needs to be examined		
2.3 Perform physical examination maneuvers that are suggested by the patient's overall presentation		
2.4 Selective observation of fine detail during the examination (where applicable)		
2.5 Selective requisition of cost-effective and high-yield laboratory work-ups (where applicable)		
Section Total (out of 20)		

Evaluation Criteria	Competency Index 1- 4	Total Points
3. Learning process and application of clinical reasoning skills:		
3.1 Appreciate the presented and implied tasks of the case		
3.2 Recognize own knowledge limitations if any, identify learning issues, acquire new knowledge to meet the assigned task		
3.3 Identify absence of findings that are 'sensitive' markers of certain conditions. Identify presence of findings that are 'specific' markers for certain conditions		
3.4 Identify presenting patterns in light of the patient's knowledge of known presentation		
3.5 Revise diagnostic hypotheses based on self-directed learning		
Section Total (out of 20)		
4. Management of the presentation:		
4.1 Discuss diagnostic impression and available treatment options with the patient in order to empower them to choose an effective and practical treatment option.		
4.2 Design appropriate management plans that ensure resolution of condition and compliance of patient with treatment plan.		
4.3 Identify and utilize community resources that may assist in resolving the presentation (where applicable)		
4.4 Involve other practitioners (consultation and/or referral) in the evaluation or management plan (where indicated)		
4.5 Design appropriate follow-up that ensures resolution of condition. Coordinate care and dissemination of information among healthcare providers within the patient's circle-of-care.		
Section Total (out of 20)		
5. Assessment of group: Includes evaluator's subjective assessment of strengths and weaknesses and suggestions for improvement.		
•		
•		
•		
•		
Section Total (out of 20)		
Competency Assessment Total Score (out of 100)		

EVALUATION OF CHARTING PRACTICE

Not only teachers and students of primary care but also naturopathic physicians and allied healthcare professionals might find this form useful for periodically evaluating charting practices in a clinical setting.

Chart Evaluation Guidelines

The statements listed below collectively represent the expected level of competency required of practice-ready primary care physicians and should be used for self-evaluation. The auditor is asked to either agree or disagree whether the chart submitted fulfills each particular statement. Circle Y or N.

Good Chart Qualities	Competency Achieved
1. The date of visit/encounter and sections written afterwards are clearly recorded.	Y / N
2. Patient identifier (name or initials) appear on each page that can accidentally be separated from the batch.	Y / N
3. Examiner's identifier (name/signature) appears at the end of each chart or sections written on different dates.	Y / N
4. There are sections titled (S) Subjective, (O) Objective, (A) Assessment and (P) Plan.	Y / N
5. Hand writing is neat and legible.	Y / N
6. The organization of the chart is chronological, focused, and obvious.	Y / N
7. All entries are in ink, corrections are stricken through and initialed without obliteration of originally recorded data.	Y / N
8. There are no overgeneralizations or omission of important data.	Y / N
9. Written style is succinct.	Y / N
10. Examiner uses language that is precise.	Y / N
11. Examiner uses medical terminology that is current, correct, and consistent.	Y / N
12. Phrases, short words, and standard medical abbreviations are used appropriately.	Y / N
13. The tone of the chart is neutral and professional.	Y / N
14. The chart does not exhibit too much detail that makes it difficult for someone else (e.g., supervisor, locum ND, auditor) to focus on pertinent issues.	Y / N
15. Diagrams and precise measurements are included where appropriate.	Y / N

Good Chart Qualities	Competency Achieved
16. Objective section captures what the examiner observed rather than what they did.	Y / N
17. Assessment section documents how the examiner arrived at their diagnostic impression.	Y / N
18. Management plan specifically relates to the examiner's diagnostic impression.	Y / N
19. The management plan adequately addresses the patient's presenting concerns.	Y / N
20. There is a clearly documented follow-up/reassessment plan.	Y / N

Several laboratory evaluations are commonly requested by naturopathic physicians in family medicine and primary care practices. Other specialized tests are requested depending on the case. Naturopathic physicians use adjunctive or specialized laboratory tests chiefly to address heavy metal toxicity, nutrient deficiency, and metabolic pathway impairment. These tests exhibit varying levels of sensitivity and predictive value. Here is a list of these tests with a brief explanation of their clinical value.

Laboratory evaluations are requested by primary care physicians to screen for, rule out, or confirm diagnoses.

Common Tests

Test	Used clinically to detect or rule-out	
EKG or ECG	Ventricular hypertrophy, coronary artery disease, rhythm disturbances, and electrolyte imbalance.	
Holter monitor	Paroxysmal rhythm disorders, functional impairment, and confirm panic attacks.	
CBC	Anemias, infections, hematologic disorders.	
Ferritin	Iron deficiency anemia, hemochromatosis, liver disease.	
WBC w/diff	Infections (detection and management), inflammatory disorders, bone marrow disorders, response to therapeutic agents (drugs, botanicals, supplements), response to toxins.	
Platelet counts	Bleeding disorders, aplastic anemia, leukemia, ITP, SLE, infectious mononucleosis.	
PT	Extrinsic clotting pathway defects, liver disease, vitamin K deficiency, warfarin therapy.	
PTT	Intrinsic clotting pathway defects, hemophilia, SLE, heparin therapy.	
BUN/creatinine	Uremia, chronic kidney disease.	
Potassium	Chronic renal failure.	
ALT	Hepatocellular disorders, hepatitis, cirrhosis.	Impaired liver function: these tests are often referred to as liver function tests (LFTs).
ALP	Obstructive jaundice, cholecystitis, pancreatitis.	
AST	Hepatocellular disorders, hepatitis, cirrhosis.	
Bilirubin	Obstructive or functional impairment of liver, nausea.	
GGT	Hepatocellular disorders, hepatitis, cirrhosis.	

LDH	Liver, heart or kidney disease.	Impaired liver function: these tests are often referred to as liver function tests (LFTs).
Albumin & total protein	Edema, ascitis, chronic renal failure.	
Amylase	Pancreatitis	Cholecystitis with or without obstruction.
Lipase	Pancreatitis	
Urobilinogen	Hemolytic anemia, hepatocellular jaundice	
Vitamin K	Bleeding disorders, liver disease, deficiency.	
Ammonia	Cirrhosis	
Imunoglobulins	Hayfever, rashes, urticaria, hives.	
Spot Urinalysis	Urinary tract infections, diabetes, occult hematuria, nephrotic and nephritic patterns.	
24 hour urine protein	Nephrotic disease, postural proteinuria, chronic kidney disease.	
Urine microscopy	Glomerulonephritis, gout, kidney stones.	
FBS, HbA1C	Diabetes (detection and monitoring).	
OGTT	Borderline diabetes, gestational diabetes.	
Serum Lipids	Dyslipidemias, (detection and monitoring), familial hypercholesterolemia.	
Electrolytes	Renal insufficiency, congestive heart failure.	
TSH, T4	Clinical and subclinical hypothyroidism and hyperthyroidism.	
Stool O& P	Parasitic infections on the GI tract.	
Gram stain	To support a diagnosis of bacterial infection.	
C&S	To identify causative bacterial pathogen and its antimicrobial sensitivity.	
Pap smear	Cervical dysplasia screening.	
Fecal Occult Blood	Colon cancer screening, small GI bleeding, anemia.	
Serum B12	Macrocytic anemias, alcoholism.	
PSA & ratio	Prostate cancer screening.	

Specialized Tests

Test	Used clinically to detect or rule-out
Bioelectrical Impedance Analysis (BIA)	Commonly used method for estimating body composition that is diagnostic or prognostic in lifestyle modification programs. This test determines the electrical impedance, or opposition to the flow of an electric current through body tissues, which can then be used to calculate an estimate of total body water (TBW). TBW can be used to estimate fat-free body mass accurately and, by difference with body weight, body fat.
Nutrient status assessment	Blood/serum tests that measure the concentrations of a variety of nutrients, vitamins, and minerals. These tests can be used to confirm a suspected deficiency or assess progress of a therapeutic regimen.
Urinary Organic Acids	Tests used to screen for inborn errors of metabolism, compromised energy production, impaired detoxification, increased intestinal microbial activity, impaired neurotransmitter metabolism, and nutrient deficiencies. The usual method of analysis is tandem mass spectrometry of a urine sample.
Urinary Indican (Obermeyer Test)	Traditional test used to screen for hypochlorhydria, bacterial overgrowth in the small and/or large intestine, maldigestion and/or malabsorption of protein. Elevated levels are considered a sensitive but not specific indicator of intestinal toxemia, overgrowth of anaerobic bacteria, malabsorption of protein, or a high protein diet.
Comprehensive Digestive Stool Analysis (CDSA)	Commonly used by functional medicine practitioners for profiling digestive effectiveness, digestive enzyme adequacy, absorption, inflammatory markers; white blood cells; occult blood; bacterial, yeast, and parasitic infections.
Breath Testing	Useful method of distinguishing bacterial overgrowth from other digestive disorders. The hydrogen and methane breath test involves using a dose of glucose or lactulose after an overnight fast in order to identify bacterial overgrowth in the small intestine. The lactose breath test screens for lactose intolerance. The urea breath test is a rapid in-office diagnostic test used to confirm infections by Helicobacter pylori, a spiral bacterium implicated in gastritis and peptic ulcer disease. Urea breath tests are recommended as a non-invasive choice for detecting H. pylori before and after PUD treatment.
Salivary Hormone Testing (SHT)	A sensitive test to screen for hormone deficiency (cortisol, sex hormones) used extensively for therapeutic monitoring of hormone replacement regimens. In integrative practices, the test is used to assess effectiveness of dietary modification and supplementation with herbal and nutritional substances on hormonal balance.
Hair Analysis	An easy and inexpensive screening test for heavy metal toxicity, drug exposure, and, to a lesser extent nutrient status. The results may be too sensitive and may not correlate with those obtained in blood testing.

Serum Heavy metals	Serum heavy metals are sensitive and specific for heavy metal burden, but may not correlate well with results obtained from tissue biopsy.
IGg food sensitivity testing	ELISA/EIA (Enzyme Immunoassays) panels test the presence of IgG antibodies in patients to numerous food allergens. The results may be too sensitive for screening purposes, but may be of limited value in therapeutic monitoring.
ALCAT	Antigen leukocyte cellular antibody test that employs a modified Coulter counter, which counts and sizes white blood cells before and after incubation with suspect foods, food additives, and food colorings, The resultant data is compared with an unreacted control (the patient's unreacted blood). This use of this test became controversial after several studies indicated that it lacks clinical utility and specificity/reliability. It may be used as crude screening tool, but must be followed with a more specific test.

I n applying standards of external evidence to primary care practices, terminology and questions about the quality of the evidence and the validity of the test are very important, as stressed by the chief medical examination boards: USMLE, MCCQE, and NPLEX.

EVIDENCE EVALUATION TERMINOLOGY

Basic scientific concepts and terms are used in evaluating test validity and study quality.

- **Test Validity**: the *accuracy* of a diagnostic test. In other words, does the test measure what it claims to measure? For example, Candida Questionnaire versus actual candida overgrowth, Depression Questionnaire versus clinical depression, MAST versus alcoholism, etc.

- **Test Reliability**: the precision, reproducibility, or consistency of any diagnostic test. If a test is reliable, then it will provide the same score if two different people administer the same test. As a primary care clinician, you should be aware of the reliability of the routine tests you use in your practice (for example, CBC, PAP smear, mammogram, PCD examinations, function tests) or anything that is used to guide your clinical reasoning process.

- **Incidence**: the number of new cases of a disease in a unit of time = absolute (or total) risk of developing a condition.

- **Prevalence**: the total number of cases of a disease (new and old) at a specific time.

- **Attributable Risk**: the number of cases of a disease attributable to one risk factor (for example, lung cancer and smoking).

- **Relative Risk**: compares the disease risk in people exposed to or harboring a certain factor with the disease risk in people who are not. This value can only be calculated from experimental or prospective studies.

- **Clinically Significant Relative Risk**: any value other than 1 is clinically significant. When a person's RR is 1.5, they are 1.5 times more likely to develop the condition in question; alternatively, if a person's RR is 0.5, they are half as likely to develop something.

- **Odds Ratio**: a less desirable method of estimating the relative risk. This value can be calculated from less rigorous studies.

As a primary care clinician, you should be aware of the reliability of the routine tests you use in your practice or anything that is used to guide your clinical reasoning process.

- **Standard Deviation**: a feature of normal or bell-shaped distributions: 1 SD holds 68% of the values, 2 SD hold 95%, and 3 SD hold 99.7% of the values.
- **Mean**: average value.
- **Median**: middle value.
- **Mode**: most common value.
- **Normal distribution**: a distribution of values where the mean = median = mode.
- **Skewed distribution**: a distribution where the data do not follow the normal bell-shaped curve.
     a. Positive skew: an excess of high values = the tail of the curve is on the right (mean > median > mode).
     b. Negative skew: an excess of low values = the tail of the curve is on the left (mean < median < mode).
- **Correlation coefficient**: measures to what degree two variables are related (ranges from −1 to +1)
- **Confidence interval**: this is the acceptable threshold for studies to be accepted by the medical community. A confidence interval of 95% indicates that the mean of the entire population is within 2 SD of your experimental mean.
- **P-value**: the chance that data were obtained by error or chance. The acceptable threshold for studies to be accepted by the scientific community is 5% or less. P-value of < 0.05 is the cutoff for statistical significance.
- **Number needed to treat (NNT)**: the number of patients who need to be treated for one patient to benefit when compared to a control group in a clinical trial. The ideal would be an NNT of 1, which means everyone benefits/improves with treatment and no one benefits/improves with control. Higher NNT = less effective treatment.
- **Number needed to harm (NNH)**: the number of patients who need to be exposed to a specific risk factor to cause harm in one patient. Low NNH = worse risk factor.

Source QUALITY OF EVIDENCE EXAMINATION QUESTIONS

The following table of questions is derived from objectives set by three examination boards: USMLE, MCCQE, and NPLEX.

MCCQE
USMLE
1. What are the differences in the quality of evidence?

Evidence Ranking: Medical evidence has been ranked from highest to lowest quality and desirability as follows:
1. Experimental studies
2. Prospective studies
3. Retrospective studies
4. Case series
5. Prevalence surveys
6. Expert opinion
7. Individual case reports

MCCQE
USMLE
2. What is an experimental study?

Experimental Studies: tend to be regarded as the 'gold standard' because they compare two equal groups, in which one variable is altered and its effect (if any) is measured. Experimental studies use double blinding and well as matched controls to ensure accurate data.

MCCQE
USMLE
3. What are prospective studies?

Prospective Studies: also known as observational, longitudinal, cohort, incidence, or follow-up studies. Generally, a sample is divided based on the presence or absence of a risk factor; the groups are then followed over time to see what diseases they develop. You can calculate relative incidence from this type of study (for example, smokers have a higher incidence of cancer of the lung, oral cavity, esophagus, larynx, pharynx, bladder, kidney, pancreas, and cervix).

MCCQE
USMLE
4. What is a retrospective study?

Retrospective study: case-control studies, in which population samples are chosen after a certain fact, based on presence (cases) or absence (controls) of disease. Retrospective studies can be used to calculate an odds ratio, but not true relative risks or incidences.

5. What are case series studies?

Source

MCCQE
USMLE

Case Series: describes the clinical presentation of people with a certain disease. This type of study is good for extremely rare diseases or a new strain of a virus, and often suggests the need for a retrospective or prospective study.

6. What are prevalence surveys ?

MCCQE
USMLE

Prevalence or Cross-sectional Surveys: look at the prevalence of a disease and the prevalence of risk factors. When used to compare two different populations (cultures, countries, socioeconomic groups, or age groups), such surveys may suggest a possible cause of a disease.

7. How is the sensitivity of a test defined? What are highly sensitive tests used for clinically?

NPLEX
USMLE
Moore,
2001

Sensitivity: the ability of a test to detect disease (the # of true positives divided by the # of people with the disease). Tests with high sensitivity are used clinically for disease screening. Remember from lab Dx the acronym SNOUT (a SeNsitive test rules OUT a suspected condition).

8. How is the specificity of a test defined? What are highly specific tests used for clinically?

NPLEX
Moore,
2001

Specificity: the ability of a test to detect non-disease or health (the # of true negatives divided by the # of people without the disease). Tests with high specificity are used clinically for disease confirmation. Remember the acronym SPIN (a SPecific test rules IN a suspected condition).

9. What is positive predictive value (PPV)?

NPLEX
USMLE

Positive Predictive Value: a calculated value that tells you the likelihood that a patient has the disease when a certain test is positive (the # of true positives divided by the total number of people with a positive test).

Source

NPLEX
Moore,
2001
MCCQE

10. How do the concepts of sensitivity, specificity, and predictive value affect interpretation of any diagnostic test result? A Bayesian 2x2 table is used for illustration.

		Disease in a community		Property	Formula
		(+)	(-)	Sensitivity	A/(A+C)
Test results	(+)	A	B	Specificity	D/(B+D)
	(-)	C	D	Positive predictive value - PPV	A/(A+B)
* A = true positives B = false positives C = false negatives D = true negatives				Negative predictive value – NPV	D/(C+D)
				Odds Ratio	(AxD)/(BxC)
				Relative Risk	[A/(A+B)]/ [C/(C+D)]
				Attributable Risk	[A/(A+B)]- [C/(C+D)]

Moore,
2001

11. What would an abnormal test result mean?

Abnormal Test Result Interpretation:

1. Patient is sick.
2. Patient is well, but a statistical outlier.
3. Patient is well, but is not of the age, sex, or race group of the reference range population.
4. Patient is well, but is carrying out a proscribed activity, such as jogging or eating, before the sample was obtained; *or*
5. Population reference range may not be the healthy reference range.

Thus, an abnormal test result may indeed be an indicator of health. That is why we recommend a clinical reasoning process based on preponderance of evidence, not just an isolated piece of data or information.

12. Is there any single test that can rule in or out a particular disease?

- No. There is no single test that exhibits sufficient SNOUT or SPIN. Even if you have a wonderfully sensitive and specific test in the 95% range, by definition 5% of normal individuals will exhibit abnormal results. So the number of "false" findings is proportional to the number of tests used. Of course, if you subject a patient to a barrage of tests (a.k.a. a panel), you are bound to find some abnormal findings there. But does the finding mean anything? Lofgren (2004) mentions that 64% of normal individuals will exhibit at least one abnormal result on a standard blood chemistry panel composed of 20 individual tests. In this case, it is indeed abnormal for anyone to have a normal "screening" by the chem-20 panel.
- Several tests in combination give you increased sensitivity (but lower specificity). To increase specificity, you need to apply tests in a sequence, for example:

  ↳ Hb shows up low on a CBC (maybe anemia, maybe not)
     ↳ Request ferritin or TIBC (rule out iron deficiency). If ferritin high suspect anemia of chronic disease or thalassemia
         ↳ Request Hb electrophoresis (rule out thalassemia)

13. What subtypes of bias may exist in a clinical study?

Bias Sub-types:
- Nonresponse bias: When people do not return printed surveys, phone calls, or return for follow-up visits.
- Lead-time bias: Due to time differentials. For example, screening tests that claim to prolong survival compared with older survival data when in fact the difference is due only to early detection, not to improved treatment or longer survival.
- Admission rate bias: When an experimenter compares outcomes from two patient populations, in which diagnostic inclusion criteria are not the same (for example, a higher rate of mortality may be due to tougher admission criteria rather than efficacy of treatment).
- Recall bias: When people inadvertently over- or underestimate risk factors because they cannot remember exactly.
- Interviewer bias: Occurs in the absence of blinding, when a scientist inadvertently categorizes an outcome "significant" in the case group and "not significant" in the control group.
- Unacceptability bias: When people do not admit to deleterious or embarrassing behavior to please the interviewer.

Examination Board References

Naturopathic Physician Licensing Examination part II (NPLEx II) blueprint. 2010. North American Board of Naturopathic Examiners (NABNE).

Brochert A. 2008. Crush Step 3. The Ultimate USMLE Step 3 Review. Third edition. Saunders Elsevier

Dugani S, Lam D, eds. 2009. MCCQE Review Notes & Lecture Series. Medical Counsel of Canada Qualification Examination Review notes. Mcgraw Hill Professional; Canadian edition.

Related References

Bickley LS. Bates' Guide to Physical Examination and History Taking. 9th ed. Philadelphia, PA: Lippincott Williams & Wilkins, 2007.

Chaput de Saintonge DM, Herxheimer A. Harnessing placebo effects in health care. Lancet 1994;344:995.8.

Dains J, Baumann L, Scheibel P. Advanced Health Assessment & Clinical Diagnosis in Primary Care. 4th ed. New York, NY: Mosby C.V. Co. Ltd., 2011.

Dixon M, Sweeney K. The Human Effect in Medicine: Theory, Research and Practice. Oxford, UK: Radcliffe Medical Press, 2000.

Edzard E, Pittler MH, Stevenson C, White A. The Desktop Guide to Complementary and Alternative Medicine: An Evidence Based Approach. London, UK: Mosby, 2001:50-55, 61-64.

Imrie R. The evidence for evidence based medicine. Complement Ther Med 2002;8:123-26.

Kaptchuk TJ. Powerful placebo: The dark side of the randomized controlled trial. Lancet 1998;351:1722.5.

Kleijnen J, de Craen AJM, van Everdingen J, Krol L. Placebo effect in double blind clinical trials: A review of interactions with medications. Lancet 1994;344:1347.9.

Lipkin M, Putnam SM, Lazare A, et al, eds. Medical Interview: Clinical Care, Education and Research. New York, NY: Springer-Verlag; 1995.

Lofgren RL. Principles of preventive maintenance and test selection. Mladenovic J (ed.). Primary Care Secrets. Philadelphia, PA: Hanley & Belfus, 2004.

Marvel MK, Epstein RM, Flowers C, Beckman HB. Soliciting the patient's agenda: Have we improved? Journal of the American Medical Association. 1999; 281:283-87.

Moore R. Hematology Laboratory Diagnosis. Hamilton, ON: McMaster University Press, 2001.

Olson KP. "Oh, by the way...": agenda setting in office visits. Fam Pract Manag. 2002 Nov-Dec;9(10):63-4.

Ontario Board of Naturopathic Medicine (BDDT-N). 2004. Policies and Guidelines. Toronto, ON, 2004.

Platt FW, Gordon GH. Field Guide to the Difficult Patient Interview. Philadelphia, PA: Lippincott Williams and Wilkins; 1999.

Sackett DL, Rosenberg WMC, Gray JAM, Richardson WS. Evidence-based medicine: What it is and what it is not. BMJ 1996;Jan 13;312:71-72.

Sackett DL, Rosenberg WMC, Gray JAM, Richardson WS. Evidence-based Medicine: How to Practice and Teach EBM. New York, NY: Churchill Livingstone, 1997.

Silverman J, Kurtz SM, Draper J. Skills for Communicating With Patients. Oxon, England: Radcliffe Medical Press Ltd; 1998.

CASE MANAGEMENT GUIDELINES

PREFACE

This clinical guide offers a series of mutually exclusive modules that develop the basic knowledge of body systems and medical conditions, clinical reasoning strategies, and therapeutic management skills needed in naturopathic family medicine primary care practice. Each module represents a body of knowledge of a system – for example, cardiology – and provides diagnostic and treatment protocols for significant conditions – for example, hypertension. At the end of each module, direct Socratic-style questions are posed to foster prompt clinical reasoning. In addition, case histories are presented for classroom discussion and for developing problem-solving skills. These are the kind of questions naturopathic medical students will face during their clerkships, clinical rotations, board examinations, and, ultimately, practice of naturopathic family medicine and primary care. Signs and symptoms and diagnostic criteria are presented in systematic lists to check off. First-line naturopathic treatment approaches are discussed in convenient charts for handy clinical reference. The first-line treatment approach, which encompasses empirical and research-based naturopathic doctrine, is referenced and critiqued in a clear manner that enables clinicians to utilize and individualize naturopathic best practices to suit their needs. Conventional treatment approaches are integrated, and emergency conditions are identified.

To enable the development of competency in the assessment and management of primary care presentations, care has been given to ensure that each module presents current research and complies with the standards of relevant medical boards and associations. The three principal bodies referenced are the study guides for NPLEX (II), USMLE, and MCCQE (II) licensing examinations:

NPLEX (II): North American Board of Naturopathic Examiners
North American Board of Naturopathic Examiners (NABNE), Naturopathic Physician Licensing Examination Part II Blueprint and Study Guide. Portland, OR: NABNE, 2005.

USMLE (II): National Board of Medical Examiners
Bouchert A. USMLE Step 2 Secrets. Philadelphia, PA: Hanley & Belfus Inc., 2000.

MCCQE: Medical Council of Canada
Molckovsky A, Pirzada KS (eds.). Review for the Medical Council of Canada Qualification Examination. Toronto, ON: Toronto Notes Medical Publishing, 2004.

Also referenced are guideline-generating national and international medical associations, such as the World Health Organization, Center for Disease Control, US Preventive Health Services Task Force, and Canadian Diabetes Association, as well as evidence-based trials, literature reviews, and expert opinion.

These primary practice guidelines, primary evidence (trials) citations, secondary sources (reviews), and published expert opinion are included as abbreviated references in the "Source" column of each module, followed by full references at the end of each module.

In sum, this section functions to prepare naturopathic medical students for their licensing board examinations by posing typical exam questions with well-reasoned answers, and offers the naturopathic primary care practitioner with a convenient clinical handbook for common presentations.

CARDIOLOGY

ELECTROCARDIOGRAM

Function

Hamption, 2003

Electrocardiogram (ECG): records the electrical activity of the heart. Various pathologies cause specific changes in the trace. The ECG is not a flawless diagnostic tool. A patient with an organic heart disorder may have an apparently normal trace, whereas a perfectly normal individual may show nonspecific abnormalities. ECG findings must be placed within the patient's clinical context. In naturopathic primary practice, ECGs may be used to screen for cardiac abnormalities where indicated (e.g., chest pain, hypertension, and COPD).

Atrial depolarization: The P waves represent atrial depolarization. The PR interval is caused by the slow propagation of the depolarization through the AVN; this allows time for the ventricles to fill. PR is measured from the start of P to the start of R. Once the depolarization reaches the ventricles, conduction must be fast. The impulse passes though the following hierarchy of structures:

AVN → Bundle of His → Right then Left bundle branches → Anterior fascicle of the left bundle branch → and finally the Posterior fascicle of the left bundle branch.

Ventricular depolarization: This is recorded as the QRS complex. In practice, the Q, R and S waves are not always present. The Q wave is defined as any initial downward deflection. The R wave is defined as any deflection upwards. The S wave is defined as any down deflection that is not Q. The T wave is the repolarization.

Interpretation

NPLEX MCCQE USMLE

1. Rate and Rhythm:
- Rate 60-100 beats per minutes (lower in athletes and those on Beta blockers).
- Sinus rhythm is considered normal when QRS is largely regular in shape and preceded by a P wave. Abnormalities of rhythm can be divided into bradycardia, tachycardia, or irregular rhythm.
- In children, sinus arrhythmia is a variant of normal, resulting in a reduced rate on inspiration.

2. Cardiac Axis: The cardiac axis is the predominant direction of ventricular depolarization. Determination of the axis is useful in the diagnosis of:
- Right ventricular hypertrophy (when the axis is >90 degrees).
- Left anterior hemiblock (when the axis is <-30 degrees).

3. P waves: The P wave is caused by the depolarization of the atria and is altered by atrial pathologies. Of note are the defective P waves caused by atrial hypertrophy:
- P pulmonale (RA hypertrophy): P pulmonale are big, tall, peaked P waves on ECG. They are associated with lung disease.
- P mitrale (LA hypertrophy): P mitrale is an ECG finding of a P wave shaped like an M. It is indicative of a hypertrophied left atrium (think mitral stenosis or LVF).

4. PR interval: The reference range for the PR interval is between 0.2 sec (each small block on ECG tracings = 0.04 sec, each large block = 0.20 sec) and 0.12 sec (3 small blocks). The PR interval represents the time taken for activation to pass from the sinus node, across the atrium, through the AV node, into the Purkinje system, and finally to activate the ventricles.

- PR interval is >0.2 seconds (5 small blocks) occurs if there is delay in the conduction pathway from the sino-atrial node to the ventricles (i.e., heart block). Remember that a finding of first-degree heart block may have no pathological significance. However it may be a sign of underlying disease.
- PR interval reduced: <0.12 seconds (3 small blocks) is always a serious pathological finding indicating Wolf-Prakinson-White (WPW) or Lown-Ganong-Levine (LGL) syndromes.

5. QRS complex:
- Normal QRS duration is never greater than 0.12 seconds (3 small blocks).
- It is prolonged (AKA "wide") in Bundle Branch Block (BBB), complete heart block, and premature ventricular contraction (PVC).

6. QT interval: Measured from the start of the QRS complex to the start of the T wave. In the normal adult it should <0.05 seconds (1 small block).
- Prolonged QT results in syncope, ventricular arrhythmia, and sudden death.
- Shortened QT interval may be due to hypercalcaemia or digoxin toxicity.

7. ST segment:
- Should be isoelectric. Myocardial infarct causes ST elevation (STEMI = S-T segment Elevation Myocardial Infarction) in the leads that reflect the area of injury and reciprocal ST depression in the leads opposite form the area of infarct.
- ST depression: indicates myocardial ischaemia, and may be associated with the discomfort of angina; rest leads to a reversal; it is not a sign of infarction; and it may be caused by hypokalemia.
- ST elevation:
- An upwardly convex and elevated ST segment indicates acute MI or less commonly variant (Prinzmetal's) angina.
- An upwardly concave, elevated and widespread ST segment indicates pericarditis (that's how you can tell pericarditis temponade from a heart attack, both have radically different treatments).

8. T waves: Mycardial ischemia (angina), necrosis (MI), and ventricular hypertrophy cause inversion of T waves due to altered repolarization. Hyperventilation may also cause inverted T waves. When it comes to T waves context matters, as they may be normally inverted in leads III + V1 in many patients, V2 in young people, V3 in people with African ancestry.
- In ventricular hypertrophy, there will be T wave inversion in the leads that represent the affected ventricle (i.e., II, V5, V6, and VL represent the left ventricle; and V1, V2, and V3 represent the right ventricle).
- Digoxin administration causes T wave inversion, particularly with sloping depression of the ST segment. Thus, it is useful to record an ECG before beginning digitalis to save later confusion about the significance of T wave changes.

MYOCARDIAL INFARCTION AND ISCHEMIA

Myocardial Infarction (MI) Presentation

NPLEX
MCCQE
USMLE

Pain
- Crushing or pressure sensation, usually not sharp.
- Poorly localized substernal pain that may radiate to shoulder (particularly in men), arm, or jaw.
- Lasts for at least half an hour and is not reproducible by palpation. If the pain is reproducible on chest palpation, the cause is in the chest wall. If the pain is related to certain foods or eating habits, it is usually gastroesophageal in origin.
- Pain is relieved by nitroglycerin in angina but not in MI (since the damage of infarction is irreversible).
- 25% of MIs are without chest pain, especially in patients with diabetic neuropathy and female patients. Instead there is CHF, shock, or confusion. This is often seen in geriatric patients.
- Notwithstanding, many primary care providers still opt for an ECG and possibly one or more cardiac enzyme assessments (such as Creatine Kinase–MB fraction, troponin I, or Lactate Dehydrogenase) to make sure that a heart attack has not occurred.

Mitake,
2010

Other MI Signs and Symptoms:
- Diaphoresis
- Anxiety
- Tachycardia
- Tachypnea
- Paleness
- Nausea and vomiting
- A large MI may cause CHF, with secondary distention of neck veins and bilateral pulmonary rales (in absence of pneumonia symptoms); S3 or S4 heart sound; new murmurs; hypotension and/or shock.

ECG Signs of MI:
- Flipped or flattened T waves
- ST segment elevation (ST depression = ischemia, while elevation = injury)
- Early segmental development of significant Q waves
- With these readings → Call an ambulance to take patient to ER immediately.

Risk Factors

NPLEX
MCCQE
USMLE

- History of angina
- Previous chest pains
- Murmurs; arrhythmias
- Risk factors for coronary artery disease (CAD)
- Hypertension
- Diabetes
- Medications, such as digoxin, furosemide, or cholesterol lowering drugs (this means that patients with Myocardial Infarction (MI) have CAD risk factors)

Source

NPLEX
MCCQE
USMLE

Common Noncardiac Causes of Chest Pain

- Gastroesophageal reflux disease (GERD) and peptic ulcer disease (PUD): There is usually a relation to certain foods (spicy, chocolate), smoking, or lying down. Pain is relieved with antacids or milk. Patient's with PUD usually test positive for *Helicobacter pylori*.
- Chest wall pain: Costochondritis and bruised or broken ribs cause well-localized and reproducible pain on chest wall palpation.
- Esophageal problems: Achalasia or esophageal spasms are difficult differential diagnoses. One has to rely on negative findings of the MI work-up and often refer for barium swallow or esophageal manometry.
- Pericarditis: This is easier to ascertain because there is usually a viral upper respiratory infection (URI) prodrome; ECG shows ST elevation; erythrocyte sedimentation rate (ESR) is elevated; and a low grade fever is present. Sitting forward often relieves this type of pain.
- Pneumonia: This is even easier to differentiate because patients will have pleuritic pain (see Pulmonology module), cough, fever, and/or sputum production.

Dains,
2011

- Aortic dissection: Memorize the following: STAR (Severe, Tearing, And Ripping) pain that may radiate to the back. Immediately refer to hospital for contrast CT to confirm. DDx from pancreatitis pain that radiates to the back but is experienced as constant, boring pain originating from LUQ. Also refer to hospital for BUN, LDH, serum glucose, AST, WBC (Ranson's Criteria) for confirmation.
- There is strong association of aortic dissection with Marfan's syndrome (tall, thin, double-jointed patients) and blunt chest traumas.

MI Management Plan

NPLEX
MCCQE
USMLE

Chest Pain Management: In primary practice, the first task when a patient complains of chest pain is to make sure it is not due a life-threatening condition. Rule out myocardial infarctions (MI) and myocardial ischemia (angina) as causative factors for the patient's complaints. An MI (heart attack) is never treated in an outpatient facility, be it allopathic or naturopathic.

Gonzales,
2009
AHA, 2006

Lifestyle Modification:
- Smoking: Smoking cessation consistently lowers blood pressure and lipids, resulting in 40% decrease in cardiovascular mortality.
- Body weight: American Heart Association (AHA) 2006 recommends primary prevention of MI by maintaining a healthy body weight.
- Diet: Rich in vegetables and fruit, whole grains, high fiber;oily fish twice per week; limit dietary saturated fat <7%, trans fat<1%, cholesterol <300mg q.d.; limit beverages and foods with added sugars; use little or no salt.
- Aspirin: United States Preventive Services Task Force (USPSTF) 2002 strongly recommends daily aspirin use (optimum dose unknown) for secondary prevention (-32% Risk Reduction for MI, -17%RR for stroke; S/E bleeding).

Age under 40: A patient under the age of 40 with no known heart disease, strong family history, or multiple risk factors for coronary artery disease (CAD) is unlikely to have an MI.

Risk Factors: Physically fit patients, consuming a healthy diet, who are without cardiac risk factors and whose HDL is high, are not likely to have heart attacks.

Source

NPLEX
MCCQE
USMLE

Angina Presentation

Angina strictly means that the heart is temporarily not getting enough oxygen. Unstable angina means a worsening of the condition of stable angina (i.e., frequency is increased). Variant or Prinzmetal angina is a rare condition, caused by coronary artery spasm.

Stable Angina Signs and Symptoms:
- Pain on exertion that is relieved by lying down and resting for a while.
- Pain is described as a squeeze or pressure behind the chest wall.
- Pain may radiate to shoulders, neck, or jaw.
- Pain lasts for less than 20 minutes and is relieved by nitroglycerin.
- Often shortness of breath, diaphoresis, and or nausea.

Unstable Angina Signs and Symptoms:
- Enzymes will be normal, but the ECG will show ST depression.
- Pain will last longer than 20 minutes, and will not be relieved by nitroglycerin.
- Pain will often begin at rest.
- If these signs and symptoms are present → Refer to ER.

Variant or Prinzmetal Angina Signs and Symptoms:
- Onset not related to exertion
- Normal enzymes
- ST elevation
- Responds to nitroglycerin.
- If these signs and symptoms are present, the recommended treatment is calcium channel blockers to reduce arterial spasms.

NPLEX
MCCQE
USMLE

Angina Management Plan

- Manage stable angina with the same measures as MI management and address risk factors for CAD.
- Prudent naturopathic management would follow best practices and opt for an ECG and possibly one or more cardiac enzyme assessments (such as Creatine Kinase–MB fraction, troponin I, or Lactate Dehydrogenase) to make sure that an MI has not occurred.
- ECG will not be remarkable unless performed during the acute attack. Everything else will be WNL.
- Routine screening of asymptomatic persons with stress ECG (exercise tolerance testing) is not advised by the American Heart Association (AHA) or the American College of Cardiology (ACC), but is recommended for stable angina patients and those at risk to help assess future risk of MI, and guide secondary prevention strategies.

Daly, 2003

Source

NPLEX

Pizzorno,
1999

Tripathi,
2009

Breslow,
2006

Zeng, 2003

Godfrey,
2010

Guidelines for First-line Naturopathic Treatment of Angina

Approach
- Reduce CAD risk factors.
- Improve excercise tolerance.
- Treat comorbid conditions.
- Provide symptom relief.
- Reduce arterial resistance.

1. Minimize obstacles to healing
- Lifestyle: Ideally, no smoking, alcohol, or caffeine. Implement a medically supervised aerobic exercise plan (start with short walks).
- Stress: Stress management (relaxation/yoga/Qi gong/behavioral therapy) 30 minutes 3X per week.
- Diet: Reduce or eliminate saturated fats, hydrogenated oils, cholesterol, fried foods, simple carbohydrates, and food sensitivities. Increase consumption of fiber, onions, garlic, vegetables, and cold-water fish.
- Risk factors: Address underlying hypertension, diabetes, or obesity if applicable.

2. Clinical nutrition
- Coenzyme Q10: 150-300 mg q.d. Reduces frequency of angina by 53%; increases exercise tolerance.
- L-carnitine: 500 mg t.i.d. Heart ischemia induces its deficiency; improves angina; and allows myocardium to be more efficient in oxygen utilization.
- Magnesium citrate: 200-400 mg t.i.d. Dilates coronary arterioles; improves myocardial energy production; reduces peripheral vascular resistance. S/E: osmotic diarrhea with higher doses.
- L-arginine: 1000 mg t.i.d. Produces nitric oxide resulting in vasodilation; scavenges free radicals released from ischemic myocardium reducing oxidative damage.
- Omega-3 fatty acids: 1g q.d. of EPA + DHA reduces risk of cardiovascular death, improves vascular reactivity, and reduces inflammation along with platelet aggregation.
- Berberine: 400-600 mg t.i.d. Enhances coronary artery blood flow.

3. Botanical medicine
- Crataegus oxyacantha: "solid extract" 100-250 mg (standardized to 10% procyanidin content) t.i.d. Excellent cardiac tonic; interacts with enzymes to enhance myocardial contractility.
- Ammi visnaga: 100 mg (standardized to 12% khellin content). Effective at relieving angina symptoms; similar in action to calcium channel blockers. S/E: may cause nausea and vomiting.
- Leonurus cardiac: 60-120 gtt tincture q.d. Increases coronary blood flow and relaxes smooth muscles.

HEART MURMURS

Source

Presentation

NPLEX
MCCQE
USMLE

Heart murmurs are exhibited by almost everyone sometime during their life. As a general guideline, those murmurs occurring without any evidence of cardiovascular abnormality are considered innocent normal variants. Murmurs that are considered normal and should not be referred to a cardiologist are:
- Functional systolic murmurs of children and young adults
- Mammary soufflé late in pregnancy and during lactation
- Aortic systolic murmur of older age

Functional Heart Murmurs: only systolic murmurs (you would be able to tell if you are taking the pulse at the same time) may be functional or flow murmurs.

Signs and Symptoms:
- Grade 2/6 (slight) systolic murmur over the aortic area.
- No chest pain, dyspnea, syncope, cyanosis, or edema.
- Normal chest radiograph and ECG results.
- Usually no other remarkable physical findings or positive family history for cardiac disease.

Management: This is a finding of no significance, which you will need to explain carefully to the concerned patient.

Adventitious Heart Sounds

NPLEX
MCCQE
USMLE

NORMAL
Murmurs are classified based on their timing and duration:
- Normal murmurs include functional systolic murmurs of children and young adults; mammary soufflé late in pregnancy and during lactation; and aortic systolic murmur of older age.
- S2 physiologic splitting on inhalation is considered benign or normal.

ABNORMAL

Auscultation	Other Findings	Diagnosis
Mid systolic click (usually) + late systolic murmur	Squatting *decreases* murmur, while valsalva increases it.	Mitral valve prolapse
Harsh systolic murmurs heard over aortic area that radiates to carotids.	Squatting *increases* murmur, while valsalva decreases it. Left ventricular hypertrophy, angina, heart failure, and syncope.	Aortic valve stenosis
Pan-systolic murmur that radiates to axilla	Left ventricular hypertrophy, pulmonary hypertension.	Mitral regurgitation

Source	Auscultation	Other Findings	Diagnosis
	Early diastolic murmur and S3 sound (resembles the rhythm of 'Tenn-es-see'); best heard at the apex.	Left ventricular hypertrophy and dilation.	Aortic regurgitation
	Late diastolic murmur and opening snap; best heard at the apex.	Atrial fibrillation, pulmonary hypertension.	Mitral valve stenosis
	S4 sound (resembles the rhythm of 'Ken-tucky'); heard just before S1.	Old age, increased resistance to ventricular filling.	Atrial Gallop

- It is good practice to take carotid pulse while listening to heart sounds. Murmurs that occur during the pulse are systolic and vice versa. S1 (LUB sound that is best heard on the right of sternum) is made when the AV valves close at the beginning of systole. S2 (DUB sound that is best heard on the left of sternum) is made when semilunar valves (aortic and pulmonic) close at the end of systole.

NPLEX
MCCQE
USMLE

Endocarditis Prophylaxis

Antimicrobial prophylaxis is considered when a patient has a known valve disease or prosthetic valves and is scheduled for surgery (dental procedures too). The idea is simple – destroy the *Staph. aureus* & *epidermidis* and *Streptococcus viridans* before the autoimmune cascade starts (again).

DEEP VENOUS THROMBOSIS

NPLEX
MCCQE
USMLE

Presentation

Signs and Symptoms:
- Hallmark is unilateral leg swelling (pitting edema), intermittent claudication, pain and/or Homan's sign present (in only 30% of DVT cases).
- Palpable cords imply superficial thrombophlebitis but not DVT.

NPLEX
MCCQE
USMLE

Risk Factors

1. Surgery (orthopedic, pelvic, or abdominal)
2. Malignancy
3. Immobilization
4. Pregnancy
5. BCPs
6. Deficiencies in anticlotting factors (e.g, antithrombin III)

Source

NPLEX
MCCQE
USMLE

Diagnosis

- Recommended diagnostic test remains Doppler ultrasound or impedance plethysmography of leg veins.
- When the diagnosis is not clear, the invasive venography is resorted to.
- If DDx edema → Refer to ER if you suspect DVT.

NPLEX
MCCQE
USMLE

Superficial Thrombophlebitis

Superficial thrombophlebitis (palpable clot cords + erthyma + edema + pain) is localized to superficial veins and is not considered a cause of pulmonary embolism.

Treatment:
- Naturopathic treatment and pressure stockings are effective at controlling or reversing the condition.
- Conventional treatment usually involves NSAIDs.

NPLEX
MCCQE
USMLE

Prognosis

DVT can cause pulmonary embolism (PE) and ascending thrombosis, requiring systemic anticoagulation therapy.

Treatment:
- IV Heparin is used to initiate treatment, then oral warfarin is used for at least 3 months.
- Naturopathic treatments may be used as adjunct or alternative treatment after the condition has stabilized.
- DVT prevention is recommended for high-risk patients, history of prior DVTs surgery, pregnancy and immobilization (long distance travel).
- DVT prevention includes frequent mobilization (scheduled walking), compression socks, and anticoagulation therapy where indicated.
- Routine screening via Doppler ultra sound is not recommended for asymptomatic patients.

Stahl, 2006
Agarwal,
2007

PULMONARY EMBOLISM

NPLEX
MCCQE
USMLE

Presentation

Signs and Symptoms:
- Classical presentation is sudden shortness of breath (due to loss of alveolar gas exchange), tachypnea (to compensate for the loss), and chest pain. → Refer to ER immediately.
- May exacerbate into lung infarction with hemoptysis, hypotension, or death.
- Ventilation/perfusion scan will show the area of diminished blood flow.
- Chest X-ray (CXR) rarely shows peripheral pleural opacities.

Source

NPLEX
MCCQE
USMLE

Causes:

- PE may follow DVT, delivery, or long-bone fractures.
- Divers who ascend too quickly (or who take flights a couple of hours after a series of deep dives) may also develop multiple air embolism (bends) as well as PE. The pulmonary arterioles act as filter to circulating emboli (e.g., thrombi, amniotic fluid, fat, or air).

DVT and Stroke

DVT can cause PE, but not stroke, because lung arterioles will act as a filter for circulating emboli. However, in the extremely rare occasion that a patient also has a patent foramen ovale or ventricular-septal defect, this argument would not hold true.

COAGULATION

NPLEX
MCCQE
USMLE

Presentation

Common Coagulation Conditions

These are the same conditions that would cause easy bruising, prolonged bleeding, and petechiae.

Condition	Prolonged Coagulation Tests	Memory Aids
Hemophilia A or B (deficiency in factor VIII or IX, respectively)	Partial Thromboplastin Time (PTT)	Mostly men are affected since it is X-linked. Common.
Von Willebrand Factor Deficiency (vWF deficiency)	PTT and bleeding time	Autosomal dominant inheritance. Common.
Liver disease	Prothrombin Time (PT) and maybe PTT	Stigmata for liver disease.
Vitamin K deficiency	PT mainly	Neonate who did not receive prophylactic vitamin K. Also malabsorption, alcoholism, and prolonged antibiotic use.

- Less common causes include uremia, vitamin C deficiency, disseminated intravascular coagulation (DIC), and prolonged corticosteroid therapy.

CONGESTIVE HEART FAILURE

Source

NPLEX
MCCQE
USMLE

Presentation

Signs and Symptoms:

"Faces"

- Fatigue
- Activity intolerance
- Cough
- Edema
- Shortness of breath (SOB on exertion)

Physical Exam Findings:

- Increased jugular venous pressure
- Rales
- S3 or S4
- Increased heart rate
- Cardiomegaly

Diagnosis:

- Reduced ventricular ejection fraction (Echo)
- Elevated levels of brain naturidic peptide (can be used for screening and prognosis)

Right Ventricular Failure

Peripheral edema; jugular venous distension; hepatomegaly; ascites; and /or cor pulmonale

Left Ventricular Failure

Orthopnea (sleeps on more than one pillow or sitting up); nocturnal dyspnea; and bilateral rales over base of lungs.

- In practice, it is usually both ventricles that are failing.

Risk Factors

- Hypertension
- Atherosclerosis
- Diabetes
- Obesity
- Metabolic Syndrome

Classification

Acute CHF: an abrupt disruption of circulation and ventilation. The common example is extensive myocardial infarction secondary to coronary atherosclerotic artery disease (CAAD).

Source

Gonzales,
2009

Chronic CHF: There are four stages of CHF, according to the American Heart Association (AHA):

- Stage I: Echocardiography shows reduced ventricular ejection + No symptoms at rest or with exercise
- Stage II: Symptom free at rest + dyspnea on moderate physical exertion
- Stage III: Symptom free at rest + dyspnea on minor physical exertion
- Stage IV: Symptoms exist at rest (peripheral edema and dyspnea)

NPLEX
MCCQE
USMLE

Conventional Treatment

Acute CHF is treated on an inpatient basis with oxygen, diuretics, and positive inotropes. Chronic CHF is treated on an outpatient basis with sodium restriction; ACE inhibitors (first-line agents that reduce mortality rates); diuretics; beta-Adrenergic blockers; andangiotensin II receptor antagonists. Advanced cases are treated with digoxin or digitoxin.

Guidelines for First-line Naturopathic Treatment of Stage I and II CHF

Approach: Naturopathic treatment is recommended for Stage I and II, but only as adjunctive therapy for Stage III and IV.

Pizzorno,
2006

1. Address underlying cause
- Reduce hypertension.
- Lose weight if obese.
- Implement a temporary medically supervised aerobic exercise plan (start with short walks) with instructions for self-monitoring.
- Stop alcohol and tobacco consumption.
- Decrease stress.

Pina, 2003

2. Dietary measures
- Encourage a low sodium healthy diet (DASH).
- Emphasize whole plant foods, fruit and nuts.
- Avoid refined, processed, and fatty foods.

3. Clinical nutrition
- L-carnitine: 300-500 mg t.i.d. for at least 6 months. Improves exercise tolerance by 16% to 25% and ventricular ejection fraction by 12% to 13%.
- Coenzyme Q10: 150-300 mg q.d. for at least 3 months. Clinical studies documented significant efficacy in improving CHF symptoms and quality of life.

Bevran-
vamd,
2011

- Taurine: 500-2000 mg t.i.d. Improves exercise capacity and cardiac function and lowers blood pressure.
- Assess and treat deficiencies in magnesium, thiamine, and arginine.

4. Botanical medicine

Saunders,
2000
Godfrey et
al, 2010

- *Crataegus oxyacantha:* 'solid extract' 100-250 mg (standardized to 10% procyanidin content) t.i.d. Used alone for early stages; combine with conventional treatment for advanced stages. Improves cardiac efficiency and work capacity.

Source

Zeng, 2003

- *Selenicerius grandifloris* (positive inotropic and negative chronotropic, Nervine) and *Convallaria majalis* (considered as a safer alternative to Digitalis) should be considered.
- Berberine: 400-600mg t.i.d. Reduces dyspnea and fatigue, improves exercise capacity, reduces systolic BP 15mmHg and 9mmHg diastolic and reduces mortality. May produce s/e of digestive upset (diarrhea, constipation).
- *Leonarus cardianca:* a traditional remedy shown in a few clinical trials to slow heart rate and increase ejection fraction. Rigorous clinical trials lacking but there is no negative evidence.

COR PULMONALE

NPLEX
MCCQE
USMLE

Presentation

Right ventricular enlargement secondary to primary lung disease (the ventricles try to increase output to overcome the imposed resistance).

Causes:
- COPD and PE
- Other less common causes include primary pulmonary hypertension and sleep apnea.
- Clinical findings may include tachypnea, cyanosis, clubbing, parasternal heave, and distinct S4 sound (over right side) in addition to signs of pulmonary disease.

CARDIOMYOPATHY

NPLEX
MCCQE
USMLE

Presentation

Term used to denote a group of primary myocardial diseases that cannot be related to coronary atherosclerosis, hypertension, valvular disease, infections, or congenital heart disease. Cardiomyopathies are considered diseases for which heart transplantation and surgical repair are recommended.

Classifications: Cardiomyopathies are classified on the basis of clinical and pathological features into three groups:
- Dilated
- Hypertrophic
- Restrictive

The most common is dilated cardiomyopathy, a systolic disorder, where progressive heart failure is caused by hypertrophy and dilation of all four chambers of the heart. This is mostly an idiopathic condition, but a minority of cases may be due to alcohol, viral myocarditis, and drugs, such as doxorubicin.

Source

Hypertrophic Cardiomyopathy: often an autosomal dominant trait, this is an idiopathic condition, where ventricular hypertrophy reduces cardiac output (diastolic dysfunction). This condition is treated conventionally with beta-blockers and calcium-channel-blockers to allow the ventricles more time to fill. Strenuous exercise should be avoided in such cases.

Causes of Restrictive and Constrictive Pericarditis

Restrictive Pericarditis: amyloidosis, sarcoidosis, hemochromatosis, and myocardial fibroelastosis may lead to restrictive cardiomyopathy. These are diagnosed by histological examination of a ventricular biopsy.

Constrictive Pericarditis: characterized by dense fibrous connective tissue that encases the heart (restricting diastolic expansion). This can be corrected by removing the abnormal pericardium. It is often idiopathic, but may follow suppurative or caseous pericarditis. Clinical signs will include a 'pericardial knock' (an early diastolic sound that represents the sudden cessation of ventricular diastolic filling imposed by the rigid pericardial sac) or S4 sound. Of course, a ventricular biopsy will not indicate any pathology.

CARDIAC ARRHYTHMIA

MCCQE
USMLE

Presentation

Normal ECG "lead II" tracing for comparison:
- Normal rhythm, called sinus rhythm, is paced from the sinoatrial (SA) node.
- The heart rate for normal sinus rhythm is from 60 to 100 beats per minute.
- Sinus rhythms show a normally oriented P wave before each QRS complex.

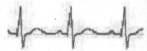

Sinus Tachycardia:
- Normal P, QRS, T, rate > 100.
- Usually no treatment is recommended.
- Treat the cause.

Sinus Bradycardia:
- Normal P, QRS, T, rate < 60.
- Usually not treated.
- Atropine is used is used in severe and symptomatic cases.

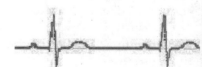

Premature Ventricular Contractions (PVCs):
- Wide QRS, unrelated to P wave.
- Usually not treated. PVCs that are increasing in frequency must be evaluated further because they may be not so benign.
- Lidocaine is used in severe and symptomatic cases.

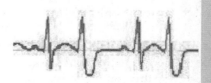

Source

Ventricular Tachycardia (VTAC):
- Bizarre, wide QRS, no P wave, rate >100.
- Emergency condition.
- Immediate Lidocaine administration is needed.

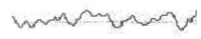

Ventricular Fibrillation (VFIB):
- Chaotic waves.
- Emergency condition.
- Defibrillate immediately.

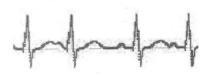

Premature Atrial Contraction (PAC):
- Premature P wave, irregular P-P interval.

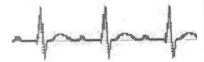

First-degree Heart Block:
- Long PR interval.
- No medical treatment is recommended.
- Beta-blockers and calcium-channel-blockers are contraindicated.

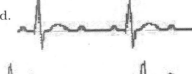

Second-degree Heart Block:
- Mobitz type I: increasing PR interval until a QRS complex is dropped.
- Usually benign but pacemaker or atropine if severe.
- Mobitz type II: multiple P waves, but when beats are conducted PR intervals are unvarying (pacemaker).

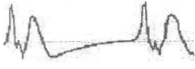

Third-degree Heart Block / with Idoiventricular (escape) Rhythm:
- Bizarre QRS, slow rate 20-40. Pacemaker is recommended.

Hypercalcemia:
- Short/absent ST segment.

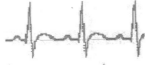

Hyperkalemia:
- Tent-shaped T wave.

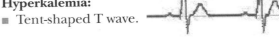

Digitalis effect:
- Scooping ST segment.

Asystole:
- Flatline.

Atrial fibrillation/flutter: Random electrical activity in the atrium + secondary irregular ventricular contractions. Acute cases are 'cardioverted' with quinidine or direct current cardioversion. Chronic cases need effective anticoagulation (since atria are acting like egg-beaters), then cardioversion. Naturopathic treatment is recommended to prevent relapses. Relapses require digoxin and sustained warfarin.

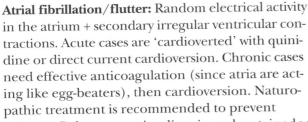

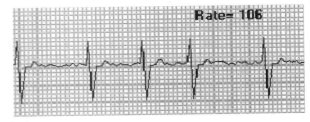

Rate= 106

Snow, 2003
AHA, 2006
Gonzales, 2009
Godfrey et al, 2010

Endocrine Disease

NPLEX
MCCQE
USMLE

Hyperthyroidism or Thyroid Storm: should always be suspected and ruled out in all presentation of sinus tachycardia or atrial fibrillation.

Source

NPLEX
MCCQE
USMLE

Wolf-Parkinson-White (WPW) Syndrome

A subtype of atrial flutter. The classical example is a child who becomes dizzy/SOB/syncope after playing, and then recovers completely with no lasting effects.

Signs and Symptoms:
- Atrial flutter is a fairly organized back-and-forth motion of electricity within the atria.
- The rate of atrial depolarization is typically 300 beats per minute.
- Usually every other atrial beat is blocked in the AV node, resulting in a typical ventricular rate of 150.
- With increasing AV block, the rate may slow to 50, 75, or 100 (if the rate is regular, it will be some fraction of 300).
- In WPW syndrome, atrial beats will be conducted 1:1, resulting in a ventricular rate of 300.

HYPERTENSION

NPLEX

Presentation

- Symptomless until vital organ damage
- High blood pressure upon testing (elevation of either systolic or diastolic)
- Traditional Chinese Medicine presentation includes:
  - Liver Fire
  - Liver Yang Rising from Yin Deficiency
  - Phlegm-Damp stagnation of the Middle Warmer
  - Yin and Yang imbalance

Macioca,
2001
Wong et
al, 1991

Hypertensive *urgency:* BP > 210/120 mmHg without symptoms.

Hypertensive *emergency:* BP > 210/120 mmHg with symptoms of end-organ damage. Examples include: acute left ventricular failure, chest pain or angina, MI, encephalopathy (headaches, confusion, papilledema, mental status change, vomiting, blurry vision, dizziness, and/or seizures), and acute renal failure.

Two-Measurement Rule: The reason for adopting the two-measurement rule is to account for normal daily fluctuations in BP (around 30 mmHg). However, most resources indicate exceptions to this rule:
- If BP is >210/120 or if end organ damage is present (see below).
- During pregnancy, where pre-eclampsia *may* be the cause of hypertension. Presentations suggestive of pre-eclampsia (proteinuria, edema, and progressive hypertension in a pregnant female) warrant prompt referral to an OB/GYN specialist for primary management.

Screening Guidelines

- Blood pressure average >140/90 mmHg, measured on two or more separate occasions taken over a period 4 weeks (two measurement rule). It follows that you should not initiate treatment until you have followed this two-measurement rule.

- Isolated elevation of either systolic or diastolic also warrants this diagnosis. For example, 145/60 mmHg and 115/95 mmHg.
- Ideally, everyone should be screened every year starting at the age of 18.
- The American Academy of Family Physicians (AAFP 2008) reports insufficient evidence for or against earlier screening, in contrast to the National Heart Lung and Blood Institute (NHLBI 2004) recommendation to check blood pressure every visit for patients ages 3-20 years. The prudent approach is to screen all asymptomatic patients every 1-2 years.

Source

Gonzales, 2009

JNC7 Classification of Blood Pressure for Adults

Classification	Systolic mmHg	Diastolic mmHg
Normal	<120	<80
Prehypertension	130-139	80-89
Hypertension		
Stage 1	140-159	90-99
Stage 2	≥160	≥100

Individuals in the prehypertension range are at increased risk for major cardiovascular events (coronary, cerebral, and renal disease as well), according to the Framingham Heart Study. The term mild hypertension is no longer considered appropriate because it may lead to a false sense of security and inaction in patients.

Associated Risk Factors

MCCQE
USMLE

- Individuals with high-normal BP are at increased risk for major cardiovascular events (coronary, cerebral, and renal disease as well), according to the Framingham Heart Study.
- Hypertension is the number-one modifiable risk factor for strokes and is a major risk factor for coronary, cerebral, and renal disease. Lowering BP significantly decreases incidence of heart disease, myocardial infarctions, atherosclerosis, renal failure, and dissecting aortic aneurysms.
- The most common cause of death among untreated patients of hypertension is the same as for the general population - coronary artery disease (CAD).

Hypertension Causes

USMLE
NPLEX
MCCQE

- Approximately 90% to 95% of hypertension cases are considered idiopathic, multifactorial, or essential hypertension.
- The remaining 5% to 10% are due to secondary causes.
- Less than 5% are traditionally considered to have curable causes for the condition (like renovascular stenosis).
- Approximately 8% may have underlying primary aldosteronism.

Most Common Causes of Secondary Hypertension (Age and Gender Specific)

Young men — Excessive alcohol intake (stop using alcohol) if it causes hypertension.
Young women — Birth control pills (stop using the pill) if it causes hypertension.

Source

MCCQE
USMLE

| *Both genders* | Renal artery stenosis (listen for bruit, request arteriogram for diagnosis). Treatment is simple balloon dilatation. |
| *Elderly* | Renal artery stenosis from atherosclerosis (diagnose as above). |

Less Common Secondary Causes of Hypertension

- *Pheochromocytoma:* wild swings in blood pressure with diaphoresis and confusion. A history of the five Ps (high BP, head pain, palpitations, perspiration, and pallor). Confirm with testing 24-hour urine sample for catecholamine degradation products (i.e., metanephrines, venyl mandelic acid, and homovallinic acid).
- *Polycystic kidney disease:* flank mass, family history (autosomal dominant pedigree), elevated serum creatinine, and blood urea nitrogen (BUN).
- *Cushing's syndrome:* moon face, buffalo hump, central obesity, peripheral wasting. Test 24-hour urine sample for free cortisol or request a dexamethasone suppression test.
- *Conn's syndrome:* aldosterone secreting adrenal tumor. Look for high levels of aldosterone, low renin, hypokalemia, metabolic alkalosis, and/or adrenal mass on CT.
- *Coarctation of the aorta:* hypertension only in upper extremities, unequal pulses, radiofemoral delay, and rib notching on CXR (associated with Turner's syndrome). Angiography establishes this diagnosis.
- *Renal failure:* from any cause. In children, be alert for post streptococcal glomerulonephritis.

MCCQE
USMLE

Laboratory Tests for Hypertension

1. Urinalysis for protein, glucose, and blood.
2. Assessment of serum levels of creatinine, potassium, glucose, calcium, and uric acid.
3. Lipid profile.
4. ECG to exclude coronary artery disease (CAD), left ventricular hypertrophy (LVH), and myocardial deterioration.

Management Plan for Hypertension

Gonzales, 2009

The following treatment strategies are presented in therapeutic order, followed by in-depth discussion of the key treatment modalities.

Stage I Hypertension Treatment (systolic BP 140-159 or diastolic 90-99 mm Hg):
1. Rule out secondary causes of hypertension.
2. Perform blood chemistry, urinalysis, lipid profile, and ECG.
3. Implement first-line dietary and lifestyle modifications for 3 to 6 months.
4. After 6 months: Re-evaluate presentation and need for adjunct treatment (clinical nutrition and/or botanical medications) for another 6 months.
5. If condition improves, re-evaluate annually.
6. With no improvement after the above 12-month period, refer to family physician for co-management.

Stage II Hypertension Treatment (systolic BP 160-179 or diastolic 100-109 mm Hg):
1. Rule out secondary causes of hypertension.
2. Perform blood chemistry, urinalysis, lipid profile, and ECG.
3. Implement first-line dietary and lifestyle modifications and adjunct clinical nutrition measures for 3 to 6 months.

4. After 3 to 6 months: Re-evaluate presentation and need for adjunct botanical medications for another 3 months.
5. If condition improves, manage as above.
6. With no improvement after the above 6 to 9 month period, refer to family physician for co-management.

Stage III Hypertension Treatment (systolic BP 180-210 or diastolic 110-120 mm Hg):
1. Rule out secondary causes of hypertension.
2. Perform blood chemistry, urinalysis, lipid profile, and ECG.
3. Implement first-line dietary and lifestyle modifications, adjunct clinical nutrition measures, and botanical medications for 1 to 3 months.
4. After 1 to 3 months: Re-evaluate presentation and need for medical treatment.
5. If condition improves, manage as above.
6. With no improvement after the above 1 to 3 month period, refer to family physician for primary management.

Urgent Hypertension Treatment: Refer to urgent care facility or to the emergency department. Once stabalized, co-manage as per Stage II above.

Guidelines for Managing Nonurgent Hypertension

- All resources recommend that the first-line treatment should always be lifestyle modifications.
- Pharmaceutical and / or botanical medications should only be started after a 3 to 6 month trial of lifestyle modifications.

Lifestyle Modifications
- Stop alcohol and tobacco consumption.
- Start the Dietary Approaches to Stop Hypertension (DASH) diet consisting of low-fat dairy, reduced saturated fat, high-fiber whole foods, increased fruits, vegetables, and nuts (expect average reduction of 11.4 mmHg systolic and 5.5 mmHg diastolic in first 11 weeks). Restrict salt and caffeine intake.
- Reduce weight (modest loss of weight of 10% or so can normalize blood pressure on its own).
- Decrease stress.
- Increase physical exercise (aerobic activity for 30 to 40 minutes at 70% of patient's Heart Rate Maximum (HRMAX) at least three times per week.

Diet and Medications
According to the 4-year Hypertension Control Program (HCP) trial, 39% of hypertensive patients successfully discontinued their medications when they followed basic nutritional intervention, which was defined as:
- Weight loss
- Salt restriction
- Alcohol avoidance

If these measures are combined with the DASH diet, a physical exercise program, and stress reduction measures, impressive outcomes may be observed. Such modest lifestyle changes can produce substantial cumulative effects.

Source

USMLE
NPLEX
MCCQE

Apple, 1997

USMLE
MCCQE
NPLEX

Apple, 1997

Stamler et al, 1987

Source

USMLE
MCCQE
CPS

Standard Pharmaceutical Medicines for Hypertension

Four classes of drugs are used as first-line therapy. Choice depends on the individual patient and the medical presentation.
1. Diuretics (Thiazide, Loop, or Potassium sparing)
2. Beta adrenergic receptor blockers (beta-blockers or BB)
3. Angiotensin converting enzyme inhibitors (ACE inhibitors or ACI)
4. Calcium antagonists

■ Treatment with a diuretic or a beta-blocker is the first-line pharmacologic strategy recommended by the Joint National Committee VI because they are the only agents that have been shown in clinical trials to reduce mortality.
■ Angiotensin-converting enzyme (ACE) inhibitors are first-line agents for congestive heart failure (they seem to reduce mortality rates).
■ In diabetes, ACE inhibitors slow progression to nephropathy and neuropathy.
■ Angiotensin receptor blockers (ARB) are used when patients do not tolerate ACIs well (e.g., Losartan Potassium "Cozaar" and Telmisartran "Micardis").

Safety Caution: Hydralazine (Apresoline) and Methyldopa (Aldomet) are considered safe for pregnant women and women of reproductive age, while Labetalol (Normodyne) is gaining acceptance. Remember that magnesium sulfate (or citrate) lowers blood pressure.

Harrison
JNC VI

Pharmaceutical Medicine Indications and Contraindications

Class	Examples	Specific Indications	Side Effects and Contraindications
Diuretics	Hydrochlorothiazide (Esidrix), Furosemide (Lasix), spironolactone (Aldactone), combination diuretics (Diazide)	Elderly, Black; CHF, central or peripheral edema.	S/E electrolyte imbalance (low serum potassium, calcium, magnesium), B vitamins depletion; C/I pregnancy, gout, and osteoporosis.
Beta Blockers	Atenolol (Tenormin), Acebutolol (Sectral), Metoprolol (Lopressor), Propranolol (Inderal)	Young, Caucasian; CHF, angina, previous MI, senile tremor, tachycardia and migraines.	C/I in diabetes (suppress symptoms of hypoglycemia), asthma, COPD, pregnancy, peripheral arterial disease (claudication), any heart block.
ACE Inhibitors	Captopril (Capoten) Enalapril (Vasotec) Lisinopril (Zestril) Ramipril (Altace)	Young, Caucasian; CHF, diabetes; impotence with other hypertension medications.	S/E electrolyte imbalance, neutropenia; C/I pregnancy, renovascular hypertension (may case acute renal failure.)

Class	Examples	Specific Indications	Side Effects and Contraindications
Calcium Antagonists	Verapamil (Isopten) Diltiazim (Cardizem) Nifidepine (Adalat) Ailodipine (Norvasc)	Elderly, Black; angina, migraines, arrhythmias, tachycardia, Raynaud's syndrome, peripheral arterial disease.	C/I heart block (verapamil or diltiazim only), sick sinus syndrome, pregnancy.

Botanical Medicines Indications and Contraindications

Botanical	Contraindications	Drug Interactions	Side Effects	Overdose
Crataegus spp.	Pregnancy	Potentiates digitalis, convallaria, and cardiac glycosides.	Nausea	Fatigue, diaphoresis, rash on hands
Piscidia erythrina	None known	None known	None known	Bradycardia, hypotension, paralysis
Viscum album	Pregnancy and lactation	Inhibits vasomotor medullary center and vagus nerve. Cholinomimetic	Lightheadedness, orthostatic hypotension	N&V; bradycardia, hypotension, vertigo, liver toxicity, central coma
Leonarus cardiaca	Pregnancy	None known	None known	N/A or None known

Source: NPLEX TNM; NPLEX, Pizzorno, 2006; Mashour, 1998; Silagy and Niel, 1994

Standard Botanical Medicines for Hypertension

- **Allium sativum:** Allicin in *Allium sativum* (garlic) exhibits moderate blood pressure lowering effect in hypertensive patients. The recommended dose is 1-2 cloves of garlic q.d. or 300 mg dried extract t.i.d.

- **Selenicerius grandifloris and Convallaria majalis:** For stable CHF patients, *Selenicerius grandifloris* (positive inotropic and negative chronotropic, nervine) and *Convallaria majalis* (considered as a safer alternative to digitalis) should also be considered.

Source

NPLEX

Guidelines for Clinical Nutrition Treatment of Hypertension

Nutritional Recommendations	Rationale	Dose (where applicable)
Restrict sodium and increase potassium intake	As the extracellular level of potassium increases, the sodium-ATP pump is activated, which causes a decrease in intracellular sodium. This is correlated by an average reduction of BP of 12-16 mmHg. Daily potassium intake and/or supplementation of 1.5-3 g decrease blood pressure about half as much as drug therapy.	Ideal K:N ratio is 5:1. Recommend fruits and vegetables relative to dietary intake.
Magnesium Citrate	Magnesium acts as a natural calcium channel blocker in clinical studies. It prevents calcium from entering vascular smooth muscles and subsequent vasoconstriction.	400-800 mg q.d. Watch for osmotic diarrhea.
Olive oil	Monounsaturated fatty acids (MUFA) in olive oil were shown in Ferrara's Mediterranean diet randomized crossover trail to reduce systolic BP by 6-8 mmHg.	Based on dietary intake.
Fish Oil	Approximately 60 clinical trials indicate that omega-3 fatty acids found in fish oils, such as eicosapentaenoic acid (EPA) and docosahexanoic acid (DHA), are effective in lowering BP. Both EPA and DHA inhibit prostaglandin synthesis in platelets and blood vessels, while EPA additionally suppresses production of thromboxane A2. Studies have shown average cumulative reduction of 10 mmHg in BP.	1-5 tsp q.d. (3-6 g q.d.)
Coenzyme Q10	Double-blind studies have indicated statistically significant average blood pressure reduction of 10.6-19.5 mmHg after 4-12 weeks of use. Coenzyme Q10 is especially indicated where there are other cardiovascular complications.	100-300 mg q.d. in divided doses, with meals.
Vitamin C	Retrospective studies show an inverse correlation between vitamin C intake and blood pressure.	Based on dietary intake.

Marz, 1999

Patki, 1990

Maizes, 2002

Ferrara, 2000

Fish oil for the heart, 1987

Digiesi, 1992

Simon, 1992

Source

Nutritional Recommendations	Rationale	Dose (where applicable)	
Pyridoxine (vitamin B-6)	One small trial indicated modest reduction of both systolic and diastolic BP with oral administration of vitamin B-6.	5 mg/kg q.d.	Ayback, 1995
Bonito protein extract	Bonito (a type of tuna) contains an oligopeptide that exhibits significant ACI activity. Three clinical trials indicate blood pressure lowering effect of at least 10 mmHg systolic and 7 mmHg diastolic without the usual ACI side effects.	Typical dose is 500 mg (isolated peptides) t.i.d.	Fujita, 2001

DYSLIPIDEMIA

Contributing author: Philip Rouchotas MSc, ND

USMLE
NPLEX
MCCQE

Presentation

Lipoproteins: lipid transporters, composed of cholesterol (or cholesteryl ester), triglycerides (TG), phospholipids, and apoprotein. The two major classes of lipoproteins are:
- TG-rich: chylomicrons and very low density lipoprotein (VLDL)
- Cholesterol-rich – low density lipoprotein (LDL) and high density lipoprotein (HDL)

Lipid Panel Report:
- TC value
- LDL-C value
- HDL-C value
- TG value
- TC: HDL-C ratio
- LDL-C : HDL-C ratio

- Dyslipidemia (a.k.a. hyperlipidemia, hypercholesterolemia, or 'high chlesterol') is one of the main known modifiable risk factors for atherosclerosis, a systemic inflammatory disease of the vascular system, which accounts for roughly half of the deaths in North America.
- The course of atherosclerosis leads invariably to coronary artery disease (CAD), cerebrovascular disease (CVD), and peripheral vascular disease (PVD).
- Atherosclerosis is the most important cause of permanent disability.

Source

NPLEX

Bugarelli,
2002

Bugarelli,
2002

NPLEX
MCCQE
USMLE

NCEP

USPHSTF
Gonzales,
2009

Risk Factors for Atherosclerosis and CAD

Classic Risk Factors: The following risk factors are additive with respect to overall risk of significant atherosclerosis and coronary heart disease. Patients with three or more risk factors have over 700% incidence of CAD compared with similar cohorts. Note that HDL levels > 60 mg/dl negate one risk factor (it is that protective).
- Low HDL < 35mg /dl
- Hypertension
- Diabetes mellitus
- Smoking > 10 cigarettes/day
- Physical inactivity
- Family history of early MI

Novel Risk Factors (gaining acceptance):
- Elevated triglycerides
- Low TC:HDL ratio
- Elevated homocysteine
- Elevated C-reactive protein (CRP)
- High serum fibrinogen
- Lipoprotein a (LPa)
- Apoprotein A-1 and B-100 LDL particle size Interleukin 6 (IL-6)

Clinical Signs of Hyperlipidemia

- Xanthelasma
- Eruptive and tendinous xanthomas
- Corneal arcus
- Lipemia retinalis (retinal blood vessels appear pink instead of red)
- Obesity

Screening Guidelines

No single protocol is universally accepted, but the following practices are the most widely followed:
1. National Cholesterol Education Program (NCEP) recommends comprehensive screening of all adults 20 years and older with a fasting lipoprotein profile (which is total cholesterol, LDL, HDL and TG) every 5 years.
2. US Preventive Health Services Task Force recommends a more reserved screening program:
   - Class A: men 35 years and older and women 45 years and older – screen via testing total cholesterol (TC) and HDL cholesterol every 5 years.
   - Class B: men & women 20 years and older with known risk factors – screen via testing TC and HDL cholesterol every 5 years.
3. Canadian Diabetes Association recommends yearly screening with a full lipoprotein profile for all adults with diabetes.

Source

Depres,
2001
Wolfret,
2004

LDL-C Risk Factor

LDL-C levels have been reproducibly correlated to increased risk of heart disease, stroke, and death:
- Levels greater than 3.9 mmol/L typically predict increased risk of disease of approximately 50%.
- Current evidence also suggests that a mere 1% decrease in LDL-C is associated with about 2% decrease in risk of coronary heart disease.

USMLE

LDL Level Calculation

LDL levels are usually calculated based on other plasma lipids measurements (this is done for economical reasons). After direct measurement is obtained for TC, HDL, and TG, LDL is estimated using the following equation:

$$LDL = TC - (HDL + TG/5)$$

This calculation is accurate, provided TG levels do not exceed 400 mg/dl. LDL levels can also be directly measured if specifically requested, but this is not routinely done in practice.

ATP III,
2004

Pre-test Fasting

- Although TC and HDL will not be significantly affected by recent food consumption, TG levels will change dramatically.
- Because routine LDL-C is calculated based on TG level, estimation of LDL-C requires a fasting sample.

ATP III Intervention Guidelines

Following the lead of the Framingham studies and algorithm for calculating lipid levels, the Adult Treatment Panel III (ATP) of the National Cholesterol Education Program (NCEP) established management guidelines in 2001, and then revised them in 2004 due to the subsequent reporting of five large clinical intervention trials utilizing statin therapy. The Canadian Cardiovascular Society (CCS) calls for a much more aggressive prescription of statin drug therapy than ATP III.

1. Regardless of the method employed (e.g., lifestyle changes, statins, niacin, fibrate), the recommended target of therapy is:

Category	Target LDL - C level
Moderate risk patients.	LDL-C < 130mg/dL
High risk patients	LDL-C < 100 mg/dL
Very high risk patients	LDL-C < 70mg/dL

2. Therapeutic lifestyle changes remain the cornerstone of the treatment of dyslipidemia.
3. Cholesterol-lowering drug therapy is recommended in high-risk patients. This category now includes diabetic individuals. It is also proposed that elderly individuals benefit from lipid lowering therapy regardless of presenting LDL-C levels.
4. Individuals with elevated triglyceride (TG) levels in addition to elevated LDL-C levels are candidates for addition of fibrates to statin therapy.

Source

5. When LDL-lowering drug therapy is employed in high-risk or moderately high-risk persons, it is advised that intensity of therapy be sufficient to achieve at least a 30% to 40% reduction in LDL-C levels.

Intervention Review:

- The NCEP established dietary guidelines as first-line interventions for the management of mild to moderate dyslipidemia in low to moderate risk individuals. The magnitude of efficacy of these interventions has been reproducibly demonstrated as 8% to10% reduction in LDL-C levels.
- A recent systematic review summarized 97 human intervention trials that cumulatively included more than 137,000 subjects in intervention groups and over 138,000 subjects in placebo groups. Relative risk for overall mortality was as follows: N-3 fatty acids 33% reduced mortality risk; statin 23% reduced mortality risk; niacin 4% reduced mortality risk; fibrates 0% reduced mortality risk.

Dietary Guidelines for Managing Dyslipedemia

Jenkins, 2002, 2003 Lamarche, 2004

Portfolio Diet: Dr David Jenkins is credited with the creation of the Portfolio diet, which is based on the hypothesis that combining various foods, each independently known to reduce LDL-C levels, would produce a magnitude of efficacy far superior to previous dietary strategies. The Portfolio diet is a meat-free diet (fish is an exception), which also restricts high-fat dairy products, and includes:

- Viscous fibers (e.g., oats, psyllium, okra,eggplant): 20 g per day
- Soy protein (e.g., soy milk, burgers, deli meats): 20 g per day
- Raw almonds: 28 g per day
- Plant sterol fortified margarine: 2000-3000 mg plant sterol per day

Efficacy: Recent studies of the Portfolio diet included three treatment groups. One group received the NCEP diet for cholesterol lowering; the second group received the NCEP diet plus therapeutic dosage of statin medication; and the third group received the Portfolio diet. The interventions have reproducibly demonstrated the following:

Treatment Group	Outcome
NCEP diet	8% reduction in LDL-C levels
NCEP diet plus statin drug	30% reduction in LDL-C levels
Portfolio diet	30% reduction in LDL-C levels

Jenkins, 2002, 2003 Lamarche, 2004 Despres, 2001

Portfolio Diet Enhancement: This diet was designed to demonstrate that "foods found in every-day grocery stores could deliver a large magnitude regarding lowering of LDL-C." To demonstrate this critical endpoint, researchers had to limit confounding variables by adhering to the following parameters:

- Subjects were prevented from losing weight by designing diets that are calorically equivalent to their pre-trial diets.
- Subjects were instructed to maintain current levels of physical activity and exercise was not encouraged.
- All aspects of the Portfolio system had to be derived from commonly consumed foods.
- No supplements of any kind were permitted.

Since clinicians are not bound by the above experimental parameters, the following strategies can be easily incorporated to enhance the magnitude of efficacy of the program:

1. Caloric restriction in any individual presenting with a BMI of greater than 25 (BMI calculated as weight in kilograms divided by height in meters squared). This intervention has demonstrated a reproducible benefit on lipid levels.
2. Low to moderate intensity exercise (like walking). A safe and effective exercise prescription is 50% to 60% of maximum heart rate (maximum heart rate = 220 minus age) four to seven times per week. This intervention has consistently demonstrated a lipid lowering effect.
3. Replace 'plant sterol fortified margarine' with a plant sterol supplement. Dose: 1500 mg per day (500 mg t.i.d., with meals). Sterol supplementation has demonstrated reproducible reduction of 10% to 14% in LDL-C.
4. Eliminating margarine would render the diet an exceptionally low-fat diet (which is known to adversely affect lipid levels). As an alternative, substitute the margarine with two tablespoons of extra virgin olive oil. The oil should be consumed raw. This intervention has been shown to reduce LDL-C levels by approximately 12%. As a side effect, it has been shown to reduce blood pressure and fasting blood glucose in diabetic individuals.
5. Inclusion of a fish oil supplement adds further benefit to the intervention. Fish oil has minimal effects on LDL-C (potentially even increasing LDL-C by 2% to 5%). However, fish oil profoundly decreases TG and significantly increases HDL-C levels. The therapeutic dose of fish oil should be no less than 2000 mg EPA/DHA combined per day. Fish oil should be consumed with meals because this increases absorption by as much as two-fold.

TC:HDL-C Ratio: Elevations of the TC: HDL ratio predict increased incidence of CAD by up to 140%. The most powerful predictor of an elevated TC:HDL-C ratio is being overweight or obese – namely, increased visceral adipose tissue (VAT). Caloric restriction, combined with exercise, results in significant decreases in VAT. Implementing caloric restriction plus exercise directly addresses the underlying cause of an increased TC:HDL-C ratio.

Hyperlipidemia Medications

Four classes of drugs are used: HMG-CoA reductase inhibitors, fibrates, niacin, and bile-acid binding resin.

Class and Examples	Mechanism of Action	Efficacy & Side Effects (S/E)
HMG CoA Reductase Inhibitors (Statins): Atrovastatin (Lipitor) Fluvastatin (Lescol) Lovastatin (Mevacor, Altocor) Pravastatin (Pravachol) Simvastatin (Zocor)	Widely used; reversibly inhibit 3-hydroxy-3-methylglutaryl coenzyme A reductase; considered first-line therapy for treating high levels of LDL cholesterol resistant to dietary control.	Can lower cholesterol by up to 35%; shown to decrease mortality risk by up to 23%. S/E: elevation of transaminases (AST, ALT), reversible myositis (with elevation of CPK), GI disturbances, nausea, headache, fatigue, insomnia, and rash.
Fibrates: Bezafibrate (Bezalip) Ciprofibrate (Modalim) Gemfibrozil (Lopid)	Fibric acid derivatives are used in hypertriglyceridemia that is unresponsive to dietary control; stimulate lipoprotein lipase; decrease TG; increase fatty acid oxidation in liver and	Ineffective in patients with elevated cholesterol but normal TG; may lower TG from 20-50% and increase HDL by 10-15%; not shown to decrease mortality risk.

Source

Lakka, 2004
Varady, 2005

St-Onge, 2003

Devaraj, 2004

Madigan, 2000

Perona, 2004

Ferrara, 2000

Harris, 1997
Sitori, 1998
Stark, 2000
GISSI-Prevenzione, 1999

USMLE
NPLEX
MCCQE
CPS

	Class and Examples	Mechanism of Action	Efficacy & Side Effects (S/E)
Source		muscle; and may decrease VLDL production.	S/E: Myositis like syndrome (especially if renal function is impaired), GI disturbances, dermatitis, impotence, headache, dizziness, and blurred vision.
	Nicotinic acid: Nicotinic acid (Niacin) Extended-release Nicotinic acid (Niaspan)	Inhibits VLDL production and thus LDL; stimulates lipoprotein lipase; decreases TG; increases HDL cholesterol; and decreases plasma fibrinogen.	Flushing side effect limits niacin's use; may lower TG by 20-50%; has been shown to reduce incidence of CAD; reduces mortality risk by 4%. S/E: flushing, dizziness, headache, palpitations, nausea, vomiting, and pruritus.
	Bile-acid-binding resins: Cholestyramine (Questran, Prevalite) Colestipol HCL (Colestid)	Basic anion exchange resins that prevent enterohepatic recirculation of cholesterol by binding bile acids in the intestine; especially useful when high LDL is the main finding.	Not absorbed systemically; have been shown to decrease mortality from CAD; relieve pruritus associated with biliary obstruction. S/E: GI disturbances are common, may aggravate hypertriglyceridemia, and interfere with absorption of fat-soluble vitamins and other drugs.

Guidelines for Naturopathic Clinical Nutrition Treatment for Dyslipidemia

NPLEX
Hu, 1997
Ascerio, 1999
Mattson, 1985
Mattson, 1985

Bugarelli, 2002
Harper, 2001

Recommendation	Rationale
Avoid eating saturated fatty acids (SFA), trans fatty acids, and undesirable polyunsaturated fatty acids (PUFA)	**Saturated fats:** very high in cholesterol content and consumption. Directly associated with increase risk of heart disease, as well as chronic degenerative diseases. SFA sources are primarily fried foods, animal and dairy products. **Trans-fatty acids**: increase LDL and decrease HDL. Associated with the highest risk of heart disease. TFA sources are margarine (some brands are TFA free), shortening, hydrogenated vegetable oils, snack foods (most brands), and deep fried foods. **Polyunsaturated fatty acids:** typically contain omega-6 fatty acids, tend to lower HDL, and promote production of inflammatory mediators and prostaglandins. Undesirable PUFA sources are corn oil, safflower oil, and cottonseed oil (used in processed food products).

Recommendation	Rationale	Source
Eat food sources of monounsaturated fatty acids (MUFA) and omega-3 fatty acids	**Monounsaturated fatty acids:** lower total cholesterol and LDL, but do not affect the level of HDL. Food sources are olives, olive oil, avocado, almonds, and cashews.	Rispin, 1992 Gore, 1994
	Omega-3 fatty acids: promote production of anti-inflammatory prostaglandins, prevent heart disease, and inhibit clot formation. Reduce risk of sudden cardiac death, arrhythmia, and hypertension. Food sources include cold-water fish (e.g., salmon, herring, mackerel, sardines, kippers), flax oil, and walnuts.	Hanaki, 1993
Increase fiber consumption	**Fiber:** in 88% of fiber interventional studies, a significant reduction in cholesterol was shown. Oat bran, oat meal, and konjac root glucomannan seem to provide the best cholesterol lowering effect, followed by psyllium and flax.	Rispin, 1992 Gore, 1994
Supplement with coenzyme Q10 (CoQ10)	**CoQ10:** depleted in patients who are taking statin drugs. CoQ10 an essential compound in mitochondrial oxidative phosphorylation, which has been demonstrated to be a strong lipid antioxidant that helps reduce symptoms of angina and improves exercise tolerance in patients with CHF. The typical supplemental dose is 100-300 mg q.d., in divided doses, with meals.	
Supplement with B vitamins	**B vitamins:** A deficiency in folic acid, vitamin B-6, and/or vitamin B-12 impairs the conversion of homocysteine (a derivative of methionine) into cysteine. Elevated plasma homocysteine levels above 10 mcg/dl is an independent risk factor for heart disease and peripheral artery disease. Supplementation with B complex vitamins has been shown to reduce this elevated risk by reversing hyperhomocystenemia.	Ubbink, 1993

Guidelines for Naturopathic Botanical Medicine Treatment for Dyslipidemia

Botanical	Evidence and Side effects	Dose
Allium sativum	Consumption of 1-2 cloves of garlic daily has been shown to reduce total cholesterol by 9-12 % and help lower blood pressure in randomized trials. The evidence is not clear regarding prepared garlic supplements.	1-2 cloves q.d. or 300 mg dried extract q.d.
Monascus purpureas	In a large clinical trial, Chinese red yeast rice demonstrated reduction of total cholesterol by 16%, reduction of LDL by 21%; and elevation of HDL by 15 %. Red yeast rice is a traditional Chinese food that exhibits HMG-CoA reductase inhibition, which is partly due to its high content of lovastatin. As with all statins, there is a potential for elevation of liver transaminases, reversible myostis, and depletion of coenzyme Q10.	1.2 g b.i.d.
Commiphora mukul	Gugulipid is the resin from the Indian myrrh tree. Randomized trials demonstrate a 10-12% reduction in TC, 25% reduction in LDL, 27% reduction in TG, and 16-20% elevation in HDL without significant side effects. There is a theoretical concern with patients on anticoagulants because they may potentiate their effects.	500 mg t.i.d. (5% guggulsterone)
Zingiber officinale	Ginger improves cholesterol levels by limiting cholesterol absorption and exhibits mild antiplatelet activity.	Taken as tea, with food, or as a standardized supplement

Examination Board References

NPLEX (II): North American Board of Naturopathic Examiners
Naturopathic Physician Licensing Examination Part II (NPLEx II) Blueprint. Portland, OR: North American Board of Naturopathic Examiners (NABNE), 2010.

USMLE: National Board of Medical Examiners
Brochert A. Crush Step 3. The Ultimate USMLE Step 3 Review. 3rd ed. New York, NY: Saunders, Elsevier, 2008.

MCCQE: Medical Council of Canada
Dugani S, Lam D, eds. 2009. MCCQE Review Notes & Lecture Series. Medical Counsel of Canada Qualification Examination Review Notes. Toronto, ON: McGraw Hill Professional, Canadian edition, 2009.

Related References

Agarwal R, Carpenter J, Davis J, Hanson CW, Iyoob S et al. Use of ultrasound for the diagnosis of deep venous thrombosis in asymptomatic inpatients. A recommendation statement from the University of Pennsylvania Health System Center for Evidence-based practice. Univerity of Pennsylvania Health System, 2007

American Heart Association. ACC/AHA/ESC Practice Guidelines for the Management of Patients with Atrial Fibrillation. Circulation 2006;114:e257-e354.

Anonymous. Dietary supplementation with n-3 polyunsaturated fatty acids and vitamin E after myocardial infarction: Results of the GISSI-Prevenzione trial. Gruppo Italiano per lo Studio della Sopravvivenza nell'Infarto miocardico. Lancet. 1999 Aug 7;354(9177):447-55.

Anonymous. Fish oil for the heart. Med lett Drugs Ther 1987;29(731):7-9.

Apple LJ, Moore TJ, Obarzanek E, et al. A clinical trial of the effects of dietary patterns on blood pressure. DASH Collaborative Research Group. N Engl J Med 1997;336:1117-24.

Ascerio A et al. 1999. Trans fatty acids and coronary heart disease. N Engl J Med 340:1994-98.

Ayback M et al. Effect of oral pyridoxine hydrochloride supplementation on arterial blood pressure in patients with essential hypertension. Arzneim Forsch 1995;45:1271-73.

Beyranvarnd MR, Kadkhodai KM, Roshan VD, Choobineh S, Parsa SA, Piranfar MA. Effect of taurine supplementation on exercise capacity of patients with heart failure. J Cardiology 2011;57(3)333-37.

Breslow JL. N-3 fatty acids and cardiovascular disease. American Journal of Clinical Nutrition. 2006;83(6):1477S-1482S.

Bugarelli R. Atherosclerosis – Complementary and Alternative Medicine Secrets. Kohatso W (ed.). Philadelphia, PA: Hanley & Belfus Inc., 2002.

Cappuccio FP et al. Does potassium supplementation lower blood pressure? J Hypertension 1991;9:465-73.

Cater NB, Garcia-Garcia AB, Vega GL, Grundy SM. Responsiveness of plasma lipids and lipoproteins to plant stanol esters. Am J Cardiol 2005 Jul 4;96(1A):23D-28D.

Compendium of Pharmaceuticals & Specialties (CPS). Toronto, ON: Canadian Pharmaceutical Association, 2005.

Dains J, Baumann L, Scheibel P. Advanced Health Assessment & Clinical Diagnosis in Primary Care. 4th edition. St Louis, MO:Mosby C.V. Co. Ltd., 2011.

Daly C, Norrie J, Murdoch DL, Ford I, Dargie HJ, Fox K. (2003). The value of routine non-invasive tests to predict clinical outcome in stable angina. European Heart Journal. 2003;23(6): 532-40.

Despres JP, Lemieux I, Dagenais GR, Cantin B, Lamarche B. Evaluation and management of atherogenic dyslipidemia: Beyond low-density lipoprotein cholesterol. CMAJ 2001 Nov 13;165(10):1331-33.

Devaraj S, Jialal I, Vega-Lopez S. Plant sterol-fortified orange juice effectively lowers cholesterol levels in mildly hypercholesterolemic healthy individuals. Arterioscler Thromb Vasc Biol 2004 Mar;24(3):e25-8.

Digiesi V et al. Mechanism of action of Coenzyme Q10 in essential hypertension. Curr Ther Res 1992;51:668-72.

Ferrara L, Raimondi AS, d'Episcopo L, et al. Olive oil and reduced need for antihypertensive medications. Arch Intern Med 2000;160:837-42.

Ferri F. Ferri's Clinical Advisor Instant Diagnosis and Treatment. St. Louis, MO: Mosby Inc, 2004.

Fujita H et al. Effect of ACE: Inhibitory agent, katobishi oligopeptide in hypertensive and borderline hypertensive subjects. Nutr Res 2001;21:1149-58.

Godfrey A, Saunders PR, et al. Principles & Practices of Naturopathic Botanical Medicine: Vol 1 Herbal Monographs. Toronto, ON: CCNM Press, 2010.

Gonzales R, Kutner J. Current Practice Guidelines in Primary Care 2009. Toronto (ON): McGraw Hill, 2009.

Gore SR et al. Soluble fiber and serum lipids: A literature review. J Am Diet Assoc 1994;94:425-468.

Grundy SM, Cleeman JI, Merz CN, Brewer HB Jr, Clark LT, Hunninghake DB, Pasternak RC, Smith SC Jr, Stone NJ; National Heart, Lung, and Blood Institute; American College of Cardiology Foundation; American Heart Association. Implications of recent clinical trials for the National Cholesterol Education Program Adult Treatment Panel III guidelines. Circulation 2004 Jul 13;110(2):227-39.

Hampton JR. ECG Made Easy. New York, NY: Churchill Livingstone, 2001.

Hanaki Y et al. Co-enzyme Q-10 and coronary artery disease. Clin Invest 1993;71(8):S112-S115.

Harper CR et al. The fats of life: The role of omega-3 fatty acids in prevention of coronary heart disease. Arch Intern Med 2001;161:2185-92.

Harris WS. n-3 fatty acids and serum lipoproteins: Human studies. Am J Clin Nutr 1997 May;65(5 Suppl):1645S-1654S.

Harrison. www.harrisonsonline.com

Heber D et al. Cholesterol-lowering effects of a proprietary Chinese red-yeast rice dietary supplement. Am J Clin Nutr 1999;69:231-36.

Hu FB, et al. Dietary fat intake and risk of CAD in women – The Nurses Health Study. N Engl J Med 1997;337:1491-99.

Jenkins DJ, Kendall CW, Faulkner D, Vidgen E, Trautwein EA, Parker TL, Marchie A, Koumbridis G, Lapsley KG, Josse RG, Leiter LA, Connelly PW. A dietary portfolio approach to cholesterol reduction: Combined effects of plant sterols, vegetable proteins, and viscous fibers in hypercholesterolemia. Metabolism 2002 Dec;51(12):1596-1604.

Jenkins DJ, Kendall CW, Marchie A, Faulkner DA, Wong JM, de Souza R, Emam A, Parker TL, Vidgen E, Lapsley KG, Trautwein EA, Josse RG, Leiter LA, Connelly PW. Effects of a dietary portfolio of cholesterol-lowering foods vs lovastatin on serum lipids and C-reactive protein. JAMA 2003 Jul 23;290(4):502-10.

Jenkins DJ, Kendall CW, Marchie A, Faulkner D, Vidgen E, Lapsley KG, Trautwein EA, Parker TL, Josse RG, Leiter LA, Connelly PW. The effect of combining plant sterols, soy protein, viscous fibers, and almonds in treating hypercholesterolemia. Metabolism 2003 Nov;52(11):1478-83.

Joint National Committee. Sixth report of the Joint National Committee on Prevention, Detection, Evaluation, and Treatment of High Blood Pressure (JNC VI). Arch Intern Med 1997;157:2413-2446.

Kamikawa T. Effects of coenzyme Q10 on exercise on exercise tolerance in chronic stable angina. AM J Cardiol. 1985;26:247.

Lakka HM, Tremblay A, Despres JP, Bouchard C. Effects of long-term negative energy balance with exercise on plasma lipid and lipoprotein levels in identical twins. Atherosclerosis 2004 Jan;172(1):127-33.

Lamarche B, Desroches S, Jenkins DJ, Kendall CW, Marchie A, Faulkner D, Vidgen E, Lapsley KG, Trautwein EA, Parker TL, Josse RG, Leiter LA, Connelly PW. Combined effects of a dietary portfolio of plant sterols, vegetable protein, viscous fibre and almonds on LDL particle size. Br J Nutr 2004 Oct;92(4):657-63.

Maciocia, Giovanni. The Foundations of Chinese Medicine. New York, NY: Churchill Livingstone, 2001.

Madigan C, Ryan M, Owens D, Collins P, Tomkin GH. Dietary unsaturated fatty acids in type 2 diabetes: Higher levels of postprandial lipoprotein on a linoleic acid-rich sunflower oil diet compared with an oleic acid-rich olive oil diet. Diabetes Care 2000 Oct;23(10):1472-77.

Maizes V. Hypertension. In: Kohatso W (ed.). Complementary and Alternative Medicine Secrets. Philadelphia, PA: Hanley & Belfus Inc., 2002.

Marz RB. Medical Nutrition from Marz. 2nd ed. Portland, OR: Omni-Press, 1999.

Mashour NH, Lin GI, Frishman WH. Herbal medicine for the treatment of cardiovascular disease. Arch Intern Med 1998;158:2225-34.

Mattson F et al. Comparison of effects of dietary saturated, monounsaturated and polyunsaturated fatty acids on plasma lipids and lipoprotein in man. J Lipid Res 1985;26:194-202.

Mills S. and Bone K. Principles and Practice of Phytotherapy: Modern Herbal Medicine. New York, NY: Churchill Livingstone, 2000.

Mikati I. Heart disease and women. Nidus Information Services. ADAM. First Consult Elsevier Inc. www.mdconsult.com, 2010.

Moore R. Hematology Laboratory Diagnosis. Guelph, ON: McMaster University Press, 2001.

Mortensen S. Long-term Coenzyme Q10 therapy: A major advance in the management of resistant myocardial failure. Drugs Exp Clin Res. 1985;11(8):581-93.

Patki PS. Efficacy of potassium and magnesium in essential hypertension. Brit J Med 1990;521-23; 301.

Perona JS, Canizares J, Montero E, Sanchez-Dominguez JM, Catala A, Ruiz-Gutierrez V. Virgin olive oil reduces blood pressure in hypertensive elderly subjects. Clin Nutr 2004 Oct;23(5):1113-21.

Pina IL, Apstein CS, Balady GJ, et al. Exercise and heart failure: a statement from the American Heart Association Committee on exercise, rehabilitation, and prevention. Circulation: Journal of the American Heart Association, 107: 1210-1225

Pizzorno JE, Murray MT. 2006. Textbook of Natural Medicine, 3rd Ed. Churchill Livingstone,Elsevier.

Pizzorno JE, Murray MT. Textbook of Natural Medicine. Vol. 1 and 2. 2nd ed. New York, NY: Churchill Livingstone, 1999.

Ripsin CM et al. Oat products and lipid lowering: A meta analysis. JAMA 1992;267:3317-25.

Saunders, PR. Herbal Remedies for Canadians. Toronto, ON: Prentice Hall, 2000.

Saynor R and Verel D. Fish oils & angina pectoris: Eskimos and their diets. Lancet 1983;1:1335.

Silagy CA, Neil HA. A meta-analysis of the effect of garlic on blood pressure. J Hypertens 1994;12:463-68.

Simon JA. 1992. Vitamin C and cardiovascular disease: A review. J Am Coll Nutr 1992;11:107-25.

Sirtori CR, Crepaldi G, Manzato E, Mancini M, Rivellese A, Paoletti R, Pazzucconi F, Pamparana F, Stragliotto E. One-year treatment with ethyl esters of n-3 fatty acids in patients with hypertriglyceridemia and glucose intolerance: Reduced triglyceridemia, total cholesterol and increased HDL-C without glycemic alterations. Atherosclerosis 1998 Apr;137(2):419-27.

Snow V, et al. Management of newly detected atrial fibrillation: a clinical practice guideline from the American Academy of Family Physicians and the American College of Physicians. Annals of Internal Medicine. 2003;139(12):1009-17.

Stahl TJ, Gregorcyk SG, Hyman NH, Buie D. Practice Parameters for the Prevention of Venous Thrombosis. Dis Colon Rectum 2006;49:1477-83.

Stamler R, Stamler J, Grimm R, et al. 1987. Nutritional therapy for high blood pressure: Final report of a four-year randomized controlled trial – the hypertension control program. JAMA 1987;257:1484-90.

Stark KD, Park EJ, Maines VA, Holub BJ. Effect of a fish-oil concentrate on serum lipids in postmenopausal women receiving and not receiving hormone replacement therapy in a placebo-controlled, double-blind trial. Am J Clin Nutr 2000 Aug;72(2):389-94.

St-Onge MP, Lamarche B, Mauger JF, Jones PJ. Consumption of a functional oil rich in phytosterols and medium-chain triglyceride oil improves plasma lipid profiles in men. J Nutr 2003 Jun;133(6):1815-20.

Studer M, Briel M, Leimenstoll B, Glass TR, Bucher HC. Effect of different antilipidemic agents and diets on mortality: A systematic review. Arch Intern Med 2005 Apr 11;165(7):725-30.

Tripathi P, Chandra M, Misra MK. Oral administration of L-arginine in patients with angina or following myocardial infarction may be protective by increasing plasma superoxide dismutase and total thiols with reduction in serum cholesterol and xanthine oxidase. Oxid Med Cell Longev. 2009:2(4):231-37.

Tripathi P, Misra MK. Therapeutic role of L-arginine on free radical scavenging system in ischemic heart disease. Indian J Biochem Biophys. 2009;46(6):498-502.

Ubbink JB et al. Hyperhomcystenemia and the response to vitamin supplementation. Clinic Invest 1993;71:993-998.

Varady KA, Jones PJ. Combination diet and exercise interventions for the treatment of dyslipidemia: An effective preliminary strategy to lower cholesterol levels? J Nutr 2005 Aug;135(8):1829-35.

Wester P and Dyckner T. Intracellular electrolytes in cardiac failure. Act Med Scand 1986; 707:33-36.

Winer N, Linas SL. Hypertension. In Mladenovic J (ed.). Primary Care Secrets. Philadelphia PA.: Hanely & Belfus, 2004.

Wolfret AL and Eckel. Abnormalities of Lipids. In: Mladenovic J. (ed.) Primary Care Secrets. Philadelphia, PA: Hanley & Belfus, 2004.

Wong ND, Ming, S, Zhou HY, Black HR. A comparison of Chinese traditional and Western medical approaches for the treatment of mild hypertension. Yale J Biol Med 1991;64:79-87.

EAR, NOSE & THROAT

HEARING LOSS

MYRINGITIS

SINUSITIS

FACIAL NERVE PARALYSIS

HEARING LOSS

Source

NPLEX
MCCQE
USMLE

Presentation

Otosclerosis: refers to otic bones fixation, which leads to hearing impairment. It is the most common cause of progressive conductive hearing loss in adults.

Presbyacusis: a gradual and progressive hearing loss that occurs as part of the normal aging process (compare presbiopia = age related vision loss) and is the most common sensorineural hearing loss in adults.

Treatment: For both presentations, supportive hearing aid is recommended.

Diagnosis: In young patients presenting with hearing loss, the following conditions should be ruled out:
- Exposure to prolonged and intense loud noise.
- Congenital TORCH infection: **T**oxoplasmosis, **R**ubella, **C**ytomegalovirus, and **H**erpes.
- Meniere's disease: deafness + severe vertigo + tinnitus + nausea/vomiting.
- Acoustic neuroma: progressive space occupying lesion manifestations.
- Labyrinthitis: may follow otitis media or meningitis.
- Side effects of drugs, such as aminoglycosides (gentamicin and streptomycin), aspirin, quinidine (class I anti-arrhythmic for NPLEX), loop diuretics, and cisplatin.
- Chronic diseases that lead to healing loss: diabetes, hypothyroidism, multiple sclerosis, and sarcoidosis.

Screening: Older adults should be routinely asked about hearing loss followed with routine whisper test (90-99% sensitivity).

Gonzales, 2009,

McGee, 2001

Common Causes of Acute Onset Deafness

Viral infection (mumps, measles, influenza, or chicken pox) constitutes the most common cause of endolymphatic labyrinthis, which manifests as relatively sudden onset sensorineural deafness. This is a self-limiting condition that usually resolves within 2 weeks.

McGee, 2001

Assessment

Weber Test: compares bone conduction in both ears (sensitivity of 54-58% makes for a poor screening tool). The normal response is to hear the vibration in the middle (or equally in both ears).
- Patients with conductive hearing loss will hear the vibration best in the affected ear.
- In contrast, patients with sensorineural hearing loss will hear the vibration best in the unaffected ear. Therefore, another test is required to investigate any perceived inequality in hearing.

Rinne Test: compares air conduction to bone conduction.

Source

- Normally air conduction is 2X greater than bone conduction (AC>BC). It follows that patients with conductive hearing will hear the vibration over the mastoid, but not next to the auditory meatus (AC<BC).
- In sensorineural hearing loss, both air and bone conduction is impaired, but the normal ratio is preserved (i.e., AC>BC). With sensitivity of 60-90% and specificity of 95-98%, it is effective at differentiating between types of hearing loss.

NPLEX
MCCQE
USMLE

Most Common Causes of Vertigo

The following conditions can cause VII cranial nerve damage and are the most common causes of vertigo:
- Meniere's disease
- Tumors
- Diabetes infections
- Multiple sclerosis

Benign Positional Vertigo: Vertigo that is associated with certain head positions, accompanied by nystagmus, and not associated with hearing loss is termed Benign Positional Vertigo. BPV is a self-limiting condition.

MYRINGITIS

NPLEX
MCCQE
USMLE

Presentation

Infectious inflammation of the tympanic membrane. Myringitis is diagnosed when otoscopy reveals vesicles + erythema on the tympanic membrane.

Cause: Infectious myringitis is most commonly caused by *Mycoplasma*, *streptococcus pneumoniae*, or viruses.

Treatment: The recommended treatment is topical antimicrobials (botanicals and/or pharmaceuticals).

PAROTID GLAND SWELLING

NPLEX
MCCQE
USMLE

Presentation

The classic example is mumps, but it may be due to neoplasms (pleomorphic adenoma), Sjogren syndrome, sialolithiasis (stone in the parotid duct), sarcoidosis, and alcoholism.

SINUSITIS

Source

Presentation: Acute Sinusitis

NPLEX
MCCQE
USMLE

An inflammation and infection of one or more of the paranasal sinuses. It is usually preceded by a URTI.

Signs and Symptoms:
- Headache
- Tenderness over affected sinuses
- Fatigue
- Purulent postnasal rhinorrhea
- Bouts of cold that last longer than 10 days is characteristic of acute sinusitis

Cause: Sinusitis is often caused by *Streptococcus spp.*, *Staphylococcus spp.*, and *H. influenza*.

Presentation: Chronic Sinusitis

NPLEX
MCCQE
USMLE

The persistent or recurrent infection and/or inflammation of one or more sinus cavities. According to the Center for Disease Control and the National Center for Health Statistics, chronic sinusitis is the most common chronic disease in the United States. Prevalence is approximately 15% in North America (that is, one in seven people in the population has chronic sinusitis).

Sub-types:
1. Type 1: persistent low-grade infection with periodic flare-ups of acute sinusitis.
2. Type 2: recurrent (at least 3 episodes within a 6 month period) sinus infection.
3. Type 3: chronic inflammation with little or no infection.

Ivker, 2002

Causes and Risk Factors:
- Common cold
- Dental infection
- GERD
- Immunodeficiency
- Nasal polyps, cysts, or deviated septum
- Emotional stress
- Air pollution
- Smoking
- Certain occupations, such auto mechanics, construction workers, painters and beauticians
- Allergies and sensitivities to pollen, animal dander, mold, dairy, and wheat
- Dry-cold air

Diagnosis: Although a definitive diagnosis sometimes requires a CT scan of the sinuses, in primary care settings, a good history and the clinical presentation suffice for reliable diagnosis. Antibiotic therapy may be considered with sinusitis ≥ 7 days in duration and in cases of acute toxic presentation. Symptomatic relief should be tried ≤ 7 days.

Gonzales 2009

Source

NPLEX

Ivker, 2002

Pizzorno,
2006

Guille-
mardin,
2010

Guidelines for Naturopathic Treatment for Sinusitis

Approach:
- Reduce Predisposing factors.
- Improve circulation/drainage of congested sinuses.
- Treat presenting infection.
- Provide symptom relief.

1. Environmental factors
- Address air pollution, the first risk factor for this condition. A thorough cleaning of living spaces (especially carpets) and heating/cooling systems (furnace, humidifier, air conditioner), installing filters on ventilation systems, using negative ion generators, and encouraging indoor plants all help to improve breathable air.
- Saline nasal spray q3h or steam inhalation b.i.d. appears to sooth inflamed mucous membranes of the nasal passages.
- Increase fluid consumption (e.g., chicken soup, ginger tea with honey and lemon). Hot showers and baths are practical hydrating methods.

2. Dietary and lifestyle measures
- Avoid dairy products, eggs, wheat, chocolate, oranges, refined sugars, and caffeine.
- Explore food sensitivities.
- Gradually progressive exercise is of great benefit in improving sinusitis, as well as preventing relapse.
- Ensure adequate periods of rest and sleep (lack of sleep leads ultimately to immune suppression).
- Recommend probiotics with meals as they modulate immune function and reduce duration of infection.

3. Clinical nutrition
- Vitamin C: 500 mg q.i.d. (or to bowel tolerance if not contraindicated)
- Vitamin E: 400 mg (mixed tocopherols are preferred) q.d.
- Zinc picolinate: 30 mg b.i.d.
- NAC (N-acetyl cysteine): 500 mg t.i.d. (mucolytic + antioxidant)
- Flaxseed oil or fish oil: 2 tbsp q.d.

4. Botanical medicine
- Grapefruit seed extract: 100 mg or 10 gtts t.i.d.
- Garlic extract or equivalent: 1200 mg q.d.
- *Echinacea spp.:* 6:1 standardized (3.5% echinacoside) solid extract: 150-300 mg t.i.d.

FACIAL NERVE PARALYSIS

Source

NPLEX
MCCQE
USMLE

Presentation

Lower motor neuron (LMN) lesion of the facial nerve causes unilateral paresis or paralyses of the whole side of the face. Lower quarter paralysis is associated with Upper Motor Neuron (UMN) lesion. Bell's palsy is the most common LMN lesion of the facial nerve. Other etiologies are viral or ischemic.

Signs and Symptoms:
- Facial paresis or paralysis
- Hyperacusis (paralysis of the stapedius → increased sense of hearing)

Causes

- Herpes infection: sometimes causes VII + VIII cranial nerve paralysis + vesicles inside ear canal or on the pinna + meningitis.
- Lyme disease: causes bilateral facial nerve palsy.
- Stroke (history of TIA is usually present)
- Middle ear or mastoid infection
- Meningitis (from any cause)
- Temporal bone fracture (for example, baseball bat hit that leads to bleeding from the ear = battle's sign)
- Tumors in the cerebellopontine space: acoustic neuroma, neurofibromatosis, and glomus vulgare.
- Occasionally follows upper respiratory tact infections, although causal association is not established.

Treatment

- Maintain lubrication to the paralyzed eye (tear drops and taping at night) to avoid corneal dryness, which causes inflammation, opacities, and ulceration.
- Almost all causes will resolve spontaneously in about 1 month, but some patients will have permanent sequelae.
- If the cause is not apparent and the medical history and neurological signs are concerning, request CT scan or MRI of the head.
- Although experimental studies are pending, supportive naturopathic measures, especially acupuncture and homeopathy, are promising in bettering the odds of developing permanent disability.

Examination Board References

NPLEX (II): North American Board of Naturopathic Examiners
Naturopathic Physician Licensing Examination Part II (NPLEx II) Blueprint. Portland, OR: North American Board of Naturopathic Examiners (NABNE), 2010.

USMLE: National Board of Medical Examiners
Brochert A. Crush Step 3. The Ultimate USMLE Step 3 Review. 3rd ed. New York, NY: Saunders, Elsevier, 2008.

MCCQE: Medical Council of Canada
Dugani S, Lam D, eds. 2009. MCCQE Review Notes & Lecture Series. Medical Counsel of Canada Qualification Examination Review Notes. Toronto, ON: McGraw Hill Professional, Canadian edition, 2009.

Related References

Dains J, Baumann L, Scheibel P. Advanced Health Assessment & Clinical Diagnosis in Primary Care. 2nd ed. St. Louis, MO: Mosby Inc, 2003.

Freise KH et al. Acute Otitis Media in Children: Comparison of Conventional and Homeopathic Treatment. Berlin, Germany: Hals-Nasen-Ohren, 1996:426-66.

Gonzales, R., Kutner, J. Current Practice Guidelines in Primary Care 2009. Toronto (ON): McGraw Hill, 2009.

Guillemardin, E., Rondu, F., Lacoin, F., Schrezenmeir, J. (2010) Consumption of a fermented dairy containing product containing the probiotic Lactobacillus casei DN-114001 reduces the duration of respiratory infections in the elderly in a randomized control trial. BR J Nutrition. 2010; 103(1):58-68.

Ivker R. Sinusitis: Complementary and Alternative Medicine Secrets. Philadelphia, PA: Hanley & Belfus Inc., 2002.

McGee, S. (2001). Evidence-Based Physical Diagnosis. Philadelphia, PA: Saunders, 2001.

Pizzorno JE, Murray MT. Textbook of Natural Medicine. Vol. 1 and 2. 2nd ed. New York, NY: Churchill Livingstone, 1999.

Pizzorno JE, Murray MT, Joiner-Bey H. The Clinician's Handbook of Natural Medicine. New York, NY: Churchill Livingstone, 2002.

Pizzorno JE, Murray MT. Textbook of Natural Medicine, 3rd ed. New York, NY: Churchill Livingstone, Elsevier, 2006.

Robert Schad Naturopathic Clinic. Policy and Procedures Manual. Toronto, ON: The Canadian College of Naturopathic Medicine, 2004.

Saunders, PR., Godfrey, A. Naturopathic Botanical Medicine: Volume I. Toronto, ON: CCNM Press, 2010.

Shapiro M. Otitis Media. In: Kohatso W (ed.). Complementary and Alternative Medicine Secrets. Philadelphia, PA: Hanley & Belfus Inc., 2002.

ENDOCRINOLOGY

Diabetes

DIABETES

Presentation

- This chronic disorder of carbohydrate, fat, and protein metabolism manifests when there is a defect in insulin secretion, insulin action, or both.
- Diabetes is characterized by chronic hyperglycemia.

New-Onset Diabetes:
- Classic presentation of new-onset diabetes is the triad:
  - Polyuria
  - Polydipsia
  - Polyphagia
- In practice, however, suspect diabetes in any patient with frank candidal infections, weight loss, or blurry vision.
- A spontaneous improvement in vision of a geriatric patient should also sound an alarm (lens swells in hyperglycemia state).

Clinical Definition

If a patient has classic symptoms of diabetes, one of the following three tests is sufficient to establish the diagnosis. In asymptomatic patients, any positive test should be repeated.
- Random plasma glucose level > 11.1 mmol/L (or > 200 mg/dL for NPLEX)
- 8-hour fasting plasma glucose (FPG) > 6.9 mmol/L (or > 126 mg/dL for NPLEX)
- 2-hour Oral Glucose Tolerance Test (OGTT) > 11.1 mmol/L, where plasma glucose is measured 2 hours after ingestion of a 75 g of glucose dissolved in water. This is the standard glucose load as defined by the WHO. This test is recommended only in the following situations:
  - To make sure a diagnosis has not been missed in patients exhibiting impaired fasting glucose (IFG), which is defined as borderline FPG values between 6.1-6.9 mmol/L.
  - To define positive urine glucose in a pregnant female as glucosuria may be perfectly normal in pregnancy (i.e., OGTT screens for gestational diabetes).

Type 1 and Type 2 Diabetes

Diabetes Type	Type 1	Type 2
Age at onset	Most commonly < 30 years of age	Most commonly > 40 years of age
Weight	Low	Normal or high
Onset	Rapid	Slow
Development of ketoacidosis	Yes	No

Source

Diabetes Type	*Type 1*	*Type 2*
Development of Hyperosmolar State	No	Yes
Level of endogenous insulin	Low or none Due to destruction of islet "B" cells	Normal or high Due to insulin resistance
Human leukocytic antigen (HLA) association	Yes	No
Islet antibody	Yes (at time of diagnosis)	No
Genetic association	Weak genetic association	Strong genetic association
Environmental factors	Post viral and possibly post toxic exposure	Obesity + inactivity
Risk for diabetic complications	Yes	Yes

Screening Guidelines

- Universal screening is *not* supported by randomized trials.
- ADA — The American Diabetes Association (ADA) recommends screening every 3 years beginning at age 45 years.
- Gonzales, 2009 — According to AAFP (2008) and USPSTF (2008) the evidence is lacking to support mandatory screening of asymptomatic pregnant women - as there is absence of high quality evidence of reduced morbidity as a result of screening. The American Diabetes Association (ADA, 2008) recommends that average risk women should be screened at 24-28 weeks, while high-risk pregnant women should be screened as soon as possible
- RSNC manual — Testing at a younger age should be considered in patients who exhibit any of following conditions, lifestyle factors, or genetic risks:
  1. Overweight
  2. First-degree relative with diabetes
  3. Belong to high-risk ethnic group
  4. Hypertensive
  5. HDL< 0.9 mmol/L (or 35mg/dL), TG > 2.82 mmol/L (or 250 mg/dL)
  6. Polycystic ovarian syndrome
  7. Acanthosis nigricans
  8. Vascular disease

NPLEX
MCCQE
USMLE

Diabetic Ketoacidosis (DKA)

Without adequate insulin administration, this condition occurs in type 1 diabetics. Absolute lack of insulin causes cellular glucose deprivation (glucose cannot enter cells without insulin) and triggers compensatory lipolysis and muscle proteolysis, which produce ketones sufficient to cause metabolic acidosis, hyperosmolar state, and ultimately coma.

- DKA is a serious emergency condition that leads to coma and death in type 1 diabetics (mortality of DKA is 10%).
- The cause is usually non-compliance with insulin therapy.

Clinical Signs and Symptoms:
- Kussmaul breathing (deep and rapid respirations)
- Dehydration
- Hyperglycemia
- Acidosis (since ketones are acidic)
- Increased ketones in the serum (causes fruity or alcohol breath odor) and urine (smells like acetone or nail polish remover)

Treatment: Acutely, this condition is treated by:
- Intravenous fluids (rehydration of DKA is probably the most effective advance in modern medicine)
- Insulin
- Electrolyte replacement

Hyperosmolar Non-ketotic State (HONK)

HONK: occurs in type 2 diabetics without adequate blood sugar control.
- HONK is an emergency condition that leads to coma and death of type 2 diabetics. If HONK presents with mental status changes, its mortality rate approaches 50%.
- Hyperglycemia and increased serum osmolality are present in absence of ketones or acidoses.
- First treatment is 'fluids, fluids, and some more fluids' and electrolytes.

NPLEX
MCCQE
USMLE

Lactic Acidotic Coma (LA)

LA has nothing to do with diabetes, but it presents very similarly to DKA in the emergency department.
- LA type I causes coma in hypoxic patients (as in shock trauma).
- LA type II is caused by impaired metabolism of lactate in the liver.

NPLEX
MCCQE
USMLE

Common Long-term Complications of Diabetes Mellitus

NPLEX
MCCQE
USMLE

All of these grim complications can be prevented or delayed indefinitely by controlling blood glucose levels.

Condition	Facts
Atherosclerosis, CAD, and MI	Diabetics often have silent heart attacks due to autonomic neuropathy.
Retinopathy	Diabetes is the number one cause of blindness for people under 50 years of age.
Peripheral vascular disease	Diabetes is the number one cause of limb amputations in the absence of trauma. It also leads to intermittent claudication and erectile dysfunction. ADA recommends aspirin therapy as prevention for all patients ≥ 40 yo or ≥ 1 cardiovascular risk factor.

Gonzales,
2009

Condition	Facts
Nephropathy	Diabetes is the number one cause of end-stage renal failure.
Peripheral neuropathy	Diabetes causes numbness of feet and silent heart attacks.
Increased risk of infections	WBCs lose function in hyperglycemic environments, but the real issue is clogged arteries (further reducing WBC presence) and inability to sense pain in uncontrolled diabetes.

Peripheral Neuropathy Complications: Peripheral neuropathy causes far more serious complications than just numb feet. These complications are:
1. Early satiety and vomiting because the stomach does not empty well
2. Erectile dysfunction
3. Cranial nerve palsies of CNIII, CNIV, and CNVI
4. Orthostatic hypotension
5. Charcot joints (refer to Rheumatology module)
6. Pressure ulcers in the feet that may progress into gangrene

Diabetic Retinopathy Treatment:
- Besides controlling blood sugar, proliferative retinopathy in diabetic patients (usually seen in type 1 DM) requires panretinal laser photocoagulation to prevent progression into blindness.
- Focal laser photocoagulation is used in non-proliferative retinopathy with macular edema.

Syndrome X

This insulin resistance syndrome is known by many names: obesity dyslipidemia syndrome, syndrome X, and metabolic syndrome.

Diagnosis: The National Cholesterol Education Program (NCEP) publishes the following diagnostic criteria for syndrome X. Three or more need to be present:
1. Abdominal obesity, which is defined as waist circumference > 40 inches in men and > 35 inches in women.
2. Hypertension or even prehypertension BP $\geq$ 130/80 mmHg.
3. FPG > 6.1 mmol/L or 110 mg/dL.
4. Dyslipidemia:
   - HDL Cholesterol < 1.0 mmol/L (40 mg/dL) for men, and < 1.3mmol/L (50 mg/dL) for women.
   - Triglycerides $\geq$ 150 mg/dL.

Assessment Guidelines

Considering the significantly increased risk for myocardial infarction, stroke, peripheral vascular disease, retinopathy, neuropathy, nephropathy, and early mortality, diabetic patients should be adequately screened for atherosclerotic disease:
1. Careful history-taking and review of systems, focusing on cardiovascular symptoms (i.e., chest pain, SOB, exertional dyspnea, and claudications).
2. Physical examination of feet (sensations, monofilament, ulcers, abnormal skin or nails), carotid bruit, and peripheral pulses.

3. Annual retinal exam by ophthalmologist
4. Dipstick (or Spot) urinalysis for albumin-to-creatinine ratio (if positive confirm with 24-hour urine collection) to screen for diabetic nephropathy + annual serum creatinine, microalbumin and eGFR.
5. Lipid profile.
6. ECG if > 40 years of age.

Management Plan for Glucose Levels

Goals:
- The goal of any approach to diabetes is to maintain postprandial (or after-meal) glucose level <11.1 mmol/L (200 mg/dL) and fasting glucose level < 6.9 mmol/L (126 mg/dL).
- Remember that the defect in diabetes also places the patient at a greater risk for hypoglycemia, which is defined as FPG < 2.5 mmol/L or 46 mg/dL. Thus, management should also maintain FPG above hypoglycemic levels.

Control and Compliance:
- Hemoglobin A1C (also known as glycosylated hemoglobin) reflects average control of plasma glucose level over the previous 2 to 3 months.
- It is recommended that hemoglobin A1C levels be monitored every 6 to 12 months for patients exhibiting good glycemic control, and every 3 months for patients with poor glycemic control.
- Rule of thumb: if you multiply the HA1C levels by 100, you will get the average blood glucose levels in mmol (multiply by 200 for mg scale).

Hypoglycemia

Occurs when blood sugar level dips below 2.5 mmol/L (which is a value that normal people would not achieve even with prolonged fasting).

Causes: The cause for hypoglycemia is usually diabetes, but endocrine defects, liver cirrhosis, and inborn metabolic defects are also factors. Addison's disease, alcoholism, and sepsis frequently exhibit fasting hypoglycemia.

Signs and Symptoms:
- Aggression
- Sweating
- Tachycardia
- Nausea
- Weakness
- Mental status changes

Treatments:
- Acute treatment: immediate glucose administration.
- Chronic treatment: identifying and circumventing the cause best addresses chronic cases.
- Blood glucose control is the desired outcome of successful treatment.

Source

NPLEX
MCCQE
USMLE

Gray, 2007
CPS

Oral Hypoglycemic Medications for Treating Diabetes Mellitus 2

If glucose control is not achieved within 2-3 months of naturopathic care or the patient develops severe hyperglycemia (HBA1c ≥9% at presentation) or diabetic symptoms, pharmacological management is indicated.

- Six classes of drugs are used in DM type 2 therapy. Choice depends on the individual patient and the medical presentation.
  - Sulfonylureas
  - Nonsulfonylureas
  - Thiazolidinediones
  - Biguanides
  - Alpha-glucosidase inhibitors
  - Combinations

NPLEX
MCCQE
USMLE

Class and Examples	Mechanism of Action	Facts and Side Effects
Sulfonylurea secretagogues: Glyburide (DiaBeta) Micronized glyburide (Glynase) Gliclazide (Diamicron) Glipizide (Glucotrol)	Widely used; stimulate pancreas to secrete insulin and somewhat increases insulin sensitivity; used alone, and with other oral agents, or insulin.	Well tolerated; taken q.d. or b.i.d.; lowers FPG by 20%. S/E: Hypoglycemia, nausea, skin sensitivity, abnormal LFTs.
Nonsulfonylureas secretagogues: Repaglinide (GlucoNorm) Nateglinide (Starlix)	Stimulate pancreas to secrete insulin; used alone and with metformin.	Taken t.i.d. or q.i.d.; selectively lowers postprandial plasma glucose. S/E: Hypoglycemia, weight gain.
Thiazolidinediones: Rosiglitazone (Avandia) Pioglitazone (Actos)	Enhance insulin sensitivity in muscle, liver, and adipose tissue by unknown mechanism; used alone and with sulfonylureas, metformin, or insulin.	Taken q.d.; long duration of action (days to weeks); can reduce HbA1C triglycerides and LDL. S/E: Dose-related weight gain, fluid retention, heart failure.
Biguanides: Metformin (Glucophage, Glucophage XR)	Insulin sensitizer; decrease glycogenolysis as well as gluconeogenesis; increase peripheral glucose utilization.	Taken q.d. to t.i.d.; lowers FPG by 20%; also lowers serum triglycerides. S/E: Metallic taste, mild anorexia, nausea, abdominal pain, bloating, diarrhea, reduced vitamin B-12 absorption (in up to 30% of patients)

Source

Class and Examples	Mechanism of Action	Facts and Side Effects
Alpha-Glucosidase inhibitors: Acarbose (Precose) Miglitol (Glyset)	Inhibit enzymes that convert polysaccharides into monosaccharides, thus limiting postprandial glucose absorption.	Taken with meals; lowers HbA1C, LDL and possibly elevates HDL. S/E: Hypoglycemia, abdominal pain, flatulence, diarrhea.
Combinations: Metformin-glyburide (Glucovance)	Combines insulin sensitization with secretion induction, leading to more insulin sensitivity, as well as production.	Practical combination; taken b.i.d.; lowers FPG by 20%; also lowers serum triglycerides. S/E: Hypoglycemia, abdominal pain, flatulence, weight gain.

Insulin

NPLEX

Indications for Insulin Use:
- Type 1 DM
- Type 2 DM, where glycemic control is poor desepite naturopathic and drug intervention.

Adverse Effects of Insulin Therapy:
- Hypoglycemia
- Hypokalemia (which causes cardiac arrhythmias and neuromuscular disturbances)
- Obesity

Types of Insulin Preparations

NPLEX
USMLE

Preparation	Class and Trade Names	Pharmacokinetics (in hours)		
		Onset	Peak	Duration
1. Regular insulin	Short acting (Novolin Toronto, Humulin-N)	0.5-1	2-4	5-8
2. Semilente insulin		1-2	2-8	12-6
3. Neutral protamine hagedorn (NPH)	Intermediate acting (Novolin, NPH, Humulin-L)	1-2	4-12	18-24
4. Lente insulin		1-3	6-14	18-24
5. Protamine zinc insulin	Long acting (Humulin-V, Lantus, Humalong)	4-8	14-20	24-36
6. Ultralente insulin		4-8	12-24	36-40

Source

NPLEX
MCCQE
USMLE

The Somogyi Effect and the Dawn Phenomenon

Somogyi effect: the body's natural reaction to hypoglycemia. If *too much NPH insulin* is given at dinnertime, the glucose level at 3 a.m. will be in hypoglycemic range. The body reacts to this condition (which occurs during sleep) by secreting glucagon, which causes a high glucose level at 7 a.m.

Dawn phenomenon: hyperglycemia caused by *too little NPH insulin* at dinnertime. The glucose level will be normal or high at 3 a.m., but will be high at 7 a.m.

NPLEX

Beta-blockers and Diabetes

Beta-blockers are generally contraindicated in diabetes because they mask the alarm symptoms of hypoglycemia (tachycardia and sweating).

Guidelines for First-line Naturopathic Treatment of Diabetes Mellitus

Approach: Dietary modifications are fundamental to the success of therapy in type 1 and type 2 DM. Evidence indicates that weight loss alone may eliminate type 2 DM completely. It reduces insulin resistance, thus circumventing the primary deficit. Although type 1 diabetics will always require insulin supplementation, better outcomes are strongly correlated with high-fiber/low-refined carbohydrate diet. Diabetic patients exhibit increased need for many nutrients and vitamins. The goal of treatment for either type is centered on improving blood sugar control, preventing or ameliorating long-term complications, and improving overall health status.

Pizzorno,
2006
Morelli
and
Zoorob,
2000

1. Dietary measures
The patient must be willing to improve lifestyle since required dietary changes are demanding, to say the least. The cornerstone of therapy is the high complex-carbohydrate diet, frequent small meals, and observance of the following:
- Eliminate simple sugars, as well as processed and concentrated carbohydrates.
- Encourage high-fiber foods, legumes, onions, and garlic.
- Avoid or eliminate saturated fats.
- Reduce weight in overweight patients (a modest 10 lb reduction in weight significantly improves metabolic control, and, in some cases, induces remission of diabetes).

Anderson,
1997

Pizzorno,
2006

Head,
2000

2. Clinical nutrition
- Chromium picolinate (or polynicotinate): 500 mcg b.i.d. Increases cell sensitivity to insulin via unknown mechanism. This dose is 350 times less than the suspected toxic dose.
- Magnesium citrate (or aspartate): 500 mg q.d. Magnesium deficiency is common in patients with DM and contributes somewhat to the development of most diabetic complications.
- Fiber (in order of preference: defatted fenugreek seeds > guar > pectin > oat bran): 20-30 g q.d. *Trigonella foenum gracum* seed fiber has been shown in clinical studies to control postprandial plasma glucose by inhibiting intestinal absorption of glucose because of a suspected alpha-glucosidase inhibitor effect.

Source
Derosa, 2010

Kilichi, 2010
Fan, 2010

Saunders, 2000

Morelli and Zoorob, 2000

La Valle, 2001

- Alpha-lipoic acid: 300-600 mg q.d. Potent antioxidant and aldose reductase inhibitor. Reduces numbness and pain in patients with peripheral neuropathy)
- Pyridoxine, biotin, and selenium. Ensure adequate intake.
- L-carnitine: 500 mg q.i.d. Reduces FPG, OGTT, HBA1C, and plasma insulin, as well as TG, TC, LDL, and BP. May delay or reduce kidney damage induced by diabetes.

3. Botanical medicine

The use of botanicals needs to be strictly controlled by the naturopathic physician so as not to precipitate hypoglycemia (especially when patient is on oral hypoglycemic drugs).

- *Mamordica charantia:* 30-60 ml fresh juice or 100-200 mg (5.1% triterpenes acids) t.i.d. Bitter melon is hypoglycemic and lowers both fasting plasma glucose and hemoglobin A1C.
- *Gymnema sylvestre:* 400-600 mcg (25% gymnemic acids) q.d. This is a potent oral hypoglycemic agent and alpha-glucosidase inhibitor that lowers plasma glucose and hemoglobin A1C and may stimulate regeneration of pancreatic insulin-secreting cells.
- *Vaccinuim myrtillus:* 80-160 mg (25% anthocyanidin content) t.i.d. This botanical is also beneficial for diabetic retinopathy.
- *Ginkgo biloba* extract: 40 mg (24% ginkgo flavoglycosides) t.i.d. Excellent for improving CNS manifestations due to peripheral vascular disease.
- *Panax ginseng:* 100 mg (5% ginsenosides) t.i.d. Reduces fasting glucose levels and helps reduce body weight in type 2 diabetes.

4. Exercise

Recommend an aerobic exercise program that elevates heart rate to 60-70 HRMAX for 30 minutes three to four times per week.

- Advise patients with well-controlled diabetes to ingest 15-30 g of carbohydrates (juice or glucose tablets) 15-30 minutes prior to beginning their exercise and every 30 minutes of exercise time to avoid exercise-induced hypoglycemia.
- Recommend complex carbohydrate snacks after completion of exercise to prevent glycogen repletion induced hypoglycemia.
- For patients on insulin, plasma glucose should be measured before, during, and after exercise.

Examination Board References

NPLEX (II): North American Board of Naturopathic Examiners

Naturopathic Physician Licensing Examination Part II (NPLEx II) Blueprint. Portland, OR: North American Board of Naturopathic Examiners (NABNE), 2010.

USMLE: National Board of Medical Examiners

Brochert A. Crush Step 3. The Ultimate USMLE Step 3 Review. 3rd ed. New York, NY: Saunders, Elsevier, 2008.

MCCQE: Medical Council of Canada

Dugani S, Lam D, eds. 2009. MCCQE Review Notes & Lecture Series. Medical Counsel of Canada Qualification Examination Review Notes. Toronto, ON: McGraw Hill Professional, Canadian edition, 2009.

Related References

American Diabetes Association. Standards of medical care for patients with diabetes mellitus. Diabetes Care 2003;26(supp 1):S50-S55.

Anderson RA, et al. Elevated intake of supplemental chromium improve glucose and insulin variables in individuals with type 2 diabetes. Diabetes 1997;46:1786-91.

Compendium of Pharmaceuticals & Specialties (CPS). Toronto, ON: Canadian Pharmaceutical Association, 2005.

Dains J, Baumann L, Scheibel P. Advanced Health Assessment & Clinical Diagnosis in Primary Care. 2nd ed. Philadelphia, PA: Mosby C.V. Co. Ltd., 2003.

Derosa G, Maffioli, P, et al. Sibutramine and L-Carnitine compared to sibutramine alone on insulin resistance in diabetic patient. Internal Medicine 2010;49:1717-1725.

Fan JP, Kim D, et al. Ameliorating effects of L-Carnitine on diabetic podocyte injury. Journal Med Food 2010;13(6): 1342-1330.

Gray J. Therapeutic Choices (5th ed.). Ottawa (ON): Canadian Pharmacists Association, 2007.

Gonzales R, Kutner J. Current Practice Guidelines in Primary Care 2009. Toronto (ON): McGraw Hill, 2009.

Head K. Natural Treatments for Diabetes. Roseville, CA: Prima, 2000.

Jonathan PC, et al. Diabetes Mellitus. In: Mladenovic J. (ed.). Primary Care Secrets. Philadelphia, PA: Hanley & Belfus Inc., 2004.

Kilicli F, Dokmetas S, et al. Inspiratory muscle strength is correlated with carnitine levels in type 2 diabetes. Endocr Res 2010;35(2):51-8.

La Valle JB, et al. Natural Therapeutics Pocket Guide. Hudson, OH: Lexi-Comp, 2001.

Marz RB. Medical Nutrition form Marz. 2nd ed. Portland, OR: Omni-Press, 1999.

Morelli V, Zoorob R. Alternative therapies. Part I: Depression, diabetes, obesity. Am Fam Physician 2000;62(5):1051-60.

NCEP: National Cholesterol Education Program. Third Report of the NCEP Expert Panel on Detection, Evaluation, and Treatment of High Blood Cholesterol in Adults (Adult Treatment Panel III). JAMA 2001;285:2486-97.

Pizzorno JE, Murray MT. Diabetes mellitus. In: Textbook of Natural Medicine. New York, NY: Churchill Livingstone, 1999.

Pizzorno JE, Murray MT. 2006. Textbook of Natural Medicine, 3rd Ed. Churchill Livingstone, Elsevier.

Saunders, PR. Herbal Remedies for Canadians. Toronto, ON: Prentice Hall, 2000.

GASTROENTEROLOGY

GASTROESOPHAGEAL REFLUX DISEASE

ESOPHAGEAL DISEASE

PEPTIC ULCER DISEASE

ACHLORHYDRIA

GASTRIC BLEEDING

DIARRHEA

CONSTIPATION

IRRITABLE BOWEL SYNDROME

INFLAMMATORY BOWEL DISEASE

LIVER DISEASE

HEPATITIS

AUTOSOMAL DISEASES

BILARY TRACT CONDITIONS

PANCREATITIS

GASTROESOPHAGEAL REFLUX DISEASE

Presentation

Gastroesophageal reflux disease simply means that stomach acid is refluxing into the esophagus. It occurs mainly due to inappropriate relaxation of the lower esophageal sphincter (LES) and/or delayed gastric emptying.

Signs and Symptoms: Patients present with heartburn, abdominal discomfort, or chest pain that is often related to eating and/or lying down.

- Heartburn
- Bloating
- Belching
- Indigestion
- Regurgitation
- Acid reflux
- Bitter taste in the mouth
- Cardiac-like pain. To differentiate GERD from MI or angina pectoris, remember that MI pain is generally made worse by movement. See the Cardiology module for guidelines.

Prevalence: The prevalence in North America is about 20% in adults. The incidence is increased significantly in patients with hiatal hernia.

Sequelae of GERD

- Esophagitis
- Esophageal stricture (which may mimic esophageal cancer)
- Esophageal ulcer
- Hemorrhage
- Barrett's metaplasia (columnar metaplasia of esophageal squamous epithelium), which often leads to esophageal adenocarcinoma

American Society of Gastrointentestinal Endoscopy (ASGE) 2006, recommends screening patients with chronic GERD for Barrett's esophagitis via endoscopy, with subsequent follow up screenings every 6-12 months in cases of positive findings (esophagitis or dysplasias).

Stomach Acid Levels in GERD

Both extremes (excess and deficiency) in stomach acid production may cause GERD:
- When acid is produced in excess (e.g., in response to *Helicobacter pylori* infection, alcohol, spicy foods, or coffee), there is a higher chance for regurgitation.

- Conversely, when stomach acid production is deficient, gastric emptying is prolonged (i.e., longer churning time is needed when acid levels are low), which in turn leads to GERD.
- Insufficient production of digestive enzymes and environmental/ food sensitivities may also play a role in GERD etiology.

Stomach Acid Levels Tests

1. Direct measurement of postprandial stomach acid after a standard meal. This is the least refuted and most invasive method for evaluating stomach acid production.
2. Direct measurement of fasting stomach pH after a standard challenge (e.g., pH sensitive telemetry capsule or GastroTest). This method is better tolerated, but its analytical sensitivity (the ability of a test method to measure what it claims to measure – postprandial versus fasting), reliability (reproducibility), and sensitivity (propensity for high false positives) remains to be seen.
3. Indirect evaluation by supplementing with betaine hydrochloride (see below) with meals and monitoring the symptoms. If GERD symptoms improve, the patient may be deficient. If the symptoms exacerbate, then stomach acid is either excessive or normal (and the supplementation is stopped).

HCl Supplementation for Managing GERD

Supplementing with betaine HCl (HCl bound to the amino acid betaine) is a documented naturopathic protocol that not only can ascertain the cause of GERD, but may even resolve the presentation altogether. Although the mechanism of action is not known, this protocol seems to restore proper stomach acid regulation.

Standard Trial HC1 Protocol:
1. The initial dose consists of one capsule containing 300-600 mg betaine HCl (often with 5-10 mg pepsin) with each meal.
2. If symptoms exacerbate, the trial is stopped.
3. If symptoms remain the same or improve, the dose is gradually increased by increments of one capsule every 2 days until the patient experiences heartburn (epigastric discomfort, heartburn, or warmth).
4. The dose is then reduced to the previously tolerated level. One capsule less than the dose that produces heartburn = therapeutic dose.
5. When the therapeutic dose starts to cause epigastric discomfort, the number of capsules per meal is again reduced by 1 capsule.
6. This protocol is continued until the initial dose starts to cause heartburn. At this point, supplementation is stopped.
7. This outcome often occurs after weeks or months of betaine HCl supplementation and indicates that stomach acid auto-regulation is achieved.

Source / NPLEX / Shapiro, 2002 / Pizzorno, 2006 / Shapiro, 2002

Source

NPLEX

Pizzorno,
2006
Marz, 1999

Guidelines for First-line Naturopathic Treatment of GERD

Recommendations	Rationale	Details
1. Avoid foods that commonly cause GERD symptoms	Coffee, alcohol, tobacco, spicy and fatty foods, and chocolate decrease lower esophageal sphincter (LES) tone and significantly stimulate HC1 production.	Trial of 1-2 months
2. Relax while eating	Relaxation favors the parasympathetic system. Have the patient sit down while eating slowly and deliberately. Prohibit television, reading, excessive chatter, or other distracting activities during meals. Focusing on chewing helps.	Always
3. Eat small meals with low fat content	High fat content has a long transit time. This increases intra-abdominal pressure and decreases the lower esophageal sphincter tone.	4-5 small meals per day
4. Increase fiber intake	Appears to decrease overall intra-abdominal pressure.	Depends on dietary intake
5. Avoid medications that aggravate the situation	Anticholinergic drugs, botanicals, and aspirin tend to decrease peristalsis and relax the LES.	Always
6. Take bitters	Bitter herbs, such as gentian, hops, angelica, and horehound, stimulate acid production and possibly increase LES tone.	1 ml of tincture or 1 oz of bitter tonics 20-30 minutes before meals
7. Take demulcents	Recommend demulcents, such as *Althea officinalis* or *Ulmus fulva*, to alleviate epigastric discomfort	With two cups of water (as needed)
8. Supplement with choline and lecithin	Anecdotal evidence of increased LES pressure. Safe in pregnancy.	Phosphatidyl choline: 500 mg q.d.
9. Weight loss (attain healthy BMI)		
10. Smoking Cessation		

- If this approach fails, evaluate the possibility of gallstones and *H. pylori* infection.
- Then try H2 blockers and proton pump inhibitors.
- Nissen fundoplication, a surgical operation, is reserved for extreme non-responsive cases.

ESOPHAGEAL DISEASE

Presentation

Signs and Symptoms:
- Difficulty in swallowing (dysphagia) and/or painful swallowing (odynophagia)
- Tendency for atypical chest pains

Hiatal Hernia and Paraesophageal Hernia

Hiatal Hernia: a sliding hernia, where the whole gastroesophageal junction moves above the diaphragm. This common and benign finding (seen on a barium study) may predispose to GERD.

Paraesophageal Hernia: a herniation of a portion of the stomach, where the gastroesophageal junction remains below the diaphragm. This is an uncommon but serious condition because the herniated portion may become strangulated. A surgical solution is recommended.

Achalasia

Signs and Symptoms:
- Intermittent dysphagia without heartburn.
- Barium swallow reveals a dilated esophagus with "bird-beak" narrowing.

Causes: Incomplete relation of a hypertensive lower esophageal sphincter (LES) and loss of peristalsis causes achalasia. It is usually idiopathic or due to CHAGAS disease (tick born *Trypanosoma cruzi* endemic to South America).

Treatment: Magnesium citrate and/or calcium channel blockers, nitrates, endoscopic balloon dilation, botulinum toxin injection. Laparoscopic myotomy with fundoplication is the most long-lasting option. Surgical myotomy represents a last resort solution.

Esophageal Spasm

Causes: Irregular, forceful, and painful esophageal contractions that cause intermittent chest pain.

Diagnosis: Esophageal manometry.

Treatment: Magnesium citrate and/or calcium channel blockers. Laparoscopic myotomy with fundoplication is the most long-lasting option. Surgical myotomy represents a last resort solution.

Scleroderma

Scleroderma (the pathogenesis of which is poorly understood) may cause aperistalsis due to esophageal muscular fibrosis. The LES becomes incompetent, and most patients will have heartburn (this is the opposite of achalasia).

Signs and Symptoms:
- Positive anti-nuclear antibody (ANA)
- Mask-like facies
- CREST syndrome = **C**alcinosis, **R**aynaud's phenomenon, **E**sophageal dysmotility, **S**clerodactyly, and **T**elangectasia

Esophageal Cancer

NPLEX
MCCQE
USMLE

Esophageal Cancer Facts:
- Usually caused by alcohol and tobacco.
- Classically seen in black men more than 40 years of age.
- Patients complain of weight loss (ominous cancer sign) and solid food "sticking" in their throat.
- Most common type is squamous cell carcinoma.

PEPTIC ULCER DISEASE

NPLEX
MCCQE
USMLE

Presentation

Signs and Symptoms:
- Chronic
- Intermittent epigastric distress (burning, gnawing, or aching pain localized and often relieved by antacids or milk)
- Epigastric tenderness on P/E
- Occult blood in stool
- Nausea and vomiting
- PUD is more common in men

NPLEX
MCCQE
USMLE

Differential Dx for Duodenal and Gastric Ulcers

Differential Feature	Duodenal Ulcers	Gastric Ulcers
% of cases	75	25
Acid secretion	Normal to high	Normal to low
Common cause	*Helicobacter pylori*	NSAIDs
Peak age	40s	50s
Ingestion of food	Initially ameliorates, then gets worse 2-3 hours after meals.	Pain is not relieved or aggravated noticeably.

Source

Gray, 2007
Lee, 2010

PUD Tests

- Endoscopy is the most sensitive evaluation (includes biopsy), but an upper GI barium study is less expensive. Evidence suggests that 80% of patients with PUD-like symptoms don't actually have PUD.
- Empiric treatment may be tried in the absence diagnostic studies studies (remote location, inability to access, financial constraints) if the symptoms are typical. However, if the complaints recur or worsen, refer to an internist for a complete workup, including endoscopy and/or an upper GI barium study.

PUD Complications

- Perforation: Look for peritoneal signs, history of PUD, and free air on abdominal radiograph. Prescribe or refer for antibiotic treatment and laparotomy with repair of the perforation.
- Gastrinoma: If ulcers are severe, atypical (e.g., located in the jejunum), or resistant to treatment, consider testing gastrin levels for Zollinger –Ellison syndrome (gastrinoma) or referring for a stomach biopsy (cancer).

Surgical Options for Ulcer Treatment

Surgical options may be considered after failure of naturopathic and medical treatment or when complications develop (perforations, bleeding). Common surgical procedures include:
- Antrectomy
- Vagotomy
- Billroth I or II

NPLEX

Guidelines for First-line Naturopathic Treatment of PUD

Pizzorno, 2006

1. Dietary measures
- Eliminate cigarette smoking, coffee, alcohol, cocaine, NSAIDs, spicy and fatty foods, and chocolate for 1-2 months.

2. Clinical nutrition
- Bismuth subcitrate: 240 mg b.i.d. before meals
- Glutamine: 500 mg t.i.d.
- Add supportive measures: Vitamins A, C, E, zinc, and flavonoids if indicated

3. Botanical medicine
Marz, 2006

Saunders, 2010

Cwikla, 2010
Eamlam-nam, 2006
Yusuf, 2004

Yasar, 2010
- Deglycerrhizinated licorice root (DGL): 380-760 mg dissolved in mouth before meals t.i.d. for 8-16 weeks
- Calendula officinalis: 30-60 gtt tincture/ 10-40 gtt fluid extract is gastroprotective and antimicrobial.
- Filipendula ulmaria: 2-4mL tincture (1:5) t.i.d. is antimicrobial against H. pylori
- Ulmus species: 1-2 tsp powdered root/1-1/2 cup water t.i.d. sooths irritated GI as demulcent
- Aloe species: gel or juice reduces gastric acid secretion and promotes healing of ulcer

If this regimen fails (uncommon) after a 2-month trial, then recommend triple therapy (usually amoxicillin, metronidazole, and bismuth) with proton-pump inhibitors and probiotics.

Source

ACHLORHYDRIA

Presentation

NPLEX
MCCQE
USMLE

Achlorhydria is the *absence* of hydrochloric acid secretion from gastric parietal cells. It is estimated that one-third of the population more than 60 years of age are achlorhydric.

Causes:
- Most commonly due to pernicious anemia, in which antiparietal cell antibodies destroy acid-secreting parietal cells, thus causing achlorhydria and vitamin B-12 deficiency.
- Often a sign of other endocrine autoimmune disorders (e.g., hypothyroidism, vitiligo, diabetes, hypoadrenalism).
- Gastric resection.

GASTRIC BLEEDING

Differential Dx Upper and Lower Gastrointestinal (GI) Bleeding

NPLEX
MCCQE
USMLE

Differential Feature	Upper GI Bleeding	Lower GI Bleeding
Location	Esophagus, stomach, or proximal small bowel	Distal small bowel, large bowel, or rectum
Common causes	Gastritis, ulcers, varices, and esophagitis	Vascular ectasia, diverticulosis, colon cancer, colitis, inflammatory bowel disease, and hemorrhoids
Stool	Tarry, black stool (melena)	Bright red blood seen in stool (hematochezia)

Radiological Imaging Studies

NPLEX
MCCQE
USMLE

- Radionuclide scans: valuable for detecting slow or intermittent bleeds if the source cannot be found with endoscopy.
- Angiography: can detect more rapid bleeds (embolization of bleeding vessels can be done during the procedure).

Management Plan for Gastric Bleeding

1. Make sure the patient is stable (ABCs, intravenous fluids, and blood if needed) before attempting to diagnose.
2. Recommend hospitalization because a nasogastric tube (NGT) aspirate needs to be obtained to determine whether you are dealing with upper or lower GI bleeding.
3. Endoscopy should follow (upper or lower depends on NGT study). Traditionally, barium x-ray studies are performed, but endoscopy is more sensitive. Endoscopically treatable conditions include vascular tears or ectasias, polyps, and varices.
4. These procedures should not be performed in an outpatient facility.

Surgery: Recommended for severe or resistant bleeds. Usually involves resection of the affected bowel (usually colon).

Diverticulosis

Mucosal sacs project through the muscular layer of the colon or rectum. It is extremely common, and the incidence increases with age. The patient is usually unaware of any ill effects unless complications occur. It is caused in part, by a low-fiber + high-fat diet.

Complications:
- GI bleeding (common cause of painless lower GI bleeding)
- Diverticulitis (inflammation of the diverticula). Signs of diverticulitis include:
  - LLQ pain
  - Fever
  - Diarrhea or constipation
  - Leucocytosis

DIARRHEA

Diarrhea

Diarrhea Etiology:
- Systemic
- Osmotic
- Secretory
- Malabsorptive
- Infectious
- Exudative
- Functional or altered intestinal transit

Systemic Diarrhea

Any illness can cause diarrhea as a systemic symptom, especially in children (e.g., otitis media).

Osmotic Diarrhea

Osmotic Diarrhea occurs when non-absorbable solutes remain in the intestines (water flows down its osmotic gradient through the semi-permeable intestinal wall). Examples include lactose or other sugar intolerances and olestra in potato chips.

Diagnosis: When the patient stops ingesting the offending substance (e.g., avoidance of milk or a trial fasting), the diarrhea stops – an easy diagnosis.

Secretory Diarrhea

Secretory Diarrhea involves too much intestinal secretion of fluid. This is an active process due to one of the following:
1. Bacterial toxins (*Vibrio cholera* and pathogenic *Escherichia coli*)
2. VIPoma (pancreatic islet tumor that secretes vasoactive intestinal peptide)
3. Bile acids after ileal resection

Diagnosis: Secretory diarrhea continues after the patient stops eating – another easy diagnosis – but remember to monitor the patient's hydration status prudently. Oral rehydration fluids are life-savers.

Common Causes of Malabsorption Diarrhea

1. Celiac sprue (look for dermatitis herpetiforms and avoid gluten in diet)
2. Crohn's disease (due to depletion of brush-border enzymes)
3. Post-gastroenteritis (also due to depletion of brush-border enzymes)

Infectious Diarrhea Signs and Symptoms

1. Fever
2. Leucocytes in stool analysis with invasive bacteria like: *Shigella* → bacillary dysentery; *Salmonella* → food poisoning; *Yersinia* → gastroenteritis; and *Campylobacter* → food poisoning in children. Leucocytes are not found in infections of toxigenic bacteria (see above).

Causes:
- Travel history: Hikers and campers drinking from lakes and streams may have *Giardia lamblia* infection. This protozoal infection usually presents with steatorrhea (fatty, greasy, malodorous stools that float) due to small intestinal involvement.
- History of antibiotic use (especially clindamycin): Consider *Clostridium difficile* → pseudo-membranous enterocolitis. Test the stool for *C. difficile* toxin.

Exudative Diarrhea Causes

Inflammation of the intestinal wall causing seepage of fluid. Mucosal inflammation is due to either IBD or cancer.

Diagnosis: As in infectious diarrhea, patients usually have fever and white blood cells in the stool, but the chronicity of symptoms and the non-bowel symptoms (see below) are clues.

Source

NPLEX
MCCQE
USMLE

Management Plan for Diarrhea

Diarrhea is a common and preventable cause of death in under-developed countries.
- Obtain a good health history (BM, diet, medication history, laxative use, and recent changes).
- Watch for dehydration and electrolyte disturbances, especially metabolic acidosis and hypokalemia.
- Look for occult blood in stool.
- Examine stool for bacteria, ova, parasites, fat content, and white blood cells.

NPLEX

Guidelines for First-line Naturopathic Treatment of Diarrhea

Gray, 2007

CATMAT,
2001

- Oral Rehydration Therapy (ORT) prevents dehydration and electrolyte loss (saves lives while you are looking for a cause).
- Recommend liberal amounts of commercially available ORT (Gastrolyte or Pedialyte). Discourage unbalanced sodium-to-glucose preparations (Jell-O, soda pop, sugary beverages, Gatorade, or other sports drinks) because they have undesirable osmotic effects. if necessary instruct patients to make their own ORT by mixing 1 level tsp (5 ml) of salt and 8 tsp (40ml) sugar to one liter of water.
- Reduce food intake (12-24 hours only).
- Stop ingestion of poorly absorbed carbohydrates (sorbitol, mannitol, xylitol, fructose, lactose) for 2 weeks.
- Encourage bland BRAT diet (low fat, low carbs, bananas, rice, unsweetened applesauce, tea + clear soup)
- Discontinue medications that may cause diarrhea (e.g., laxatives, antacids, antibiotics, diuretics, prostaglandins, acarbosem orlistatt)
- Prescribe probiotics (esp. Lactobacillus, S. boulardii)
- Psyllium increases fecal water holding capacity and may bind bacterial toxins (i.e. C. difficile)
- Discourage antibiotic use (except for Traveller's diarrhea) due to self-limiting nature of most diarrheas, cost of treatment, potential for promoting antibiotic resistance, and potential adverse drug reactions.

CATMAT,
2001

- Support use of Bismuth salts (subcitrate "compounded" or subsalicylate "Pepto-Bismol") as they are shown to be effective in idiopathic diarrhea and microscopic colitis - use with caution as the salicylates may cause damage to GI mucosa particularly in patients who are also using ASA or NSAIDS; black stools due to bismuth may be confused with melena.

Gray, 2007

- Be cautious of commercially available synthetic opioids (e.g., Loperamide "Imodium") because they are very effective antimotility agents, which is an undesirable effect if diarrhea is caused by micro organisms (toxic megacolon). These agents have undesirable side effects (sedation, nausea, abdominal cramps) and tolerance occurs with chronic use.

Hemolytic Uremic Syndrome

HUS occurs when a GI infection produces toxic substances that destroy red blood cells and, in turn, causes kidney injury.

Diagnosis: Test for hemolytic anemia (evident on CBC and blood smear), thrombocytopenia (CBC), and acute renal failure (BUN and creatinine clearance).

Treatment: Treatment is supportive (in a hospital) because patients may need dialysis or transfusions.

CONSTIPATION

Source

NPLEX

Pizzorno, 2006

Presentation

Subjective Definition: patient complains of infrequent BM and stools that are hard and difficult to expel. Symptoms of constipation include bloated-uncomfortable feeling and sluggishness.

Objective Definition: While the concept of ideal bowel movement frequency is a topic of debate in naturopathic circles, the objective signs of clinical constipation are clear:
1. Less than 3 bowel movements per week
2. More than 3 days without a bowel movement
3. If average daily stools weigh less than 35 gm on an adequate diet

Common Causes of Constipation

- Not enough fiber in the diet. The most common reason by far is a diet typically low in vegetables, fruits, and whole grains and high in fats found in cheese, eggs, and meats.
- Not enough liquids and/or lack of exercise.
- Medications, such as calcium channel blocker and codeine containing drugs.
- Medical conditions, such as colon cancer (causing bowel obstruction), rectal fissures, hypothyroidism, diverticulitis, and irritable bowel syndrome.
- Changes in life or routine, such as pregnancy, older age, and travel.
- Abuse of laxatives. If patients are accustomed to laxatives (natural or otherwise), they will be adaptively constipated without them.
- Ignoring the urge to have a bowel movement (common in children).
- As sequelae of CNS conditions, such as stroke (common).

NPLEX
MCCQE
USMLE

Assessment

1. Obtain a good health history (BM pattern, diet, medication history, laxative use) and inquire about any contributing lifestyle changes.
2. Assess dietary intake and composition.
3. Physical exam: check for weight loss, assess abdomen; do a rectal exam and anoscopy (to rule out fecal impaction, anal fissures, and/or hemorrhoids).
4. If the this strategy is unproductive, run the following tests:
   - Fecal occult blood or hem screen (to rule out colon cancer)
   - Sensitive TSH (to rule out hypothyroidism)
   - CBC (to rule out diverticulitis)

Source

NPLEX
Pizzorno,
2006

Guidelines for First-line Naturopathic Treatment of Constipation

Approach: Treatment will vary according to causative factors. However, the following generalizations are recommended for lifestyle/dietary induced and chronic idiopathic constipation.

1. Dietary measures
- Increase vegetable, fruit, and fiber (flaxseed, oat bran, guar gum, and pectin) intake.
- Avoid saturated fats, cholesterol, sugar, animal protein, and fried foods.
- Experiment with elimination diet for 3 weeks.
- Ensure adequate hydration: 2 liters of water daily.

2. Lifestyle changes
- In younger patients, recommend an aerobically adequate exercise program.
- For older patients, a daily leisurely walk should be adequate.

3. Clinical nutrition
- Vitamin B complex, high potency formulation: 100 mg q.d.
- Vitamin C: 1000 mg t.i.d. or to bowel tolerance
- Bulk forming laxatives: To help produce a bowel movement within 12 to 24 hours:
  - 5 g q.d. of combination fiber (guar gum+ pectin+ psyllium+ oat bran) in three divided doses with meals OR
  - 3-4 g q.d. of glucomannan (water-soluble dietary fiber that is derived from konjac root)
- Magnesium citrate 400-800 mg q.d.
- Probiotics 1-25 billion CFU q.d. (4-12wks)

Guerrara,
2009
Chmie-
lewska,
2010

4. Botanical medicine (adjunctive short-term stimulant laxatives)
- *Cascara sagrada:* 20-30 mg of cascarosides q.d. for < 8-10 days. C/I pregnancy, Crohn's disease, and appendicitis.
- *Aloe vera:* 50-200 mg of latex q.d. for < 10 days. C/I pregnancy, breast-feeding, and IBD.
- *Cassia senna:* 20-60 mg of sennosides OR 1-5 ml of 1:5 tincture q.d. < 10 days. C/I first trimester of pregnancy.

Source

IRRITABLE BOWEL SYNDROME

Presentation

NPLEX
MCCQE
USMLE

Signs and Symptoms: Irritable bowel syndrome is considered a common psychosomatic GI complaint:
- Anxiety
- History of diarrhea (also bloating, abdominal pain, and/or mucus in stool) aggravated by stress
- Relieved by defecation

Gray, 2007

Diagnostic Criteria:
- Recurrent abdominal pain/discomfort for 3 days + ≥2 Sx:
  - Improvement with defecation
  - Onset associated with a change in frequency of stool
  - Onset associated with a change in form of stool

Assessment

NPLEX
MCCQE
USMLE

- Look for psychological stressors in the history and negative findings in physical exam and lab tests.
- IBS is a diagnosis of exclusion: basic lab tests, rectal exam, stool exam, and sigmoidoscopy can be ordered. It is the most likely diagnosis if all of these tests give you negative results, especially in young adults.
- There is a 3:1 female to male incidence ratio.

Guidelines for First-line Naturopathic Treatment of IBS

Pizzorno, 2006

1. Dietary measures
- Increase fiber-rich foods.
- Implement hypoallergenic diet.
- Avoid refined sugars.

2. Clinical Nutrition
- *Lactobacillus acidophilus:* 1-2 billion eq. per day.
- Enteric-coated volatile oil preparations (peppermint/caraway): 0.2-0.4 ml b.i.d. between meals.
- 5-HTP 50-300 mg t.i.d. May be helpful in constipation predominant IBS, though it may worsen symptoms in diarrhea-IBS.

Evans, 200
Shuffle-
botham,
2006
Gershon,
2007
Sikaneler,
2009

3. Lifestyle: Leisurely walks, 20 minutes daily.

4. Counseling
- Stress reduction program
- Biofeedback

Source

NPLEX
MCCQE
USMLE

Gray, 2007

INFLAMMATORY BOWEL DISEASE

Differential Dx

Differential Feature	Crohn's Disease (CD)	Ulcerative Colitis (UC)
Origin of lesion	Distal ileum and proximal colon	Rectum
Extent of inflammation	Transmural (throughout)	Limited to mucosa and submucosa
Progression	Irregular (skip-lesions)	Continuous (no skip-lesions)
Location	From mouth to anus	Only involves the colon, rarely extends into ileum
Bowel habit changes	Obstruction and abdominal pain	Bloody diarrhea
Classic lesions	Fistulas/abscesses, cobblestoning, and string sign (on barium x-ray)	Pseudopolyps, lead-pipe colon (on barium x-ray), and toxic megacolon
Colon cancer risk	Somewhat increased	Significantly increased Colonoscopy surveillance recommended to commence 7 years after diagnosis
Surgery	Not recommended (may make it worse)	Recommended (proctocolectomy, ileoanal anastomosis, and pouch formation)
Common signs and symptoms	Fever; profuse, constant loose stools; anorexia; apathy; prostration; abdominal signs are normal; distended abdomen; and possibly rebound tenderness.	

Source

NPLEX
MCCQE
USMLE

Extra-gastrointestinal Manifestations of IBD

Both CD and UC can cause:

- Uveitis
- Arthritis
- Ankylosing spondylitis
- Erythema nodosum or multiforme
- Primary sclerosing cholangitis
- Failure to thrive in children
- Toxic megacolon (markedly distended colon, common in UC)
- Anemia
- Fever

NPLEX
MCCQE
USMLE

Toxic Megacolon

This condition may be precipitated by the use of motility suppressor antidiarrheal medications (e.g., Imodium-loperamide hydrochloride). This is classically seen with IBD and infectious colitis, especially *Clostridium difficile.* That is why antidiarrheal medications for any diarrhea with fever (infectious diarrhea) should not be recommended.

- Patients present with a high fever, leukocytosis, abdominal pain, rebound tenderness, and a dilated segment of colon (by palpation and radiograph).
- This is an emergency condition requiring prompt hospitalization. Instruct the patient not to eat. → Send to ER.

NPLEX
MCCQE
USMLE

Gray, 2007

Conventional Treatment of IBD

- Emergency treatment and hospitalization in some patients. The goal is to achieve remission, which, once attained, can be maintained by conservative therapy. As treatment is complex, refer to gastroenterologist for initial assessment and remission planning.
- Steroids during severe flare-ups.
- Corticosteroids (hydrocortisone, Methylprednisone, Budesonide, Prednisone) are recommended during flare-ups and to induce remission in CD and UC (70% response rate) but not for maintenance therapy. Prednisone 40-60mg QD for 12-16 weeks is the most common prescription. Long term systemic use may lead to S/E osteoporosis, Cushing's syndrome, avascular necrosis of femoral head.
- 5-aminosalicylic acid (5-ASA), Salofalk, Pentasa, Sulfasalazine, and Asacol) are used widely to maintain remission. 5-ASA is much more effective in maintenance therapy of UC than in CD. S/E profile includes nausea, headaches, rashes, hemolytic anemia, hepatotoxicity, and oligoispermia. A recent systematic review concluded that 5-ASA maintenance therapy had no benefit on CD.
- Short courses of antibiotics (metronidazole, or ciprofloxacin) are useful in patients with Crohn's disease and perianal fistula.
- Adjunctive immune suppression via use of Azathiopine, 6-mercaptopurine (6-MP) or methotrexate is used in refractory Crohn's disease to control symptoms or to reduce the dose of prednisone (S/E bone marrow suppression, cytopenias, infections).
- Biologic response modifiers "Infliximab" are antibodies directed toward TNF-α are gaining acceptance as remission inducers in CD and UC that is refractory to above treatment options. Side effects range from headaches, flushing, and lightheadedness to ANA Lupus-like Syndrome, opportunistic infections and lymphoma.
- NSAIDs should be avoided as they can precipitate or worsen symptoms

Guidelines for First-line Naturopathic Treatment of IBD

Approach:
- First-line treatment starts with comprehensive dietary modifications.
- Maintain remission.
- Reduce inflammation.
- Provide symptom relief.

1. Dietary measures
- Eliminate all possible food sensitivities (wheat, corn, dairy, carrageenan-containing foods)
- Provide a diet high in complex carbohydrates and fiber, low in sugar and other refined carbohydrates.
- Elemental diet (e.g., Peptamen, Nutren, Mediclear) is a proven effective alternative to corticosteroids to induce remission of acute IBD.
- Hypoallergenic (oligoantigenic) diet usually maintains remission once attained.
- Smoking cessation

2. Clinical nutrition
- Glutamine: 500 mg t.i.d.
- Modified Robert's Formula (Bastyr's formula): 2-3 '00' capsules (or equivalent in tincture) t.i.d. with meals
- Quercetin: 400 mg t.i.d. 20 minutes before meals
- Evaluate and correct deficiencies in vitamins A and E, magnesium, and zinc.
- Evaluate and correct deficiencies in vitamins A, D, E and K, magnesium, calcium, iron, and zinc

LIVER DISEASE (HEPATITIS)

Presentation: Acute Hepatitis

Signs and Symptoms of Acute Liver Disease :
- ↑ Liver Function Tests (LFTs): AST (SGOT for NPLEX), ALT (SGPT for NPLEX), bilirubin, ALP, prothrombin time or international normalized ratio (INR)
- Jaundice
- Nausea and vomiting
- RUQ tenderness
- Hepatomegaly (liver span)

Causes of Acute Liver Disease:
- Alcohol
- Medications
- Infection (hepatitis)
- Reye's syndrome
- Biliary tract disease

Presentation: Chronic Hepatitis

Signs and Symptoms of Chronic Liver Disease:
- LFTs will be elevated but not to the same levels seen in acute Liver Disease
- There may be jaundice, nausea, vomiting
- RUQ tenderness

Stigmata:
- Gynecomastia
- Testicular atrophy
- Palmar erythema
- Spider angiomas
- Ascites

Causes of Chronic Liver Disease:
- Alcohol
- Infection (Hepatitis)
- Metabolic disease

Source

NPLEX
MCCQE
USMLE

Metabolic Disorders Resulting From Liver Failure

Metabolic Disorders	*Rationale*
1. **Coagulopathy:** PT (prothrombin time) or even PTT (partial thromboplastin time) are prolonged.	The liver is responsible for synthesis of coagulation factors. Vitamin K is useless because the liver cannot utilize it in its failed state. Symptomatic patients must be given fresh frozen plasma to survive.
2. **Jaundice/ hyperbilirubinemia**: Elevated conjugated and unconjugated bilirubin.	Liver is responsible for the metabolism of both by-products of hemoglobin degradation (DDx with biliary tract disease).
3. **Hypoalbuminemia**	Liver makes albumin.
4. **Portal Hypertension**	Always seen with cirrhosis or chronic liver disease. This leads to hemorrhoids, varices, and caput medusae.
5. **Ascites**	You add portal-hypertension to hypoalbuminemia; the result is always ascites. On physical exam, shifting dullness and fluid wave.
6. **Hyperammonemia**	The liver detoxifies ammonia into uric acid. Treat with decreased protein intake and a substance that decreases ammonia absorption (lactulose).
7. **Hepatic Encephalopathy**	High bilirubin and ammonia in turn cause irritation of brain tissue. Look for coarse tremor (asterixis) and mental status changes.
8. **Hepatorenal Syndrome**	Idiopathic causality relationship, where liver failure induces kidney failure.
9. **Hypoglycemia**	Glycogen is stored in the liver.
10. **Disseminated Intravascular Coagulation (DIC)**	Normal liver cells usually remove activated clotting factors. In liver failure, this is not done, leading to this end-stage emergent condition.

HEPATITIS

Alcoholic Hepatitis Abnormality

NPLEX
MCCQE
USMLE

- ↑ AST (SGOT) that is more than twice the value of ALT (SGPT), although both maybe elevated.
- GGT will be markedly elevated.

Hepatitis A

Signs and Symptoms:
- Anti-hepatitis A immunoglobulin (IgM) is positive during or shortly after jaundice episode.
- No significant long-term sequelae of infection with the exception of rare cases of acute liver failure.
- Transmission is through fecal contamination (e.g., day-care center or restaurant food).

Hepatitis B

Infection Sources:
- Shared needles
- Sexual contact
- Perinatal transmission (mother to baby)
- Transfused blood (a risk factor in the past but all blood banks now test for HBV and HCV)

Prevention: Best treatment is preventive vaccination, community education, condoms, etc.

Risk: 10% of patients will develop chronicity that predisposes to hepatobiliary cirrhosis and hepatocellular cancer.

Serology of Hepatitis B Infection

NPLEX
MCCQE
USMLE

- Hepatitis B surface antigen (HBsAg) is positive only with unresolved acute or chronic infection.
- Hepatitis B surface antibody (HBsAb) is positive when patient is immune (recovered or vaccinated). It never appears if the patient has chronic hepatitis.
- Hepatitis B 'e' antigen (HBeAg) is a marker for infectivity, which means that if a patient exhibits anti-hepatitis B 'e' antibody (HBeAb), the likelihood of them spreading the disease is low.
- The first antibody to appear is the IgM hepatitis B core antibody (HBcAb) during the "window phase" when both HBsAg and HBsAb are negative.
- Screening (HBsAg) is recommended for all pregnant women, high risk groups, and patients from Asia, Pacific Islands, Africa and endemic countries.

Gonzales, 2009

Possible Sequelae of Chronic Hepatitis B or C

NPLEX

- Cirrhosis
- Hepatobiliary cancer

Source

NPLEX
MCCQE
USMLE

Hepatitis B Treatment

Hepatitis B immunoglobulin should be given to individuals exposed to hepatitis within 48 to 72 hours of exposure. Examples include newborn babies, whose mothers are HepB positive, and health-care workers after a needle-stick injury (even if they are vaccinated, unless their HBsAb titer is known).

Hepatitis C

Causes:
- Post-transfusion hepatitis (most likely cause). Screening for HCV was developed recently.
- Positive hepatitis C antibody means that the patient has had an infection in the past, but does not mean the infection has been cleared.

Risk Factor: Hepatitis C is 8 times more likely than hepatitis B to progress into chronicity, cirrhosis, and cancer.

Gonzales,
2009

Screening for HCV is recommended only in high-risk patients; drug users, healthcare workers after needle stick injuries, children of HCV-positive mothers, chronic liver disease patients, chronic hemodialysis, and blood or organ recipients before 1992 (i.e., before mandatory HCV surveillance).

Prevention: Treatment is not usually successful; thus, prevention is paramount.

NPLEX
MCCQE
USMLE

Hepatitis D

- Hepatitis D is seen only in patients with hepatitis B. Not only does it piggyback on it, but also the co-infection may become chronic.
- Transmission is similar to HBV.
- IgM antibodies to hepatitis D antigen indicate resolution of a recent infection.
- Positive hepatitis D antigen indicates chronicity.

MCCQE
USMLE

Hepatitis E

- Via fecal contamination of food sources, like HAV.
- Uniquely, there is no chronic state.
- It is often fatal in pregnant women.

MCCQE
USMLE

Drug-induced Hepatitis

- Acetaminophen
- Tuberculosis drugs: isoniazid, rifampin, and pyrazinamide
- Halothane (anesthetic)
- Carbon tetrachloride
- Tetracycline
- HMG-CoA reductase inhibitors (e.g., cholesterol lowering agents, such as Lipitor)

Source

NPLEX
MCCQE
USMLE

Conventional Treatment for Acute Viral Hepatitis

Acute viral hepatitis is extremely debilitating (fever, headaches, GI discomfort, nausea and vomiting, diarrhea, arthralgia, drowsiness, malaise, and itching) requiring bed-rest and 9 to 16 weeks for recovery.

- Supportive treatment, bed-rest.
- Limited use of interferon alpha-2a or alhpa-2b in chronic cases of HBV or HCV.
- Avoid contact with others during contagious phase (3 weeks before and after onset of acute symptoms).

Guidelines for First-line Naturopathic Treatment of Acute Viral Hepatitis

NPLEX

1. Dietary measures
- Avoid alcohol and hepatotoxic medications.
- Acute:
  - Replace fluids (vegetable broth, diluted vegetable juices, herbal teas).
  - Restrict solid food intake to brown rice, steamed vegetables, and lean protein.
- Chronic:
  - Avoid saturated fats, simple carbohydrates, oxidized fatty acids, and animal fat.
  - Recommend a calorically adequate diet that is primarily vegetarian.

Pizzorno, 2006

2. Clinical nutrition
- Vitamin C: to bowel tolerance and maintain 1000 mg t.i.d. in chronic cases
- Bovine liver and thymus extracts (received some favorable literature review thus far)
- L-carnitine: 500-1000 mg t.i.d. may be beneficial for patient with hepatitis C experiencing fatigue
- Taurine: 2 g t.i.d. (minimum 3 months) for chronic hepatitis ($\downarrow$ ALT, $\downarrow$ AST, $\downarrow$ triglyceride, $\downarrow$ cholesterol)

Anty, 2011

Hu, 2008

3. Botanical medicine
- *Glycyrrhiza glabra* (standardized to 5% glycyrrhetinic acid): 250-500 mg t.i.d. for 9-16 weeks (with increased potassium-rich foods and weekly monitoring for possible hypertension side effect)
- *Silybum marianum* (standardized to silymarin content): 140-210 mg silymarin t.i.d. for 9-16 weeks
- *Curcuma longa*: 300 mg t.i.d. In vitro studies demonstrated antiviral properties toward hepatitis B and C. Given the safe side effect profile of turmeric, a trial therapy may be tried.

Kim, 2009
Kim, 2010

Idiopathic Autoimmune Hepatitis

NPLEX
MCCQE
USMLE

This condition is classically seen in 20- to 40-year-old women with anti-smooth muscle or anti-nuclear antibodies, and no risk factors or lab markers for other causes of hepatitis.
Treatment: Corticosteroid therapy.

Source

AUTOSOMAL DISEASES

NPLEX
MCCQE
USMLE

Presentation: Hemochromatosis

Primary hemochromatosis is an autosomal recessive trait, where excessive iron is deposited in the liver, pancreas, heart, skin, and joints (see Hematology module).

Signs and Symptoms:
- Iron deposition leads to cirrhosis and/or hepatocellular carcinoma, diabetes, dilated cardiomyopathy, "bronze diabetes" skin pigmentation, and arthritis.
- Men are symptomatic earlier and more often than women due to menstrual loss of iron.

Treatment: Phlebotomy: weekly or biweekly removal of 500 ml of blood until iron levels return to normal.

Secondary Hemochromatosis: caused by iron overload, which is classically due to ineffective erythropoiesis (e.g., thalassemia), hemolysis, and excessive iron intake.

Dugani,
2009
Gray, 2007

Screening: Screening of asymptomatic patients is not recommended. Screen symptomatic patients or those with family history via blood testing for serum ferritin + transferrin saturation index, if elevated recommend confirmation via C282Y genetic test or liver biopsy.

Wilson's Disease

Wilson's disease (hepatolenticular degeneration) is another autosomal recessive disease, where excessive copper is deposited mainly in the liver and to some extent in the CNS.
- Serum ceruloplasmin (copper binding protein) is low, but serum copper may be normal. Liver biopsy is confirmatory and will show excessive copper deposition in the liver.
- Think of Wilson's disease in patients with liver disease, CNS manifestations (tremor), psychiatric manifestations (psychosis), and Kayser-Fleischer rings in the iris.

Dugani,
2009

Screening: recommended for relatives of patient's with Wilson's disease.

Treatment: Copper chelation with penicillamine or other copper chelating agents.

NPLEX
MCCQE
USMLE

Alpha-1 Antitrypsin Deficiency Relatives

Alpha-1 Antitrypsin Deficiency Diagnosis: Young adult with cirrhosis and emphysema without risk factors for either. This is another rare autosomal recessive disease (i.e., look for an autosomal recessive family history because it skips generations).

BILIARY TRACT CONDITIONS

Source

Presentation

MCCQE
USMLE

Biliary Tract Obstruction Signs and Symptoms:
- Very high ALP
- Elevated conjugated bilirubin (more than unconjugated bilirubin because the liver still functions normally)
- Pruritus
- Clay-colored stool
- "Coca cola" dark urine (unconjugated bilirubin is never excreted in urine because it is tightly bound to albumin)

Types of Biliary Tract Obstruction:
- Bile duct obstruction
- Cholestasis
- Cholangitis
- Primary biliary cirrhosis
- Primary sclerosing cholangitis

Causes of Common Bile Duct Obstruction

MCCQE
USMLE

Gallstone (Choledocholithiasis)

- This is the most common cause. Look for the five Fs: female, forty, fertile, fair complexion, and obese.
- Most gallstones are silent until they either produce cholecystitis or common bile duct obstruction.
- Ultrasound is often diagnostic, if not, endoscopic retrograde cholangio-pancreatography (ERCP) is recommended.

Pancreatic Cancer

- Clinical diagnosis is delayed because in most cases the symptoms are non-specific.
- Look for weight loss; dull abdominal pain; jaundice; palpably enlarged gall bladder (Courvoisier sign); and migratory thrombophlebitis (Trousseau syndrome).
- The etiology of pancreatic cancer is unknown, and to complicate matters, there is no satisfactory prevention or treatment. CT or ultrasound is often diagnostic.

Source

NPLEX

Pizzorno,
2006

Guidelines for First-line Naturopathic Treatment of Gallstones

Approach: Treatment varies slightly based on gallstone composition (80% are mixed, 20% are exclusively mineral). However, the following generalizations are adequate for both types:

1. Dietary measures
- Increase vegetable, fruit, and fiber (flaxseed, oat bran, guar gum, and pectin) intake.
- Avoid saturated fats, cholesterol, sugar, animal protein, and fried foods.
- Use elimination diet for 12 weeks.
- Ensure adequate hydration: 2 liters of water daily.

2. Clinical nutrition
- Phosphatidylcholine: 500 mg q.d.
- L-Methionine: 1 g q.d.
- Combination fiber (guar gum+ pectin+ psyllium+ oat bran): 5 g q.d. in three divided doses with meals

3. Botanical medicine
Duration of treatment should be no less than 12 weeks:
- *Taraxicum officinalis* (4:1): 250-500 mg t.i.d.
- *Peumus boldo:* (1:1) 0.5-1.0 ml t.i.d.
- *Silybum marianum* (standardized to silymarin content): 140-210 mg silymarin t.i.d.
- *Phyllantus niruri* Chanca piedra(10:1): 500 mg b.i.d.

MCCQE
USMLE

Common Causes of Cholestasis

- Birth control pills
- Pregnancy
- Obesity

NPLEX
MCCQE
USMLE

Primary Biliary Cirrhosis

Signs and Symptoms:
- Seen in middle-aged women with no risk factors for liver or biliary disease.
- Marked pruritus, jaundice, and positive antimitochondrial antibodies. The rest of the work-up will be negative.
- Unfortunately, the only treatment recommended is liver transplantation.

MCCQE
USMLE

Cholangitis

Cholangitis: inflammation of the bile duct that is usually caused by gallstone dislodgment in the common bile duct.

Primary Sclerosing Cholangitis: occurs in young adults with IBD (usually UC). It presents like regular cholangitis.

Symptoms and Diagnosis: Fever + RUQ pain + jaundice = Charcot's triad (diagnostic signs).

Treatment: Recommended treatment is surgical excision and antimicrobial treatment.

PANCREATITIS

Presentation

Acute Pancreatitis Signs and Symptoms:
- Epigastric abdominal pain that radiates to the back
- Nausea and vomiting without relief of pain
- Leucocytosis
- Elevated levels of serum Amylase and Lipase
- Cullen's sign – blue-black umbilicus; and/or Grey Turner's sign – blue-black flanks. These patients need to be hospitalized.
- Perforated ulcers are also associated with elevated serum amylase. However, patients usually have free air on abdominal radiographs and history of PUD.

Acute Pancreatitis Causes:
- >80% are due to alcohol and gallstones.
- Less common causes include:
  - Hypertriglyceridemia
  - Mumps
  - Trauma
  - Hypercalcemia
  - Steroid medications
  - Scorpion bites

Complications of Acute Pancreatitis

- Pseudocyst formation
- Abscess formation
- Infection
- Chronic pancreatitis

Chronic Pancreatitis

Chronic Pancreatitis Causes: Chronic pancreatitis is almost always caused by alcoholism and repeated acute pancreatitis. Gallstones do not cause chronic pancreatitis (only acute).

Treatment: Recommended treatment is alcohol abstention, oral pancreatic enzymes, and fat-soluble vitamins (i.e., A, D, E, and K).

Source

NPLEX
MCCQE
USMLE

COLORECTAL CANCER (CA)

Presentation

- Colon cancer is the 3rd most common cancer in Canada and the 2nd leading cause of death from cancer. Fortunately, the death rate is declining, partially due to earlier screening and diagnosis.

Symptoms:

Because the location of the cancer varies among patients, so do the symptoms. Refer for colonoscopy patients presenting with rectal bleeding, blood in stool, severe anemia, and changes in bowel habits (e.g., constipation alternating with frequent diarrhea). Low ferritin or anemia in postmenopausal women or men needs to be assessed with FOBT .

Screening Guidelines for Adults ≥ 50 yo (average risk)

Dugani,
2009
Beers,
2006
Gonzales,
2009
CCS, 2011

Annual FOBT screenings reduce cancer mortality by 33% (although there is no evidence that all cause mortality is reduced).

- Fecal Occult Blood Test annually OR
- Flexible sigmoidoiscopy every 5 years OR
- Colonoscopy every 10 years
- Earlier screening (begin at 40 yo), including genetic testing, is recommended for higher risk individuals. Individuals with FHx of CA in 1st degree relative >60 yo (or two 1st degree relatives with CA) should have colonoscopy done at 40 yo, followed with colonoscopy every 5 years.
- Diet: high in animal products, fats, and refined carbohydrates, while low in fiber
- Genetics: FHx of colorectal cancer and/or polyps
- PMHx: IBD, colon polyps
- Age: ≥50 yo
- Radiation: ≥30 Gy of radiation to whole abdomen (e.g., CT scan of entire abdomen)

Risk Factors:

- Personal history of IBD, familial adenomatous polyopsis (FAP), Lynch syndrome, Peutz-Jeghers syndrome, other cancer
- Racial and ethnic: African or ashkenazi (eastern European Jewish) descent
- Lifestyle: sedentary, obesity, smoking, alcohol consumption, night shiftwork
- Type II diabetes
- Previous radiation therapy

Examination Board References

NPLEX (II): North American Board of Naturopathic Examiners
North American Board of Naturopathic Examiners (NABNE), Naturopathic Physician Licensing Examination Part II Blueprint and Study Guide. Portland, OR: NABNE, 2005.

USMLE (II): National Board of Medical Examiners
Bouchert A. USMLE Step 2 Secrets. Philadelphia, PA: Hanley & Belfus Inc., 2000.

MCCQE: Medical Council of Canada
Molckovsky A, Pirzada KS (eds.). Review for the Medical Council of Canada Qualification Examination. Toronto, ON: Toronto Notes Medical Publishing, 2004.

Related References

Anty R, Marjoux S, Bekri S, DeGalleani L, Dainese R, Gelsi E, Cherikh F, Tran A, Piche T. Plasma carnitine is associated with fatigue in chronic hepatitis C but not in the irritable bowel syndrome. Aliment Pharmacol Ther. 2011;33(8): 961-68.

Beers MH, Porter RS, Jones TV, Kaplan JL, Berkwits M. The Merck Manual of Diagnosis and Therapy. 18th ed. Whitehouse Station, NJ: Merck Research Laboratories , 2006.

Canadian Cancer Society. Colorectal Cancer Statistics at a Glance, 2011. Online at http://www.cancer.ca

Cutler P. Problem Solving in Clinical Medicine: From Data to Diagnosis. 3rd ed. Baltimore, MD: Lippincott Williams & Wilkins, 1998.

Chmielewska A, Szajewska H. Systematic review of randomized controlled trials: probiotics for functional constipation. World Journal of Gastroenterology. 2010;16(1): 69-75.

Cwikla C, Schmidt K, Matthias A, Bone KM, Lehmann R, Tiralongo E. Investigations into the antibacterial activities of phytotherapeutics against Helicobacter pylori and Campylobacter jejuni. Phytotherapy Research. 2010;24(5):649-56.

Dugani S, Lam D. Toronto Notes: Comprehensive Medical Reference & Review for MCCQE & USMLE II. 25th ed. Toronto (ON): Toronto Notes for Medical Students, Inc., 2009.

Eamlamnam K, Patumraj S, Visedopas N, Thong-Ngam D. Effects of Aloe vera and sucralfate on gastric microcirculatory changes, cytokine levels and gastric ulcer healing in rats. World Journal of Gastroenterology. 2006;12(13): 2034-39.

Evans BW, Clark WK, Moore DJ, Whorwell PJ.. Tegaserod for the treatment of irritable bowel syndrome and chronic constipation. Cochrane Database Systematic Review. 2007;4:CD003960.

Ferri F. Ferri's Clinical Advisor Instant Diagnosis and Treatment. New York, NY: Mosby, 2009.

Gershon MD, Tack J. The serotonin signaling system: from basic understanding to drug development for functional GI disorders. Gastroenterology. 2007;132(1): 397-414.

Gonzales R, Kutner J. Current Practice Guidelines in Primary Care 2009. Toronto ON: McGraw Hill, 2009.

Gray J. Therapeutic Choices. 5th ed. Toronto, ON: Canadian Pharmacists Association, 2007.

Guerrera MP, Volpe SL, Mao JJ. Therapeutic uses of magnesium. American Family Physician, 2009;80(2):157-62.

Hirota WK, Zuckerman MJ, Adler DG, Davila RE, Egan J, Leighton JA, Qureshi WA, Rajan E, Fanelli R, Wheeler-Harbaugh J, Baron TH, Faigel DO. Standards of Practice Committee, American Society for Gastrointestinal Endoscopy. ASGE guideline: the role of endoscopy in the surveillance of premalignant conditions of the upper GI tract. Gastrointest Endosc. 2006;63(4):570-80.

Hu YH, Lin CL, Huang YW, Liu PE, Hwang DF. Dietary amino acid taurine ameliorates liver injury in chronic hepatitis patients. Amino acids. 2008; 35(2):469-73.

Kim K, Kim KH, Kim HY, Cho HK, Sakamoto N, Cheong J. Curcumin inhibits hepatitis C virus replication via suppressing the Akt-SREBP-1 pathway. FEBS Lett. 2010;584(4):707-12.

Kim HJ, Yoo HS, Kim JC, et al. Antiviral effect of Curcuma longa Linn extract against hepatitis B virus replication. Journal of Ethnopharmacology. 2009;124(2): 189-96.

Lee L. Peptic ulcer disease. First Consult Elsevier Inc., 2010. Online at www.mdconsult.com

Marz RB. Medical Nutrition form Marz. 2nd ed. Portland, OR: Omni-Press, 1999.

Murray M. Encyclopedia of Nutritional Supplements. Rocklin, CA: Prima Publishing, 1996.

Pitchford P. Healing with Whole Foods. Asian Traditions and Modern Nutrition. 3rd ed. Berkley, CA: North Atlantic Books, 2002.

Pizzorno JE, Murray MT. Textbook of Natural Medicine. Vol. 1 and 2. 2nd ed. New York, NY: Churchill Livingstone, 1999.

Saunders PR, Godfrey A. Naturopathic Botanical Medicine: Volume I. Toronto (ON): CCNM Press, 2010.

Shapiro M. Gastroesophageal Reflux. In: Kohatso W (ed.). Complementary and Alternative Medicine Secrets. Philadelphia, PA: Hanley & Belfus Inc., 2002.

Sikander A, Rana SV, Prasad KK. Role of serotonin in gastrointestinal motility and irritable bowel syndrome. Clin Chim Acta. 2009;403(1-2): 47-55.

Shufflebotham J, Hood S, Hendry J, et al. Acute tryptophan depletion alters gastrointestinal and anxiety symptoms in irritable bowel syndrome. American Journal of Gastroenterology. 2006;101(11): 2582-87.

Yasar B, Abut E, Kayadibi H, Toros B, Sezikli M, Akkan Z, Kaskin O, Kurdas OO. Efficacy of probiotics in Helicobacter pylori eradication therapy. Turksih Journal of Gastroenterology. 2010;21(3): 212-17.

Yusuf S, Agunu A, Diana M. The effect of Aloe vera A. Berger (Liliaceae) on gastric acid secretion and acute gastric mucosal injury in rats. Journal of Ethnopharmacology. 2004;93(1): 33-37.

GERIATRICS

Contributing author: Lorinda Sorenson, ND

COGNITIVE FUNCTION

PHYSICAL FUNCTION

CARDIOLOGY

DIABETES

GI SYSTEM

CANCER

GERIATRICS

Presentation

The most common issues that geriatric patients present with are:

- Malnutrition
- Physical disability. When compounded by lack of means of transportation, this can lead to dependence, immobility, and social isolation.
- Under- diagnosed and untreated conditions, such as depression and hearing loss.
- Polypharmacy issues. The average North American elderly patient is on four to six pharmacologic agents with the potential for dietary restriction, and a significant risk of interaction between prescribed and OTC pharmaceutical, nutritional and botanical agents.
- Cognitive decline and age-related dementia is probably the most significant challenge. Cognitive decline, combined with social isolation, often leads to mood disorders, depression, aggression (or psychosis), problems with diet, problems with compliance with prescriptions, and sexual issues.

Epidemiology and Longevity

- 8% of the world's population is above the age of 65. In the USA and Canada, about 15% of the population is over age 65, and this group is exhibiting the most rapid growth in numbers percentage-wise.
- On a global level, the 85-and-over population is projected to increase 151% compared to a 104% increase for the 65-and-over population, and a 21% increase for the population under age 65.
- According to Canadian Census (2006), 84.5% of seniors (65+) live in private households, while 7.5% (up from 7.4% in 2001) live in nursing homes, health care facilities, or similar collective dwellings. In Canada, seniors represent 61% of the population living in collective dwellings.
- In the United states 5% of seniors (65+) live in nursing homes, representing 89% of the population living in collective dwellings.

Consequences for Primary Care:

As longevity increases so does the need for healthcare provision; for example, in Canada:

- 65+ age group: N=4,335,000; 324,000 (7%) live in a collective dwelling Vs 4,011,000 (93%) living at home
- 75+ age group: N=2,047,000, 276,000 (13%) live in a collective dwelling Vs 1,771,000 (87%) living at home. There is an increase in the number and the % share of seniors living in collective dwellings between 2001 and 2006 due to the growing share of persons aged 75 and over within the senior population.

This fact has serious consequence for primary care providers, who are expected to care for the unique needs of seniors within the community rather than in nursing homes. Beyond the age of 72, for example, health needs of seniors increase exponentially, and access to primary care providers remains constrained.

Source

NPLEX
MCCQE
USMLE

Special Nutritional Needs of the Elderly

- Older people in general need fewer calories because they tend to be less active and their body composition changes. Daily energy requirements per kg generally decline with age, specifically between 30 and 90-year-old, due to loss of muscle mass. For example, at age 80, the average elderly patient will have half of the lean body mass of the average 30-year-old.
- However, there are specific nutrients that elderly patients will need more of, such as calcium, vitamin D, vitamin B-12, folate, and iron.

NPLEX
MCCQE
USMLE

Digestion and Malnutrition

- Digestion can be impaired in the elder population due to less food intake (financial issues, social issues, less taste receptors); decreased mastication from poor fitting dentures; less muscle tone in masseter muscle; dysphagia; decreased gastric HCL secretion; gastric dysmotility; slowed gastric emptying leading to earlier satiety; and decreased efficiency of absorption (malabsorption). Another reason for eating less may be due to taking multiple prescription pharmaceuticals (polypharmacy) and being worried about interactions.
- When you add diet restriction, malabsorption, increased demands for certain nutrients, age-related social and psychological issues, it is easy to see why most elderly people suffer from malnutrition and its manifestations (reduced muscle mass, weight loss, osteoporosis, muscle weakness, sensory decline and impaired mobility).

NPLEX
MCCQE
USMLE

Hearing and Vision Changes

On average, some predictable vision and hearing loss will be experienced by older patients:

Presbycusis: almost 100% of the population will have some hearing loss by age 85. High pitch goes first and earlier in men (decreased hearing w/ diminished acuity and discrimination. Screen patients for hearing loss and recommend annual visits to an audiologist. Hearing aids help prevent social isolation.

Presbyopia: by age 50, 88% of people need assistance with reading due to loss of elasticity of the lens. Think bifocal glasses when you think of presbyopia. Screen for vision and recommend annual visits to an optometrist.

These sensory changes are not normal when the symptoms are sudden or associated with pain.

COGNITIVE FUNCTION

Source

Brain atrophy

MCCQE
NPLEX

Cerebral atrophy is a non-specific finding that can result from brain injury or degeneration and occurs normally in aging. However, many disease processes result in distinctive patterns of atrophy due to differential involvement of different areas of the brain; for example, hippocampal, amygdalar, and global brain atrophy on brain MRI have been proposed as early markers of Alzheimer's disease.

Undifferentiated Dementia

NPLEX
MCCQE
USMLE

Prevalence: 5-8% of all people over the age of 65 have some form of dementia, and this number doubles every 5 years above that age. It is estimated that as many as half of people 85 or older suffer from dementia.

Dains,
2011

Memory Loss: Memory loss is the most common cognitive complaint of elder patients. In undifferentiated dementia, it may appear as:

- Disorientation for dates
- Naming difficulties *(anomia)*
- Recent recall problems
- Difficulty copying figures
- Decreased insight
- Social withdrawal
- Irritability, mood changes
- Problems managing finances
- Difficulty learning and retaining new information
- Personality alterations
- Irritability, anxiety
- Depression

Alzheimer Disease (AD) or Senile Dementia of the Alzheimer Type (SDAT)

Alzheimer disease is the most frequent cause of dementia, accounting for 70% of all cases of dementia in seniors 71 and older. AD is a progressive neurodegenerative disorder characterized by the development of β-amyloid plaques and neurofibrillary tangles in frontal, temporal and parietal cortex.

Harrison,
2008

Diagnosis:
- Anterograde amnesia (can't learn new things)
- One of following:
  - Aphasia (trouble with speech production and comprehension)
  - Apraxia (motor difficulties)
  - Agnosia (can't recognize objects)
  - Disruption of executive functions (planning, organizing, sequencing, abstracting)

**See the Neurology module for more information.

Source

NPLEX
MCCQE
USMLE

Harrison,
2008

NPLEX
MCCQE
USMLE

NPLEX
MCCQE
USMLE

Harrison,
2008

Vascular Dementia

- Vascular dementia is the second most common form of dementia in North America and Europe after Alzheimer disease, but it is the most common form in some parts of Asia. The prevalence is 1.5% in Western countries and approximately 2.2% in Japan.
- The prevalence rate of dementia is 9 times higher in patients who have had a stroke than in those who have not had a stroke. One year after a stroke, 25% of patients develop new-onset dementia. Within 4 years following a stroke, the relative risk of incident dementia is 5.5%.
- The condition is not a single disease, but a group of syndromes relating to different vascular mechanisms (e.g., lacunar infarcts, vascular compromise).

Organic Diseases that Present with Dementia

- Parkinson disease
- Dementia with Lewy body
- Persistent alcohol dementia
- Neurosyphilis
- B-12, folate, thiamine deficiency
- Hypothyroidism
- Chronic infection
- Brain tumor
- HIV dementia
- Pick's disease: a type of fronto temporal dementia (FTD). In people under age 60, FTD is the most common cause of dementia. FTD affects approximately 6.7 people per 100,000 in the 45-64 age group. The term *Frontotemporal dementia* is increasingly used to describe the clinical syndrome, while *Pick's disease* is used to classify patients in whom the pathology shows classic Pick bodies (only a minority of patients with the clinical features of FTD).

Pseudodementia

- Depression in the elderly can manifest in impairment in thinking, withdrawal from social interactions, memory loss, and apathy that resembles dementia (thus "pseudo" dementia).
- Scrutinize every dementia presentation for depression markers (e.g., loss of spouse, terminal or debilitating disease, frequent crying, suicidal thoughts). The good news is once the depression is treated, pseudodementia goes away.

MONTREAL COGNITIVE ASSESSMENT (MOCA)
Version 7.1 Original Version

NAME :
Education :
Sex :
Date of birth :
DATE :

VISUOSPATIAL / EXECUTIVE

Copy cube

Draw CLOCK (Ten past eleven) (3 points)

POINTS

(E) End (A) (5) (B) (2) (1) Begin (D) (4) (3) (C)

[ ]

[ ]

[ ] Contour [ ] Numbers [ ] Hands

___/5

NAMING

[ ]   [ ]   [ ]

___/3

MEMORY
Read list of words, subject must repeat them. Do 2 trials, even if 1st trial is successful. Do a recall after 5 minutes.

	FACE	VELVET	CHURCH	DAISY	RED	No points
1st trial						
2nd trial						

ATTENTION
Read list of digits (1 digit/ sec.).

Subject has to repeat them in the forward order	[ ] 2 1 8 5 4	
Subject has to repeat them in the backward order	[ ] 7 4 2	___/2

Read list of letters. The subject must tap with his hand at each letter A. No points if ≥ 2 errors
[ ] F B A C M N A A J K L B A F A K D E A A A J A M O F A A B ___/1

Serial 7 subtraction starting at 100   [ ] 93   [ ] 86   [ ] 79   [ ] 72   [ ] 65   ___/3
4 or 5 correct subtractions: **3 pts**, 2 or 3 correct: **2 pts**, 1 correct: **1 pt**, 0 correct: **0 pt**

LANGUAGE
Repeat : I only know that John is the one to help today. [ ]
The cat always hid under the couch when dogs were in the room. [ ]   ___/2

Fluency / Name maximum number of words in one minute that begin with the letter F   [ ] _____ (N ≥ 11 words) ___/1

ABSTRACTION
Similarity between e.g. banana - orange = fruit   [ ] train – bicycle   [ ] watch - ruler   ___/2

DELAYED RECALL

Has to recall words WITH NO CUE	FACE [ ]	VELVET [ ]	CHURCH [ ]	DAISY [ ]	RED [ ]	Points for UNCUED recall only	___/5
Optional Category cue							
Multiple choice cue							

ORIENTATION
[ ] Date   [ ] Month   [ ] Year   [ ] Day   [ ] Place   [ ] City   ___/6

© Z.Nasreddine MD   www.mocatest.org   Normal ≥ 26 / 30   TOTAL ___/30
Add 1 point if ≤ 12 yr edu

Administered by: _____

Source

NPLEX
MCCQE
USMLE

Gonzales,
2008

NPLEX
MCCQE
USMLE

NPLEX
MCCQE
USMLE

NPLEX
MCCQE
USMLE

Assessing Cognitive Function in the Elderly

Assessing cognitive function in the elderly is part of assessing mental status. Any impairment in being able to function in the real world is associated with reduced quality of life (of patients and their care givers – remember most live at home) and an increased economic burden. This can ultimately result in the loss of the ability to live independently. Early detection of functional impairments in the elderly should be practiced preventatively to provide early treatment if needed.

Mini-mental Status Exam (MMSE): has a high sensitivity and specificity in evaluating memory loss and cognitive impairment. However, the MMSE cannot itself diagnose dementia or delirium, and results should be considered in the context of hearing, vision problems, physical disabilities, age, educational level, and cultural influences.

Short Test of Mental Status (STMS): more effective than MMSE in differentiating between the cognitively healthy and the cognitively impaired.

Montreal Cognitive Assessment (MoCA): designed as a rapid objective screening instrument for mild cognitive dysfunction. It assesses different cognitive domains: attention and concentration, executive functions, memory, language, visuoconstructional skills, conceptual thinking, calculations, and orientation. Another simple test is the clock drawing task with a simple three-item word recall.

Psychosis

Psychosis in the elderly may manifest as suspiciousness, delusions, and hallucinations. These experiences may predispose an elderly person to aggression, tend to be socially isolating, and are often disabling. Up to 2% to 5% of elderly persons living in the community exhibit some degree of psychosis. Rule out dementia, adverse side effects of drugs, or incompatible drug interactions.

Hepatic Encephalopathy

Hepatic encephalopathy or portal systemic encephalopathy (PSE) should be considered when patients with advanced liver disease exhibit a change in mental status.

Signs and Symptoms: forgetfulness, personality changes, problems becoming aroused or alert or other loss of consciousness, cognition changes, motor function changes and flapping tremors (asterixis). Infection, gastrointestinal bleeding, medications, and increased protein intake are common precipitants of encephalopathy.

Diagnosis: can be elucidated during physical examination by checking for fetor hepaticus and asterixis, and evaluating mental status. Diagnoses confirmation via liver function tests.

Renal Encephalopathy

Also called uremic encephalopathy. Consider this in patients with renal disease, especially kidney failure, who have alterations of consciousness and cognition. When seen with kidney failure it is manifested when creatinine clearance (CrCl) levels fall and remain below 15 mL/min.

Signs and Symptoms: vary from mild (lassitude, fatigue) to severe (seizures, coma). Severity and progression depend on the rate of decline in renal function; thus, symptoms are usually worse in patients with acute renal failure.

PHYSICAL FUNCTION

Syncope

Sycope is the most common cause of 'passing out', defined as a sudden, transient loss of consciousness and postural tone from transient and sudden reduction of blood flow to the brain. The common pathophysiologic mechanism responsible for most syncopal spells is a transient reduction in cerebral blood flow and hypoperfusion.

Causes:
- Vasovagal syncope (a.k.a. neurocardiogenic) is the most common neural type, especially in the young and usually follows situations of emotional stress, but can also occur in geriatric patients.
- Carotid sinus syndrome
- Orthostatic hypotension
- Cardiac syncope
- Cerebrovascular syncope
- Psychiatric syncope
- Post prandial syncope
- Drugs

Assessment: Work-up includes history and physical (especially any cardiac hx), orthostatic BP, ECG, R/O and cardiac cause. Treatment will depend on cause, but will need to reduce risk factors, evaluate for incompatible drug interactions, treat underlying illness, and assess for the risk of falls and comorbidity.

Vertigo

Vertigo is usually due to a disturbance in the vestibular system that provides conscious awareness of head position and movement. When the dysfunction is primarily in the vestibular system, the problem can involve either its end organ (labyrinth), nerve, or central connections. The vertigo is associated with jerk nystagmus and is frequently accompanied by nausea, postural unsteadiness, and gait ataxia. Since vertigo increases with rapid head movements, patients tend to hold their heads still.

Common Causes:
- Benign paroxysmal positional vertigo
- Acute vestibular neuronitis or labyrinthitis
- Ménière's disease
- Migraine
- Anxiety disorders

Treatment will depends on the etiology; however, benign paroxysmal positional vertigo is a common cause and has several treatment recommendations.

Source

NPLEX
MCCQE
USMLE

Benign Paroxysmal Positional Vertigo (BPV)

Benign paroxysmal positional vertigo (BPV) is the most common cause of relapsing vertigo. It affects people increasingly as they age and can severely affect balance in the elderly, leading to potentially injurious falls. It appears as short episodes of vertigo with certain head positions usually accompanied by nausea and nystagmus.

Diagnosis: based on characteristic symptoms, on nystagmus as determined by the Dix-Hallpike maneuver (used to diagnose benign paroxysmal positional vertigo).

Treatment: canalith repositioning procedure (Epley maneuver or a Modified Epley maneuver). Often, the adverse effects of drugs worsen dysequilibrium.

NPLEX
MCCQE
USMLE

Osteopenea and Osteoprosis

Osteopenia: the condition of decreased bone density and bone mass due to inadequate synthesis.

Osteoporosis: the condition of decreased bone mass (density or volume), cortical thickness, and number and size of cancellous trabeculae and defined by a T score 2.5 SD below the mean peak value of young adults.

Risk Factors: lower body weight (<70 kg) is the single best predictor of low bone mineral density, and no current use of estrogen therapy is incorporated with age in the 3-item Osteoporosis Risk Assessment Instrument (ORAI).

Screening: bone density measured at the femoral neck by Dual Energy X-ray Absorptiometry (DEXA). This is the best predictor of hip fracture.

Treatment: weight bearing exercises for fall prevention, calcium, vitamin D, bisphosphonates, and hormone replacement where indicated.

CARDIOLOGY

Hypertension

All elderly people should be screened for hypertension at every healthcare visit and at least annually. For most elderly patients, hypertension does not have a reversible cause and is asymptomatic. Isolated systolic hypertension, a common form of hypertension in the elderly, is defined as systolic BP >= 140 mm Hg and diastolic BP < 90 mm Hg.

CHF

Heart failure is common among persons over 65 years, and is very common among hospitalized patients.

Signs and Symptoms:
- Dyspnea
- Fatigue (particularly with exertion)
- Orthopnea
- Dependent edema
- Jugular venous distention
- Hepatojugular reflux

Elderly patients may also have other symptoms, such as somnolence, confusion, disorientation, weakness, fatigue, failure to thrive. On auscultation course, wet inspiratory rales can be heard, particularly in the lower lung fields.

Diagnosis: based on clinical findings. In elderly persons, a fourth heart sound (S_4 gallop), particularly if soft, does not necessarily indicate clinically significant heart disease. Confirm your suspicion via echocardiography.

**See Cardiology and Neurology section for more information on management.

DIABETES

Increased Risk:

- The elderly are at a higher risk for diabetic complications because of their long-term exposure to elevated glucose levels and the high prevalence of the comorbidities of hypertension and dyslipidemia.
- In patients over 65, risk factors are similar to the rest of the population: obesity; sedentary lifestyle; family history of DM; history of impaired glucose regulation; gestational DM or delivery of a baby > 4.1 kg; history of hypertension or dyslipidemia; polycystic ovary syndrome; and black, Hispanic, or American Indian ethnicity.

Hyperglycemia:

- In the elderly, hyperglycemia may manifest subtly as urinary incontinence, lethargy or fatigue, depression, cognitive impairment (including dementia), falls, chronic pain, or unexplained weight loss.
- Many elderly patients with type 2 DM are not obese; in these patients, insulin secretion is severely impaired and peripheral insulin resistance is mild or nonexistent.
- Drugs can cause or exacerbate hyperglycemia in the elderly; corticosteroids, β-blockers, some fluoroquinolone antibiotics (which may also cause hypoglycemia), 2nd-generation antipsychotics, high doses of thiazide diuretics, and therapeutic doses of niacin.

Screening:

Patients over 60 years old should be screened regardless of whether additional risk factors are present. Fasting blood glucose should be measured at least once every 3 years if levels are normal and at least annually if levels are elevated, indicating impaired glucose regulation. Most elderly patients can be treated as aggressively as younger patients, but some require modifications based on their life expectancy, functional status, cognitive abilities, preferences, and other presenting constraints.

** See Gastroenterology section for more information about managing DM.

GI SYSTEM

Heartburn

NPLEX
MCCQE
USMLE

Gastroesophageal reflux disease and esophagitis are thought to be more common in the elderly but true incidence is unclear.

Symptoms: atypical symptoms are rare in the elderly, but constitutional/nonspecific sx are more common and can have more problems long term: vomiting, anorexia, weight loss, and anemia. Because the presentation of GERD in the elderly is different than in younger patients, the condition may be missed.

Assessment:
Endoscopy should be done in all elderly patients who present that are suspected of having GERD. Barium studies/radiograph can be helpful in differentiating hiatal hernia, achalasia, ulcers, strictures and Baretts's esophagus.
Treatment goal is to provide relief of symptoms, to address predisposing issues, prevention of complications (e.g., Barret's metaplasia).

**See Gastrointestinal section for more information about management of GERD.

CANCER

Breast Cancer

NPLEX
MCCQE
USMLE

Increased Risk: Breast cancer risk increases with age, with incidence of disease peaking in the eighth decade of life. More than 25% of breast cancer mortality is from women who are over 80 years old. Most speculate that mammography has a definite benefit in older women, but sensitivity and specificity of mammography reaches its maximum in the ninth decade.

Prostate Cancer

NPLEX
MCCQE
USMLE

Incidence: prostate cancer is common in older patients. Oddly, more men die with prostate cancer than from it, as the course can be protracted and many patients are asymptomatic. The incidence increases with age; approximately 75% of prostate cancer is diagnosed in men over 65 years old.

Symptoms: the most common symptom present is obstructive uropathy, and in advanced cases some symptoms related to distant metastases, such as weight loss, bone pain, or neurologic symptoms may be present.

Source

NPLEX
MCCQE
USMLE

Screening:

- Many cases are diagnosed by screening with digital rectal examination (DRE) and serum prostate-specific antigen (PSA).
- The American Cancer Society and the American Urological Association recommend annual screening with DRE and PSA for men over 50 years with a life expectancy of over 10 years. PSA levels less than 4 ng/mL are considered normal, levels of 4 to 10 ng/mL have a 25% positive predictive value for prostate cancer, and levels over 10 ng/mL have a 67% positive predictive value. Thus, even at high levels, the test is not specific. Plus, other conditions, including prostatitis and a recent prostate biopsy, can elevate PSA levels.
- If an abnormal DRE and/or an elevated PSA are detected, a transrectal ultrasound (TRUS)-guided prostate biopsy is recommended.

Staging: Once diagnosed, prostate cancer is staged using the Gleason system, which assesses the microscopic appearance of the prostate gland as a whole (glandular architecture) more so than the individual cells. The Gleason score is reported as two numbers and their final sum. The first number represents the most prevalent pattern in the biopsy, and the second number represents the second most prevalent pattern. A final sum of 2 to 4 is considered less aggressive; 5 to 7, moderately aggressive; and 8 to 10, most aggressive.

OTHER CONDITIONS

NPLEX
MCCQE
USMLE

Impotence and Lack of Sexual Desire

Lack of sexual desire in the elderly is not normal and should be investigated and managed. Things to consider would be drug side effects (polypharmacy) and depression. Females may see a reduction in both sex and intimacy due to a shorter life expectancy of males in the same age group. The need for intimacy and sexual desire is a normal part of everyone's life and is not determined by age.

Pressure Ulcers in Immobilized Patients

Treatment:
- Indentify patients at risk: incontinence, disability and dysmotility, malnourishment, mental disability
- Decrease pressure, friction and skin folding
- Keep skin clean and dry
- Avoid excessive bed rest
- Change position at least every two hours to relieve pressure.
- Avoid oversedation
- Provide good nutrition and hydration
- Do not massage the area of the ulcer. Massage can damage tissue under the skin.
- Doughnut-shaped or ring-shaped cushions are not recommended. They interfere with blood flow to that area and cause complications.

Sleep Habits

- Older patients, in general, will exhibit increased need and duration of total daily sleep (includes napping through the day).
- There is a decreased time in stages 3 and 4 and less deep quality sleep with more transitions between REM and stages 1 and 2. Encourage going to bed early and scheduled naps during the day.

Examination Board References

NPLEX (II): North American Board of Naturopathic Examiners
Naturopathic Physician Licensing Examination Part II (NPLEx II) Blueprint. Portland, OR: North American Board of Naturopathic Examiners (NABNE), 2010.

USMLE: National Board of Medical Examiners
Brochert A. Crush Step 3. The Ultimate USMLE Step 3 Review. 3rd ed. New York, NY: Saunders, Elsevier, 2008.

MCCQE: Medical Council of Canada
Dugani S, Lam D, eds. 2009. MCCQE Review Notes & Lecture Series. Medical Counsel of Canada Qualification Examination Review Notes. Toronto, ON: McGraw Hill Professional, Canadian edition, 2009.

Related References

Canadian Census 2006 Housing Series: Issue 10—The Housing Conditions of Canada's Seniors. Housing in Canada Online on the CMHC website, at www.cmhc.ca

Cleveland Clinic Website: http://my.clevelandclinic.org/disorders/dementia/hic_types_of_dementia.aspx

Dains J, Baumann L, Scheibel P. Advanced Health Assessment & Clinical Diagnosis in Primary Care. 4th edition. St Louis, MO: Mosby C.V. Co. Ltd.

Fauci AS, Braunwald E, Kasper DL, Hauser SL, Longo DL, Jameson JL, Loscalzo J, eds. Harrison's Principles of Internal Medicine. 17th ed. New York, NY: McGraw-Hill Companies, Inc., 2008.

Ferri FF. Ferri's Clinical Advisor. Philadelphia, PA: Elsevier, 2009.

Gonzales R, Kutner J. Current Practice Guidelines in Primary Care 2009. Toronto, ON: McGraw Hill, 2009.

Pizzorno JE, Murray MT. Textbook of Natural Medicine. 3rd ed. New York, NY: Churchill Livingstone, Elsevier, 2006.

GYNECOLOGY

Contributing authors: Zeynep Uraz, ND, and Alan Vu, ND

PELVIC INFLAMMATORY DISEASE

SEXUALLY TRANSMITTED INFECTIONS

CONTRACEPTION

AMENORRHEA

ADENOMYOSIS

DYSFUNCTIONAL UTERINE BLEEDING

POLYCYSTIC OVARIAN SYNDROME

LEIOMYOMAS

MENOPAUSE

BREAST ISSUES

PELVIC PROLAPSE

PREGNANCY

PELVIC INFLAMMATORY DISEASE (PID)

Source

MCCQE
NPLEX

Gala, 2010
Ferri, 2010
CDC PID
Treatment
Guidelines,
2010

Katz, 2007

Gray, 2007

Presentation

PID refers to inflammatory and/or infectious processes that ascend from the vaginal canal to any or all of the upper genital organs: endometrium (endometritis), fallopian tubes (salpingitis), pelvic peritoneum (peritonitis), and any adjacent organs.

Infertility:
PID is the most common cause of preventable infertility in the United States and Canada. The risk of infertility can range from 8% to 75% depending on the severity and frequency of PIDs. Other PID sequelae include tubal scarring, susceptibility for ectopic pregnancy, development of a tubo-ovarian abscess, sepsis, and chronic pelvic pain.

Signs and Symptoms:
- Symptoms can range from non-existent (silent PID) to extremely severe.
- The most common symptom is pelvic pain.
- The most common presentation is a female aged 13-35 with PID Minimal Criteria = abdominal pain + adnexal tenderness + cervical motion tenderness and at least one of the following: temp > 38C, elevated ESR, elevated CRP, leucocytosis, purulent cervical/vaginal discharge, WBCs on wet mount of vaginal secretions, or laboratory findings consistent with cervical infection with *Chlamydia trachomatis* or *Neisseria gonorrhea*.

Management Plan

- On suspicion of PID, prescribe or refer for empiric antibiotics, test for STIs to confirm suspicion, request blood work (CBC, ESR, beta hCG), midstream urinalysis and microscopy.
- Refer PID presentations to hospital in cases of suspected or confirmed pregnancy, severe pain, vomiting, abdominal guarding or rebound tenderness, or adnexal swelling.

Conventional Antimicrobial Drug Treatment

In outpatient settings, the recommended empirical treatment is combination antimicrobials that cover most of the implicated organisms (e.g., *Chlamydia trachomatis, Neisseria gonorrhea, Gardnerella vaginalis, Escherichia coli, Bacteroides spp*):
- Fluroquinilone ± Nitroimidazole:
  - Levofloxacin 500 mg PO q.d. ± metronidazole 500 mg b.i.d. X 14 days; OR
  - Olofloxacin 400 mg PO q.d. ± metronidazole 500 mg b.i.d. X 14 days; OR
- Cephalosporin + Tetracycline ± Nitroimidazole:
  - Ceftriaxone 250 mg IM single dose + Doxycycline 100 mg PO b.i.d. X 14 days ± metronidazole 500 mg b.i.d. X 14 days; OR

Source

- Cefotaxime 1 g IM single dose + Doxycycline 100 mg PO b.i.d. X 14 days ± metronidazole 500 mg b.i.d. X 14 days.

Reassess in 48-72 hours; if no improvement, refer to hospital. Watch for progression into sepsis or tubo-ovarian abscess (palpable on exam and/or visible on ultrasound). An unruptured abscess may respond to antibiotics alone. A ruptured abscess is an emergent condition and requires prompt surgical laparotomy and excision of affected tube (unilateral disease) or may rarely necessitate bilateral slapingo-oopherectomy in severe bilateral disease.

Abad, 2009
Wiesen-feld, 2003

Probiotics

Naturopathic care for PID is adjunctive and involves the use of oral and/or vaginal probiotics. Evidence suggests that specific strains of *Lactobacillus spp.* (*L. rhamnosus* GR-1, *L. reuteri*, and other peroxide producing lactobacilli) reduce the risk of bacterial vaginosis, maintain acidic environment, and are protective against PID.

NIAID, 2009
Gala, 2010

Patient Education

Crucial for preventing infection and re-infection:
- Avoid intercourse until partner has been successfully treated
- Avoid douching
- Reduce number of sexual partners
- Examine and question partners for STI risk
- Use of barrier contraceptives (when possible)
- Monitor closely for future infertility

SEXUALLY TRANSMITTED INFECTIONS (STIs)

Ferri, 2010

Causative Organism	Findings	First-line Treatment
Chlamydia trachomatis Primary chlamydia	Most common STI, dysuria, dyspareunia, rectal pain, post coital bleeding, clear mucoid discharge, can be asymptomatic in females, positive culture or antibody test	Azithromycin single dose OR Doxycycline X 7 days. Povidone-iodine 1:100 retention douche daily is beneficial. Zinc sulfate (1 tbs 2% solution in 1 pint of water) is an alternative
Chlamydia trachomatis Secondary chlamydia (Lymphogranuloma venerium)	Unilateral inguinal lympha-denopathy; coalescence of affected nodes "bubo" with external fistulae formation that drains purulent or bloody discharge; fever, fatigue, headache,	Azithromycin OR Doxycycline. Incision and drainage of bubos may be necessary.

Causative Organism	Findings	First-line Treatment
	anorexia, nausea, backache; ulcerative proctitis (with anal transmission); may be asymptomatic; serology (rising antibody titer against C. trachomatis L1-3	
Neisseria gonorrhea	Mucopurulent discharge, cervicitis, can be asymptomatic, positive culture, gram negative diplococcic on gram stain	Ceftriaxone single dose OR Cefixime + Azithromycin or Doxycycline for presumed Chlamydia coinfection
Bacterial Vaginosis polymicrobial (*Prevotella sp., Mobiluncus sp., G. vaginalis*, Ureaplasma, Mycoplasma	Thin grey/white malodorous "fishy" discharge, fishy smell on KOH preparation (positive whiff test), clue cells, can be asymptomatic	Metronidazole oral or vaginally OR Clindamycin vaginally + probiotics (*L. rhamnosus* and *Lactobacillus reuteri*). Povidone-iodine 1:100 retention douche daily is beneficial
Trichomonas vaginalis	Foul-smelling "rancid" frothy yellow-green discharge; pruritus, "strawberry cervix," vaginal erythema, dysuria, post coital bleeding, can be asymptomatic, motile flagellated organisms and WBC seen under microscope	Metronidazole OR Tinidazole single oral dose.
Candida albicans	Thick white "Cottage cheese" discharge; vaginal erythema, dysuria, dyspareunia, KOH test will show pseudohyphae, common in uncontrolled diabetes patients, post antibiotic therapy, and during pregnancy.	Topical derivatives better than nystatin e.g., clotrimazole, miconazole. Single dose and 1-3 regiments effective in uncomplicated cases.
Herpes simplex virus (HSV 1 or HSV 2)	Multiple, shallow, grouped vesicles on erythematous base; painful ulcers; recurrence and resolution; dysuria possible; prodrome of malaise, fever, and regional lymphadenopathy.	Early treatment on suspicion with Acyclovir, valacyclovir, and famciclovir decreases the possibility of ongoing transmission. Treatment does not eradicate virus but helps symptomatically.

Causative Organism	Findings	First-line Treatment
Treponema pallidum Primary syphilis	Localized painless ulcer with indurated base chancre. No discharge or pain; spirochetes seen on dark-field microscopy; RPR, VDRL or treponemal tests can be used to confirm	Penicillin G
Treponema pallidum Secondary syphilis	Condyloma lata, macupapular rash on palms and soles; generalized lymphadenopathy, serology is positive, RPR, VDRL or treponemal tests can be used to confirm	Penicillin G
Haemophilus ducreyi Chancroid	Localized PAINFULL ulcer with soft base "soft chancre"; looks like syphilitic ulcer but painful; gram stain shows characteristic appearance of organisms "school of fish."	Azithromycin OR Ceftriaxone
Human papillomavirus HPV	Venereal warts, koilocytosis on pap smear	Many treatment exist for warts (acid, cryotherapy, laser, podophyllin)
Molluscum contagiosum	Multiple 1-5mm flesh-colored, dome-shaped, dimpled centre, pearly lesions; intracellular inclusions under microscope	Many (curettage, cryotherapy, laser, coagulation)
Pediculosis pubis Crabs	Lice "crabs" or Nits "eggs" visible on pubic hair, itching, small blue spots on skin where bitten, skin irritated and erythematous	Topical agents permethrin or pyrethrins with piperonyl butoxide. Lindane is a second line treatment due to concerns of toxicity. Bedding and linens should be laundered thoroughly.
Sarcoptes scabei Scabes	Intense pruritus especially at night, external genitalia erythema; microscopy of skin scrapings may identify the mite	Permethrin cream OR oral Ivermectin. Pruritis takes up to 2 weeks to resolve after successful treatment. Bedding and linens should be laundered thoroughly.

CONTRACEPTION

Source

NPLEX
USMLE

Kliegman,
2011
Gray, 2007
Canadian
Contracep-
tion
Guidelines,
2004

Efficacy

When educating patients about efficacy of a contraceptive method, it is important to consider two types of efficacy. Efficacy rates determined by clinical trials are considered "perfect use efficacy rates" and are measured as the percentage of women who do not conceive in the first year of use. "Typical use efficacy rates" correspond to the observed percentage of women in the general population who do not conceive in the first year when using the method of contraception. The methods that involve the least amount of patient involvement often have the highest typical use efficacy rates.

Method	Efficacy	Contraindications (CI) vs Cautions (CA)	Side Effects vs Advantages
Intrauterine Devices(IUD) Copper-T IUD, Nova-T, Flexi-T	Typical 95% Perfect 95%	CI: Pregnancy, undiagnosed vaginal bleeding, stenosed cervix, current PID or STI, cervical or endometrial cancer uterine anomaly, copper allergy. CA: Risk for PID and tubal infection is too high for nullipara; condoms needed for STI protection.	SE: spotting in first 3 months; uterine perforation on insertion (rare); endometrial embedding. Salpingitis, menorrhagia, pain, infection, ectopic pregnancy. ADV: Can remain in place for 10 years; Rapidly reversible action; no contraceptive routine required; hormone free. Decreases risk for endometrial and cervical cancer.
Progestin-only Intrauterine System (IUS) Levonogestral 20 ug q.d. day; Mirena	Typical 99.8% Perfect 99.8%	CI: Pregnancy, undiagnosed vaginal bleeding, stenosed cervix, current PID or STI, cervical or endometrial cancer, uterine anomaly + postpartum endometriosis, acute liver disease, hematological malignancies. CA: Condoms needed for STI protection; inserted within 7 days of onset of menses to be effective immediately.	SE: Spotting for first 3 mo; uterine perforation on insertion(rare); menstrual changes (eg., reduced flow, amenorrhea; uncomfortable/painful insertion. ADV: Can remain in place for 5 years; Rapidly reversible action; No contraceptive routine required; may reduce dysmenorrhea & endometriosis.

Method	Efficacy	Contraindications (CI) vs Cautions (CA)	Side Effects vs Advantages
Progestin-only Injectable Contraceptive Depot-Medroxy-progesterone Acetate (DMPA)	Typical 97% Perfect 99.7%	CI: Pregnancy, undiagnosed vaginal bleeding, current breast cancer, known hyper sensitivity + Severe cirrhosis, acute viral hepatitis, liver tumors CA: Condoms needed for STI protection; consider other option for women with risk factors for osteoporosis; injected within first 5 days of onset of menses.	SE: Breast tenderness, insomnia or somnolence, fatigue, mood changes (e.g., depression, irritability), weight gain, menstrual irregularities, decreased bone density, slow reversibility of action (up to 10 months) low libido, skin sensitivity reactions, hyperprexia acne. Adv: each injection is effective for 3 months; good for women who should avoid high estrogen doses, such as migraine sufferers.
Progestin-Only oral "Mini-pill" Norethindrone, Micronor	Typical 92% Perfect 99.7%	CI: Pregnancy, current breast cancer, known hyper sensitivity + acute viral hepatitis, liver tumors. CA: Condoms needed for STI protection; consider other option for women with risk factors for osteoporosis; injected within first 5 days of onset of menses.	SE: Higher incidence of ectopic pregnancy compared to COCs. Irregular bleeding in 12% of users in first mo, 3% in 18 mo. Adv: Preferred contraception in lactating women; recommended for women with contraindication to estrogen contraception.
Combined Estrogen + Progestin Oral Contraceptives (COCs) Ovral, Brevicon, Ortho, Select, Diane, Cyclen, Loestrin, Marvelon, Othro-Cept, Demulen, Minestrin, Alesse, Linessa, Synphasic, Tri-Cyclin,	Typical 92% Perfect 99.9%	Absolute CI: history of MI, CAD, Stroke, TIA, valvular heart disease, ischemic heart disease, history of venous thromboembolism, sever cirrhosis, liver tumour, breast cancer, migraines with aura, <6wk post partum, >35 yr old smoker (>15 cig per day), hypertension ≥160/100mmHg; known coagulation deficiency. Relative CI: Diabetes, estrogen hypersensitivity, gallbladder disease, obesity, high BMI/weight.	Major SE: Thromboembolism rare), stroke, retinal artery (thrombosis, myocardial infarction, benign liver tumour, cholelithiasis, hypertension. Common SE: breakthrough bleeding, amenorrhea, nausea/vomiting, bloating chloasma, breast tenderness, mood changes (e.g., depression), headaches. ADV: Method of choice for most young couples, especially for teens, if combined with

Method	Efficacy	Contraindications (CI) vs Cautions (CA)	Side Effects vs Advantages
Triophasil, Triquiar		CA: Condoms needed for STI protection; daily tablet (have to remember); patients with diarrhea or spotting at higher risk of COC failure; monitor INR in patients on oral anticoagulants	condoms. Lower dose estrogen has increased safety and decreased side effects.
Transdermal Contraceptive Patch Evra	Typical 99.1% Perfect 99.3%	CI: Same as COCs CA: condoms needed for STI protection, patch applied on first day of withdrawal bleeding once per week for 3 weeks, followed by a patch free week. 1 wk	Major SE: Same as COCs. Common SE: Breast discomfort in 19% of users in first 2 mo, headache 22%, skin reaction under patch 20%, nausea 20%, dysmenorrheal. Adv: No daily contraceptive routine (only weekly); helps regulate menses, decreases menstrual flow; decreases dysmenorrheal; eliminates mittleschmerz; can decrease PMS, hirsutism, no interference with intercourse.
Vaginal Contraceptive Ring NuvaRing	Typical 98.8% Perfect 99.3%	Absolute CI: Same as COCs Relative CI: uterovaginal prolapse, vaginal stenosis. CA: Condoms needed for STI protection, ring is self-inserted in vagina for 3 weeks then removed for 1 week; effect starts in 3 days; Concurrent use of vaginal tampons not recommended; can be expelled, can be expelled during severe straining.	Major SE: Same as COCs Common SE: vaginal discomfort, vaginitis (5%), headache (5%), leukorrhea, decreased libido, nausea breast tenderness. Adv: No daily contraceptive routine (only every 3 weeks).
Diaphragm Ortho Diaphragm	Typical 80% Perfect 94%	CI: Inability to achieve proper fit, marked uterine prolapse, large cystocele or rectocele, vaginal anomaly, recurrent UTI	SE: Hypersensitivity to latex and or spermicide. Infection if not used or cleaned properly, toxic shock syndrome, urinary

Method	Efficacy	Contraindications (CI) vs Cautions (CA)	Side Effects vs Advantages
Coil, Wide Seal		CA: Condoms needed for STI protection; Inserted up to 6 hours prior to intercourse; used with spermicide to increase efficacy.	tract infection. Adv: Suited to infrequent intercourse, can be used in breastfeeding women; silicone diaphragms available for women with latex allergy.
Sponge Protectaid, Sponge, Today	Typical 71% Perfect 82%	CI: Inability to achieve proper fit, recurrent UTIs CA: Condoms needed for STI protection; Inserted prior to intercourse; used with spermicide to increase efficacy; not to be used during menstruation; 20% better efficacy in nulliparous women.	SE: May enhance HIV transmission by damaging vagina mucosa; toxic shock syndrome (rare). Adv: suited to infrequent intercourse, can be used in breastfeeding women.
Cervical Cap	Typical 60% Perfect 76%	CI: Cervical deformity, inability to obtain suitable fit, current PID or STI, cervical or endometrial cancer, dysplasia, recurrent vaginal urinary or cervical infections. Abnormal cervical cytology, chronic cervicitis, recurrent salpingitis. CA: Condoms needed for STI protection; not to be used within 6 wks of delivery; used with spermicide to increase efficacy; 20% better efficacy in nulliparous women; must be inserted prior to intercourse.	SE: Vaginal discharge, vaginal odour, cervical or fornices ulceration, hypersensitivity, infection if not used or cleaned properly, vaginitis, toxic shock syndrome (rare). Adv: Suited to infrequent intercourse, can be left in place for up to 48 hrs; can be used in breastfeeding women.
Male Condom	Typical 86% Perfect 97%	CI: hypersensitivity to latex, polyurethane, or lanoline. CA: may use with separately provided vaginal spermicide to increase efficacy, use water based lubricants as latex condoms degraded by oil based products.	SE: Hypersensitivity to latex in either partner. Adv: Protects against STIs including HIV; best suited for infrequent intercourse.

Method	Efficacy	Contraindications (CI) vs Cautions (CA)	Side Effects vs Advantages
Female Condom	Typical 80% Perfect 95%	CI: Hypersensitivity to polyurethane, vaginal anatomical abnormalities that make fitting difficult. CA: Not to be used with male condoms (higher risk of displacement); inserted up to 8 hr prior to intercourse and removed immediately.	SE: Discomfort. Adv: Suited for women who find spermicide irritating or who dislike messiness of other vaginal barrier methods.
Sterilization, Tuba Ligation	Typical 99.5%	CI: Pregnancy, conditions that can aggravated by general anesthesia, pelvic infection. CA: Reversible only if salpingectomy not performed and sufficient length of undamaged tubal remnants remain.	SE: 0.7% ectopic pregnancy likelihood. Adv: Method of choice for couples with completed family.
Sterilization, Vasectomy	Typical 97.8%	CI: Infectious diseases, local infection, sexual dysfunction, local genital abnormalities (e.g., hernias). CA: Reversible if <10 yr since procedure.	SE: Local pain, scrotal ecchymosis, swelling. Adv: Method of choice for couples with completed family.
Spermicides Vaginal Contraceptive Film, others	Typical 74% Perfect 94%	CI: Hypersensitivity CA: Less effective if used alone. Not effective against HIV or STI; increase risk of genital leasions resulting in increased risk of HIV transmission.	SE: Hypersensitivity Adv: Used to enhance efficacy of condoms, diaphragms and cervical caps.
Sympto-thermal Control; Calendar Method; Fertility Awareness Method (FAM)	Typical 80% Perfect 91%	CI: Irregular cycle CA: High pregnancy rates; use when pregnancy is an acceptable outcome; Requires high motivation and discipline; depends on identification of mucus and	SE: None Adv: Readily available, inexpensive, no pharmacological agent or local irritant.

Method	Efficacy	Contraindications (CI) vs Cautions (CA)	Side Effects vs Advantages
		basal body temperature to identify fertile time; intercourse is avoided on fertile days.	
Coitus interruptus	Typical 73% Perfect 96%	CI: None CA: High pregnancy rates; use when pregnancy is an acceptable outcome; Requires high motivation and discipline of both partners; if doubt occurs as to whether withdrawal was effective, emergency contraception should be considered.	SE: None Adv: Readily available; inexpensive, no pharmacological agent or local irritant.

AMENORRHEA

Source

Brotchert,
2008

Presentation & Assessment

Primary Amenorrhea:
Any female who has not menstruated by age 16 has primary amenorrhea. In practice, to evaluate a primary amenorrhea presentation:
- Order a pregnancy test (pregnancy can cause primary amenorrhea)
- If negative, conduct a physical exam to screen for abnormalities, such as absent uterus or turner syndrome
- If unproductive, request or prescribe progesterone
- If menses occurs within 2 weeks, conclude that estrogen and an intact uterus are present
- If bleeding does not occur, conclude that estrogen is not present or that the patient has an anatomic abnormality

Remember that a phenotypic female with normal breast development, with no axillary or pubic hair, with primary amenorrhea and no induced menses after progesterone administration, is very likely a case of androgen insensitivity syndrome in a genotypical male.

Secondary Amenorrhea:
By contrast, any previously menstruating female whose menses ceases has secondary amenorrhea.
- Order a pregnancy test (all secondary amenorrhea patients are assumed pregnant until proven otherwise)
- If negative obtain a history and conduct a physical exam:
  - If unproductive, request or prescribe progesterone
  - If menses occurs within 2 weeks , conclude she has sufficient estrogen, then
    - Check luteinizing hormone (LH) level
      - If LH is high, patient has polycystic ovarian syndrome. Treat accordingly.
      - If LH is low or normal patient has pituitary adenoma, hypothyroidism or low gonadotropin levels (drugs, stress, exercise, anorexia nervosa. Check serum prolactin, TSH, and refer to gynecologist and/or endocrinologist
  - If menses does not occur with 2 weeks, conclude that she does not have sufficient estrogen, then
    - Check follicle stimulating hormone (FSH)
      - If FSH is high, patient has premature ovarian failure or menopause. Screen for undiagnosed causes such as autoimmune disorders, history of chemotherapy, genetic disorders. Refer to gynecologist and/or endocrinologist.
      - IF FSH is low or normal, the patient may have a neoplasm affecting the hypothalamus. Refer for a brain MRI and an endocrinology consult.

Source

NPLEX
MCCQE
USMLE

Katz, 2007

Fritz, 2011

Fritz, 2011

ENDOMETRIOSIS

Presentation

Endometriosis is ectopic endometrial tissue (glandular and stromal tissue) outside the uterus.
- Endometriosis is the most likely cause of infertility in menstruating women over the age of 30.
- Patients with endometriosis are usually nulliparous, over the age of 30 with new onset or worsening dysmenorrhea + dyspareunia + dyschezia (painful defecation) and/or perimenstrual spotting.

Assessment

On physical examination watch for common signs of tender adnexae in a patient without PID (this is a clue), nodularities of the uterosacral ligaments and a retroverted uterus.
- On suspicion request laparoscopy, which is diagnostic upon visualization of raised flat brown ``powder-burns,`` blood filled ``chocolate cysts," or raised blue ``mulberry spots.``

Management Plan

Appropriate management of endometriosis depends on the severity of symptoms, the desire for fertility, and the risk of gastrointestinal or urinary tract obstruction. Conventional options are listed in order of recommendation:

First-line Treatment
- Try for 3 months before consideration of other therapies:
- NSAIDS +
- Low dose oral contraceptives (COCs) cyclical or more commonly continuous use of low-dose monophasic COCs relieve symptoms in 75 to 100% of cases, reduce menses, suppress ovulation, and delay recurrence of disease.
- Progestin-only contraceptives suppress GnRH secretion, inhibit ovulation, induce hpoestrogenic hormonal environment
- Medroxyprogestrone acetate (MPA) depot injection significantly reduces pain and induces amenorrhea. Not to be used with younger females who wish to become pregnant after treatment.
- Levonogestril (LNG) intrauterine system (IUS) provides an effective management option for mild to moderate symptomatic endometriosis for up to 3 years. See above for details on LNG IUS.

Second-line Treatment
- Danazol an androgen derivative, inhibits the production of LH. The overall effect of danazol is a high-androgen, low-estrogen anovulatory state that inhibits the growth of endometriosis. Common side effects include weight gain, fluid retention, hirsutism, acne, fatigue, decrease breast size, atrophic vaginitis, emotional lability and hot flushes.
- GnRH analogues (nafarelin, goserelin, leuprolide) suppress the production of FSH and LH. Treatment usually yields pain relief and involution of implants. Side effects include hot flushes, vaginal dryness, decreased libido, depression, changes in skin texture, bone mineral depletion (up to 1% annually), headache, irritability and fatigue.

- Conservative surgery
  - Laparoscopy or laparotomy excision of implants and adhesions is the most minimally invasive approach. Used in endometriosis-associated infertility; and
  - Uterosacral nerve ablation (LUNA) is considered as adjunct to relieve endometriosis-associated pelvic pain
  - Presacral neurectomy (PSN) is another adjunct to conservative surgery considered for relieving severe midline dysmenorrhea associated with endometriosis
- Hysterectomy is considered in cases of intractable pain that has not responded to more conservative measures.
- Hysterectomy plus salpingo-oophorectomy is considered for treatment-resistant endometriosis-associated pelvic pain or adnexal masses in women with extensive extra-uterine disease.

Source

Grodstein, 1993
Brune–Tran, 2010
Ziaei, 2005

Infertility

One of the most clinically relevant long-term outcomes of endometriosis is its association with infertility. It is estimated that 20% to 40% of infertile women have endometriosis. Treatment of infertility related to endometriosis involves various methods of assisted reproductive technology (ART) including insemination with washed sperm in combination with clomiphene citrate or exogenous gonadotropins, in-vitro fertilization (IVF), and laparoscopic removal of lesions. Pregnancy rates are highest in the one year following surgical removal of endometrial lesions (see infertility section for more details).

NPLEX

Guidelines for First-line Naturopathic Treatment of Endometriosis

Approach: Depends on symptoms and patient goals. If the preservation of fertility is a priority, discussing early child-bearing is worthwhile. Because there is some evidence suggesting a correlation between the exposure of dioxin-like polychlorinated biphenyls (PCBs) and endometriosis, advise parents to avoid early-life exposure of female children
Counsel all patients on benefit of reduced exposure at any age.

Dietary measures
- Education regarding diet and lifestyle factors are relevant in endometriosis.
- Because there is some evidence that indicates that that consumption of caffeine is related to endometriosis in a dose dependent fashion, patient's should be advised to keep consumption below 5 g of caffeine per month.

Clinical nutrition
- Some research supports the use of 200-500 IU of vitamin E to alleviate the pain of primary dysmenorrhea. Depending on the mechanism of action, this may also be useful and relevant in the treatment of dysmenorrhea secondary to endometriosis.

Source

NPLEX
MCCQE
USMLE

Katz, 2007

ADENOMYOSOSIS

Presentation

Adenomyosis is ectopic endometrial (glandular and stromal tissue) in muscular layers of the uterus. This proliferation of ectopic tissue within the myometrium causes a diffuse or focal enlargement of the uterus. Patients with adenomyosis are usually over the age of 40 with secondary dysmenorrhea + new onset or worsening menorrhagia.

Assessment

- Physical examination may reveal a symmetrically enlarged and boggy uterus in diffuse adeno-myosis, or an area of focal enlargement in focal adenomyosis.
- Clinically, it is difficult to distinguish this condition from leiomyoma on physical exam. Notwith-standing, refer for dilation and curettage to rule out endometrial cancer. Confirm suspicion with ultrasonography (83% sensitivity, 85% specificity) or MRI (more sensitive and specific than US).
- Often a definitive diagnosis of adenomyosis is only made with histological examination of uterine tissue after hysterectomy.

Management Plan

There is no current medical cure for adenomyosis. NSAIDs and hormonal contraceptives are recommended to reduce endometrial proliferation and blood loss. GnRH agonists and levonogestrel intrauterine systems (LGN-IUS) show promising symptoms relief in women with menorrhagia associated to adenomyosis. With severe and life threatening menorrhagia presentations, hysterectomy remains the recommended management option.

DYSFUNCTIONAL UTERINE BLEEDING (DUB)

Brotchert, 2008

Presentation

Uterine bleeding that is not associated with menstruation, pregnancy, inflammation or tumor is termed dysfunctional uterine bleeding (DUB). This is diagnosis of exclusion and is the most common cause of abnormal uterine bleeding. 70% of cases are associated with unopposed estrogen leading to annovulatory cycles. DUB is common and considered physiologic during the few months immediately following menarche and those preceeding menopause. The most common pathologic cause of DUB is polycystic ovary syndrome (PCOS).

Assessment

In women over 35, always refer DUB presentations for dilation and curettage to rule out endometrial cancer. Order a complete blood count to asses for anemia (secondary to excessive blood loss). Rule out PCOS first then move on to uncommon causes (infections, endocrine, coagulation defects, and estrogen producing tumors.

Management Plan

If you find the cause, treat it, otherwise manage bleeding as follows:
- NSAIDs are considered first line management option for DUB; and
- COCs are also considered first line management option for menorrhagia and DUB; or
- Progesterone which is used in cases of severe bleeding

POLYCYSTIC OVARIAN SYNDROME (PCOS)

Presentation

Polycystic ovarian syndrome is the most common endocrine disorder in reproductive age women (7% prevalence) and the most likely cause of infertility in women under 30. The classic presentation is a patient who is overweight, hirsut, and amenorrheic.
- The primary pathology is LH:FSH ratio greater than 2:1, insulin resistance, androgen excess and unopposed estrogen, which increases risk for endometrial hyperplasia and carcinoma.
- PCOS also predisposes women to abdominal obesity, type II Diabetes, dyslipidemia, and hypertension. Early recognition and appropriate management can thus significantly improve mortality and morbidity.

Assessment

- The most common chief concerns associated with a diagnosis of PCOS are hirsutism (90%) + menstrual irregularity with anovulation (90%) + infertility (75%).
- Confirm your suspicion by requesting serum LH, FSH, DHEAS, Prolactin, TSH, 17-hydroxyprogesterone and an ovarian ultrasound (multiple ovarian cysts visualized).
- Rule out hyperprolactinemia, hypothyroidism and 21-hydroxylase deficiency, which may mimic or compound presentation.

Management Plan

- The first-line treatment for PCOS is nutrition and exercise. At least 50% of women with PCOS are obese and even a small reduction in weight (2% to 5% of overall body weight) can result in improved menstrual regularity and metabolic function.
- Recommended conventional treatment are birth control pills, cyclic progesterone, or androgen receptor antagonists (spironolactone or flutamide). If the patient desires pregnancy, refer to a

Source

Nestler,
2009

NPLEX

Marsh,
2009
Fulghesu,
2002
Thys–
Jacobs,
1999
Rashidi,
2009

reproductive endocrinologist or gynecologist for a trial clomiphene citrate therapy (induces ovulation).

- Metformin can also be used in combination with clomiphene citrate as an insulin sensitizing agent to improve ovulation rates in some women.
- The last resort is ovarian drilling, a surgical procedure that destroys some of the follicles of the ovary, and ultimately decreases androgen production, and ideally leads to regular ovulation.

Guidelines for First-line Naturopathic Treatment of PCOS

Approach: Early identification of illness (at menarche) may be the most important role a naturopathic physician can play. It provides an opportunity for education regarding potential possible outcomes of PCOS, such as metabolic syndrome and infertility. This may motivate patients to make healthy lifestyle choices early on to circumvent undesirable PCOS sequelae. Educate patients about risk of associated illnesses and available approaches to mitigate those risks, including lifestyle modification and weight loss.

Dietary measures
Dietary therapy should focus on a low glycemic index/load diet, with the ultimate goal of decreasing abdominal obesity and overall BMI (to 20-24).

Clinical nutrition
- There is some promising research showing that 1200 mg of D-chiro-inositol, administered for 6-8 weeks in obese women with PCOS significantly increases the action of insulin, and thus improves ovulatory function and decreased serum androgens, blood pressure, and plasma triglyceride concentrations (3).
- N-acetyl-cysteine (NAC) has also been shown to improve insulin sensitivity and ovulatory function in women with PCOS in some studies .
- Some preliminary research has also shown that supplementation with calcium and vitamin D can improve ovulatory outcomes in women with PCOS. The research is preliminary, but appears to be most relevant in obese women with PCOS .

LEIOMYOMAS

Source

Presentation

Fritz, 2011
Katz, 2007
Brutchert,
2008

Leiomyomas (fibroids) are benign uterine tumors that arise from the smooth muscle cells of the myometrium. More than 45% of women have uterine fibroids by the fifth decade of life. The incidence of fibroids increases with age and varies by population studied, but prevalence can be as high as 80% in older women of African decent.

- Large and symptomatic uterine leiomyomas are the most common indication for hysterectomy and account for one third of all hysterectomies.
- Malignant transformation is very rare <1% and some experts believe it does not occur.
- It is difficult to recognize fibroids in practice, as most do not cause any symptoms. About a third of women with leiomyomas will become symptomatic.
- Common presentation is menorrhagia, metrorrhagia, and pelvic pain, heaviness or pressure.
- Other indicators may include a palpable firm pelvic mass, bloating, and symptoms associated with physical compression of adjacent structures (e.g., constipation, urinary frequency and urgency).
- Watch for rapid growth during pregnancy or use of estrogen (e.g., birth control pills) or regression after menopause.
- Fibroids are a very uncommon cause of infertility, and are a culprit only when they are mechanically obstructing sperm transport to the ovum, or implantation due to location and size.

Fritz, 2011

Assessment

Pizzorno,
2009

- Request pelvic or transvaginal ultrasound to confirm your diagnostic suspicion.
- Refer all women over 40 with menorrhagia or metrorrhagia for dilation and curettage to rule out endometrial cancer.

Management Plan

NPLEX
MCCQE
USMLE

There are several options for treatment of uterine fibroids:
- Medical treatment consists of progestin-only contraceptives, and monitoring growth with ultrasound.
- Adjunctive hormonal treatment with GnRH agonists as a way to block the ovarian production of steroid hormones is also an option. Although this is often an effective therapy for decreasing the size of fibroids, the side effects can be severe (decreased bone mass, vasomotor symptoms, headache, mood changes, vaginal dryness, joint pain and depression).
- Surgical management can range from uterine artery embolization (blocking of the arteries that supply fibroids), myomectomy (removal of the fibroid), and hysterectomy.
- Naturopathic treatment of uterine fibroids usually aims to manage the symptoms caused by fibroids (e.g., menorrhagia and iron deficiency anemia) until a woman reaches menopause and fibroids subsequently shrink.

MENOPAUSE

Source

NPLEX
MCCQE
USMLE

Katz, 2007

Gray, 2007

Hillman,
2004

Presentation

Physiologic menopause is defined as cessation of menstruation for 12 months or more between the ages of 45 to 55, with the average age being 51.
- Natural (physiologic) menopause occurs as a result of genetically programed ovarian failure.
- Menopause may also be medically or surgically induced or may occur prematurely (known as premature ovarian failure).
- There is a gradual hormonal shift that occurs in menopause, which usually begins 5 to 7 years before the permanent cessation of ovarian function. During this period, there is a gradual increase and then decrease in estrogen production by the ovaries, and a decrease in progesterone caused by occasional anovulatory cycles.

Signs and Symptoms:
The most common symptoms of menopause are vasomotor symptoms (hot flushes) and vaginal atrophy. Other symptoms include:
- Irregular menstrual cycles
- Psychological changes (anxiety, depression, insomnia, difficulty concentrating, nervousness, irritability)
- Decrease in libido
- Urinary incontinence and atrophy of urinary tract epithelium
- Fatigue
- Dry, thinning skin
- Weight gain
- Osteoporosis
- Increase risk cardiovascular disease (unknown if directly related to menopause)
- Increase risk of breast cancer and colon cancer

Assessment

Diagnosis can be made when the clinical history is highly suggestive of menopause. If there is any doubt that symptoms may be a result of another underlying condition, it would be prudent to rule out other causes.
- FSH and estrogen confirm diagnosis of menopause (i.e., FSH will be significantly elevated and estrogen will be significantly depressed). TSH and prolactin may be relevant to order if other causes of amenorrhea are suspected.

Other tests to consider involve those that are relevant to long- term prevention:
- Mammography: Yearly to rule out breast cancer in all post-menopausal women
- Cholesterol panel : Screening at regular intervals according to guidelines for long-term risk of cardiovascular disease
- Bone density studies: Screening at regular intervals according to guidelines to rule out decreasing bone density
- Transvaginal sonography: If bleeding occurs in a post-menopausal woman (after complete cessation of menses for >1 year). To assess for endometrial hyperplasia and potential risk of carcinoma.

Source

NPLEX
MCCQE
USMLE

Sood, 2011

Carmi-
gnani,
2010
Jerri, 2002
Stahl, 1987
Wuttke,
2003

NPLEX

Management Plan

Management of menopause with hormone replacement therapy has been controversial in recent years. Prior to publication of the findings of Women's Health Initiative Study in 2002 (and the early termination of the study), hormone therapy (HT) was widely prescribed. When the results of the study began to emerge, it showed that women on HT had an increased cardiovascular disease risk and were at a greater risk for breast cancer. These results significantly reduced the number of women who opted for HT during their transition into menopause. As more data continue to emerge, the pendulum is swinging back as evidence indicates that women who exhibit vasomotor symptoms or urogenital atrophy, and those who start HT during their transition into menopause (2 to 3 years after menopause), also exhibit a cardioprotective effect from HT. The North American Menopause Society (NAMS 2010) issued a position statement that stipulates that although there is an increased risk of venous thromboembolism with the use of HT in any population, the magnitude of risk is low. They further published guidelines for the use of HT in menopause, as follows:

- Unopposed systemic estrogen therapy (ET) increases the risk of endometrial cancer, and is not recommended without adequate progestogen therapy to oppose the effects of ET on the uterine tissue
- Women without a uterus should not be prescribed progestogen with systemic ET
- Progestogen therapy is not indicated with low dose local ET for vaginal atrophy, or for ultra-low dose transdermal application for the prevention of osteoporosis
- HT is not recommended in women with a history of endometrial cancer
- HT is likely not safe to use in breast cancer survivors
- The lowest therapeutic dose of ET should be initiated with an appropriate progestin dose
- HT should be initiated soon after onset of symptoms related to menopause and should not be initiated after the age of 60
- Each individual woman should make an informed decision regarding the risks and benefits of HT

Alternative treatment options for symptoms related to menopause exist and may be sought out by patients. Depending on jurisdiction, some practitioners prescribe bio-identical hormone therapy. Contrary to popular belief, the term ``bio-identical hormones`` refers to synthetic hormones that are identical in structure to naturally occurring hormones rather than hormone like substances that occur naturally in plants. It follows that all therapeutic uses of hormones carry some risk and some benefit. Although some evidence suggests that bioidentical hormones have a lower risk profile than conventional HT, more good quality studies are needed before widespread use can be supported.

Guidelines for First-line Naturopathic Treatment of Menopause Symptoms

Approach: Menopause may be a prime opportunity for education about a healthier diet and lifestyle (sleep hygiene exercise, meditation, avoidance of smoking and limiting alcohol intake). As the patient ages, she may be more motivated to make the changes that will decrease the risk for chronic disease and improve long-term quality of life.

The following options may be used as adjunctive or alternative to conventional care depending on patient goals and individual symptoms:

Botanical medicine

- Soy isoflavone: There are some quality studies supporting the use to reduce the frequency and severity of vasomotor symptoms.
- Trifolium pretense: Two clinical trials support the use of red clover to decrease the severity and frequency of hot flashes.
- Cimicifuga racemosa: Mixed results with the use of black cohosh to reduce hot flashes. Some studies show a decrease in severity and frequency of hot flashes when compared to estrogen therapy and others have not.

BREAST ISSUES

Presentation

Breast Discharge :

Discharge can be caused by birth control pills, antipsychotic medications, hormone therapy, and hypothyroidism. Do not suspect breast cancer if the discharge is bilateral and non-bloody. The patient likely has a prolactin producing adenoma, or another endocrine disorder; confirm by measuring prolactin level. In practice, if the discharge is unilateral and_ or is associated by a mass always consider breast cancer in your differential diagnosis; request a biopsy to rule it out.

Breast Mass in women under 35:

This unlikely to be breast cancer. It is likely one of the following:

1. Fat necrosis with a history of trauma
2. Fibrocystic disease if breast palpation exhibits multiple, bilateral, tender (premenstrually), cystic masses
3. Fibroadenoma if breast palpation exhibits painless, discrete, sharply circumscribed, rubbery, mobile mass. Excision is curative but not often required unless the patient desires or there is clinical concern for cancer.
4. Mastitis/abcess if patient presents with painful, reddish, fluctuant mass

Mammography is not indicated in this age group as breast tissue is too dense. In the rare occasion that cancer is suspected, request a breast ultrasound then proceed to biopsy if findings are not reassuring.

Breast Mass in women 35 or over

This can be breast cancer, so always rule it out:

1. Fat necrosis with a history of trauma
2. Fibrocystic disease as above. However in this age group, aspiration of cyst fluid and baseline mammography are recommended. If the cyst fluid is bloody, proceed to biopsy to rule out cancer
3. Fibroadenoma as above. However in this age group, get a baseline mammogram and request a biopsy to rule out cancer. Monitor progress in future visits
4. Breast Cancer classically presents with a discrete, unilateral, hard, fixed mass with nipple retraction, or peau d`orange. Notwithstanding, many breast cancers do not exhibit these features especially early on. In the absence of classic features of fat necrosis or fibrocystic

Source

disease, when faced with a new breast mass in a woman 35 or older, always request a base line mammogram and a biopsy.

Breast mass in post menopausal women:
This is considered breast cancer until proven otherwise. Mammography and ultrasound are indicated. Ultrasound and MRI are secondary tools. In this age group, determine need for biopsy based on risk factors, physical exam findings and imaging characteristics.

PELVIC PROLAPSE

Presentation

NPLEX
MCCQE
USMLE

Pelvic organ prolapse refers to the protrusion of any of the pelvic organs (urinary bladder, urethra, uterus, bowel) into or out of the vaginal canal. Visual inspection can guide diagnosis. Prolapse occurs as the pelvic floor muscles are no longer able to support the pelvic organs in their correct anatomical positions. Symptoms depend on the structures that are prolapsed as well as the extent of prolapsed. It is important to note that affected patients are often asymptomatic.

Gala, 2010

Physical exam finding	Type	Structure prolapsed	Common Symptoms
Bulge in the upper anterior vaginal wall	Cytocele	Urinary bladder	Urinary urgency, frequency and incontinence
Bulge in the lower anterior vaginal wall	Urethrocele	Urinary bladder and urethra	Urinary urgency, frequency and incontinence
Uterus descends or bulges into the apexl/center of vaginal canal	Uterovaginal	Uterus Vaginal vault	Bleeding/discharge due to ulceration
Loops of bowel bulging in upper posterior vaginal wall	Enterocele	Small bowel	Bowel symptoms including incomplete voiding
Rectum bulges in lower posterior vaginal wall	Rectocele	Rectum	Difficulty in defecating

Katz, 2007

Gala, 2007

Risk Factors

- The most common and relevant contributing factor to pelvic organ prolapse is previous vaginal delivery of a term infant, especially difficult deliveries involving forceps and vacuum extraction.
- Other risk factors include anything that may chronically increase intra-abdominal pressure (chronic cough, ascites, repeated lifting of heavy weights, frequent straining due to constipation) as well as advanced age, smoking, high impact sports, diabetes, and connective tissue disorders.

Ferri, 2010
Katz, 2007

Source

Assessment

- Diagnosis.is based on clinical abdominal and pelvic exam. Special techniques with a speculum can be used to determine site of prolapse and pelvic organs that may be involved.
- If prolapse is suspected and significant treatment is required, referral to a gynecologist is required., diabetes, constipation).

Management Plan

Braekken, 2010
Hagen, 2004

- The nature of treatment for vaginal prolapse depends on the degree to which the patient is bothered by her symptoms and not necessarily related to the severity of prolapse.
- It is ideal to address the issue of prolapse preventatively where possible, by attempting to reduce any potential sources of increased intra-abdominal pressure. Controlling conditions that may be contributing to pelvic organ weakness is also important (e.g., asthma).
- When prolapse is mild, a woman may benefit from perineal/Kegel exercises and other lifestyle modifications (eg. smoking sessation and weight loss).
- In more moderate cases of prolapse and in women who are not eligible for surgery, a pessary can be used. A pessary is a firm, ring-shaped device that is inserted into the vaginal canal as a means of supporting the structures that have the potential to prolapse. Pessaries are individually sized and are inserted by a physician, and should be removed and cleaned regularly by either the patient or the practitioner.
- Topical application of estrogen is often used to decrease the incidence of urinary tract infections in post menopausal women and to improve urogenital atrophy, which is especially useful with the combined use of pessaries.
- For refractory or severe cases, surgery is indicated. Surgical procedures to correct vaginal prolapse depend on which organ is prolapsed. Often, more than one type of prolapse is repaired at the same time. Surgical procedures involve repositioning organs in their proper place, and the securing them with surgically shortened ligaments.
- Naturopathic treatments include lifestyle modification and adjunctive management of contributing factors. Education includes advocating for a dietary plan that leads to weight loss (if needed) and regular bowel movements that are easy to pass. Kegel exercises that mimic the actions of stopping urination may be beneficial in strengthening the pelvic support structures and reducing symptoms. Physical therapy with a trained professional in addition to home exercises may be beneficial as well. Adjunctive care to manage contributing conditions and factors is considered in the integrative management of patients (e.g., addressing chronic cough, diabetes, smoking, and heavy lifting).

PREGNANCY

In practice, consider that all women of reproductive age are pregnant before treating any condition. Do not recommend or prescribe a substance that is teratogenic or of uncertain effect on pregnancy unless pregnancy is indeed impossible. X-rays and and CT scan should only follow confirmation of absence of pregnancy. A female patient who is on the birth control pill may still be pregnant (compliance, efficacy).

Signs of Pregnancy:
1. Amenorrhea
2. Morning sickness
3. Hegar sign (softening of the lower uterine segment)
4. Chadwick sign (dark discoloration of the vulva and vaginal walls)
5. Linea nigra (vertical line of increased pigmentation in the midline of lower abdomen)
6. Melasma ``mask of pregnancy`` (photodistributed macular hyperpigmentation midline)
7. Increased pigmentation of the nipples and areola
8. Quickening, the mother's first perception of fetal movements, should not be expected before 18 weeks gestation for a primigravida (16 wks for a multigravida)

On suspicion of pregnancy, request a quantitative serum human chorionic gonadotropin (test can estimate age of pregnancy). Urinary HCG tests (including readily available commercial versions) are good screening tools; however, any positive results need to be confirmed with a serum HCG test.

Examination Board References

NPLEX (II): North American Board of Naturopathic Examiners
Naturopathic Physician Licensing Examination Part II (NPLEx II) Blueprint. Portland, OR: North American Board of Naturopathic Examiners (NABNE), 2010.

USMLE: National Board of Medical Examiners
Brochert A. Crush Step 3. The Ultimate USMLE Step 3 Review. 3rd ed. New York, NY: Saunders, Elsevier, 2008.

MCCQE: Medical Council of Canada
Dugani S, Lam D, eds. 2009. MCCQE Review Notes & Lecture Series. Medical Counsel of Canada Qualification Examination Review Notes. Toronto, ON: McGraw Hill Professional, Canadian edition, 2009.

Related References

Abad CL, Safdar N. The role of lactobacillus probiotics in the treatment or prevention of urogenital infections–a systematic review. J Chemother. 2009 Jun;21(3):243-52.

Albertazzi P, Pansini F, Bonaccorsi G, Zanotti L, Forini E, De Aloysio D. The effect of dietary soy supplementation on hot flushes. Obstet Gynecol. 1998 Jan;91(1):6-11.

Black A. Francoeur D, Rowe T et al. SOGC clinical practice guidelines: Canadian Contraception Consensus. J Obstet Gynaecol Can 2004;26(3):219-96.

Braekken IH, Majida M, Engh ME, Bø K. Can pelvic floor muscle training reverse pelvic organ prolapse and reduce prolapse symptoms? An assessor-blinded, randomized, controlled trial. Am J Obstet Gynecol. 2010 Aug;203(2):170.e1-7.

Bruner-Tran KL, Osteen KG. Dioxin-like PCBs and endometriosis. Syst Biol Reprod Med. 2010 Apr;56(2):132-46.

Bruner-Tran KL, Ding T, Osteen KG. 2010. Dioxin and endometrial progesterone resistance. Semin Reprod Med. 2010 Jan;28(1):59-68. Epub

Carmignani LO, Pedro AO, Costa-Paiva LH, Pinto-Neto AM. The effect of dietary soy supplementation compared to estrogen and placebo on menopausal symptoms: a randomized controlled trial. Maturitas. 2010 Nov;67(3):262-9.

Dains J, Baumann L, Scheibel P. Advanced Health Assessment & Clinical Diagnosis in Primary Care. 4th ed. St Louis, MO: Mosby C.V. Co. Ltd., 2011.

Etlik Zubeyde Hanim Women's Health Teaching and Research Hospital, Gynecology Clinic, Ankara, Turkey. Epub 2010 Nov 12.

Ferri FF. Ferri's Practical Guide to the Care of the Medical Patient. 8th ed. St Louis, MO: Mosby Elsevier, 2010.

Fritz MA, Speroff L. Clinical Gynecologic Endocrinology and Infertility. 8th ed. Philedelphia, PA: Lippincott Williams & Wilkins, 2011.

Fulghesu AM, Ciampelli M, Muzj G, Belosi C, Selvaggi L, Ayala GF, Lanzone A. N-acetyl-cysteine treatment improves insulin sensitivity in women with polycystic ovary syndrome. Fertil Steril. 2002 Jun;77(6):1128-35.

Gala RB. Patient Encounters - The Obstetrics and Gynecology Work-Up. Philedelphia, PA: Lippincott Williams & Wilkins, 2010.

Gonzales R, Kutner J. Current Practice Guidelines in Primary Care 2009. Toronto (ON): McGraw Hill, 2009.

Gray J. Therapeutic Choices. 5th ed. Ottawa, ON: Canadian Pharmacists Association, 2007.

Grodstein F, Goldman MB, Ryan L, Cramer DW. Relation of female infertility to consumption of caffeinated beverages. Am J Epidemiol. 1993;1371353-60.

Guay MP, Dragomir A, Pilon D, Moride Y, Perreault S. Changes in pattern of use, clinical characteristics and persistence rate of hormone replacement therapy among postmenopausal women after the WHI publication. Pharmacoepidemiol Drug Saf. 2007 Jan;16(1):17-27.

National Institute of Allergy and Infectious Disease (NIAID) http://www.niaid.nih.gov/topics/pelvicInflammatoryDisease/Pages/default.aspx

Neville Hacker, J. George Moore, Joseph Gambone. 4th ed. Essentials of Obstetrics and Gynecology. New York, NY: Elsevier, 2004.

Hagen S, Stark D, Maher C, Adams E. Conservative management of pelvic organ prolapse in women. Cochrane Database Syst Rev. 2004;(2):CD003882.

Hillman JJ, Zuckerman IH, Lee E. The impact of the Women's Health Initiative on hormone replacement therapy in a Medicaid program. J Womens Health (Larchmt). 2004 Nov;13(9):986-92.

Jeri AR. The use of an isoflavone supplement to relieve hot flashes. Female Patient. 2002;27:35-37.

Katz VL. Comprehensive Gynecology. 5th ed. St Louis, MO: Mosby Elsevier Inc., DATE.

Kliegman RM, Stanton B, St. Geme J, Schor N, Behrman RE. Nelson Textbook of Pediatrics. 19th ed. Philadelphia, PA: Saunders, 2011.

Lehmann-Willenbrock W, Riedel HH. Clinical and endocrinologic examinations concerning therapy of climacteric symptoms following hysterectomy with remaining ovaries. Zentralbl Gynakol. 1988;110:611-18.

Masha A, Manieri C, Dinatale S, Bruno GA, Ghigo E, Martina V. Prolonged treatment with N-acetylcysteine and L-arginine restores gonadal function in patients with polycystic ovary syndrome. J Endocrinol Invest. 2009 Dec;32(11):870-72.

Marsh KA, Steinbeck KS, Atkinson FS, Petocz P, Brand-Miller JC. Effect of a low glycemic index compared with a conventional healthy diet on polycystic ovary syndrome. Am J Clin Nutr. 2010 Jul;92(1):83-92.

Nestler JE, Jakubowicz DJ, Reamer P, Gunn RD, Allan G. Ovulatory and metabolic effects of D-chiro-inositol in the polycystic ovary syndrome. N Engl J Med. 1999 Apr 29;340(17):1314-20

The North American Menopause Society (NAMS). 2010. POSITION STATEMENT. Estrogen and progestogen use in postmenopausal women. The Journal of the North American Menopause Society. 2010;17):242-55.

Ozdegirmenci O, Kayikcioglu F, Akgul MA, Kaplan M, Karcaaltincaba M, Haberal A, Akyol M. 2011. Comparison of levonorgestrel intrauterine system versus hysterectomy on efficacy and quality of life in patients with adenomyosis. Fertil Steril. 2011 Feb;95(2):497-502.

Pizzorno JE, Murray MT. Textbook of Natural Medicine. 3rd ed. New York, NY: Elsevier, 2006.

Rashidi B, Haghollahi F, Shariat M, Zayerii F. The effects of calcium-vitamin D and metformin on polycystic ovary syndrome: a pilot study. Taiwan J Obstet Gynecol. 2009 Jun;48(2):142-47.

Sood R, Shuster L, Smith R, Vincent A, Jatoi A. Counseling postmenopausal women about bioidentical hormones: ten discussion points for practicing physicians. JABFM. 2011 March-April; 24(2).

Stoll W. Phytopharmaceutical influences of atrophic vaginal epithelium: double-blind study on Cimicifuga versus an estrogen preparation. Therapeutikon. 1987;1:23-32.

Thys-Jacobs S, Donovan D, Papadopoulos A, Sarrel P, Bilezikian JP. Vitamin D and calcium dysregulation in the polycystic ovarian syndrome. Steroids. 1999 Jun;64(6):430-5.

Upmalis DH, Lobo R, Bradley L, Warren M, Cone FL, Lamia CA. Vasomotor symptom relief by soy isoflavone extract tablets in postmenopausal women: a multicenter, double-blind, randomized, placebo-controlled study. Menopause. 2000 Jul-Aug;7(4):236-42.

Van de Weijer PH, Barentsen R. Isoflavones from red clover (Promensil) significantly reduce menopausal hot flush symptoms compared with placebo. Maturitas. 2002;42:187-93.

Warnecke G. Influence of a phytopharmaceutical on climacteric complaints. Med Welt. 1985;36:871- 74.

Wiesenfeld HC, Hillier SL, Krohn MA, Landers DV, Sweet RL. Bacterial vaginosis is a strong predictor of Neisseria gonorrhoeae and Chlamydia trachomatis infection. Clin Infect Dis. 2003 Mar 1;36(5):663-68.

Wuttke W, Seidlova-Wuttke D, Gorkow C. The Cimicifuga preparation BNO 1055 vs. conjugated estrogens in a double-blind placebo-controlled study: effects on menopause symptoms and bone markers. Maturitas. 2003;44(suppl 1):S67-S77.

Ziaei S, Zakeri M, Kazemnejad A. A randomized controlled trial of vitamin E in the treatment of primary dysmenorrhoea. BJOG 2005;112(4):466-69.

Ziaei S, Faghihzadeh S, Sohrabyand F. A randomised placebo-controlled trial to determine the effect of vitamin E in treatment of primary dysmenorrhea. BJOG 2001;108:1181-83.

HEMATOLOGY

ANEMIA

BLEEDING DISORDERS

MONONUCLEOSIS

ANEMIA

Presentation

Anemia involves a decrease in number of RBCs or Hb content caused by blood loss, deficient erythro-poiesis, excessive hemolysis, or a combination of these changes. The term anemia denotes a complex of signs and symptoms, rather than a diagnosis. There are several categories of anemia, the majority of which are due to blood loss, excessive red blood cell destruction, and deficient red blood cell production.

- In most cases seen in clinical practice, anemia presents as a sign of blood loss (through menses or gastrointestinal bleeding) or nutrient deficiency (e.g., iron, folate, and/or B-12).
- Iron deficiency is by far the most common nutritional cause of anemia.

Symptoms:
- Fatigue
- DOE (dyspnea on exertion)
- Light-headedness, dizziness
- Syncope
- Palpitations
- Angina
- Claudications

Signs:
- Pallor (better seen in palpebral conjunctiva and mucous membranes)
- Tachycardia (compensation)
- Systolic ejection murmurs (compensation)
- Clues to underlying pathology (e.g., jaundice in hemolytic anemia)

Diagnostic criteria: Call it anemia only if CBC indicates the following:
- Men: RBC < 4.5 million/μL, Hb < 14 g/dL, *or* Hct < 42%
- Women: RBC < 4 million/μL, Hb < 12 g/dL, *or* Hct < 37%

Diagnostic History

When diagnosing a possible case of anemia, inquire about the following history:
- Blood loss: trauma, surgery, melena, hematemesis, and menorrhagia
- Chronic diseases
- Family history: hemophilia, thalassemia, sickle cell disease, glucose-6-phosphatase deficiency (G6PD)
- Alcoholism: may lead to iron, folate, and B-12 deficiencies, as well as GI bleeds
- Medications

Source

NPLEX
MCCQE
USMLE

Pizzorno,
2006

Assessment

Tests for Anemia:

- Complete blood count (CBC) with red blood cell indices:
  1. First, the hemoglobin and/or hematocrit must be below normal.
  2. Second, the mean corpuscular volume (MCV) indicates whether the anemia is Microcytic (MCV <80), Normocytic (MCV =80-100), or Macrocytic (MCV >100).
  3. Third, the reticulocyte count is elevated in hemolysis because the bone marrow tries to compensate for RBC loss. Conversely, it is decreased when the bone marrow is not responding properly.
- CBC interpretation: A peripheral blood smear is performed whenever the CBC or RBC indices return an abnormal result. Look for classic findings of specific diagnoses:

Blood Smear Results and Interpretations

Findings	Interpretation	Findings	Interpretation
Sickeled cells	Sickle cell	Howell-Jolly bodies	Sickle cell disease or asplenia
Hyper-segmented neutrophils	Folate/B-12 deficiency	Teardrop-shaped RBCs	Myelofibrosis
Hypochromic microcytic RBCs	Iron deficiency	Schistocytes, helmet cells, and fragmented RBCs	Intra-vascular hemolysis
Parasites in RBCs	Malaria or babesiosis	Spherocytes and elliptocytes	Hereditary spherocytosis and elliptocytosis
Heinz bodies	G6PD	Acanthocytes and spur cells	Abetalipoproteinemia
Bite Cells	G6PD or other hemolytic anemias	Target cells	Thalassemia or liver disease
Iron inclusions in RBCs	Sideroblastic anemia	Polychromasia and reticulocytosis	Hemolysis
Basophilic stippling	Lead poisoning	Burr cells or echinocytes	Uremia; chronic renal failure

Source

NPLEX
MCCQE
USMLE

Marz, 1999

Causes of Microcytic, Normocytic, and Microcytic Anemia

Category	With low reticulocyte count	With normal or elevated reticulocyte count
Microcytic	Lead poisoning Sideroblastic anemia Anemia of chronic disease Iron deficiency	Thalassemia Hemoglobinopathy Sickle cell disease
Normocytic	Cancer or dysplasia Acute leukemia Bone marrow suppression Medications (bone marrow suppressors) Anemia of chronic disease Aplastic anemia Endocrine (thyroid or pituitary failure) Renal failure	Acute blood loss Hemolysis (multiple of causes) Medications (inducers of anti-RBC antibodies, see above)
Macrocytic	Folate deficiency Vitamin B-12 deficiency Medications (e.g., methotrexate, phenytoin)	None

NPLEX
MCCQE
USMLE

Medications that Cause Anemia

Many medications can cause anemia as a side effect. While the etiological mechanisms vary considerably, the following generalizations can be made:

Drug	Rationale
Methyl dopa Penicillins	Induce production of RBC antibodies, which leads to hemolysis.
Sulfa drugs	Induce production of RBC antibodies, which leads to hemolysis. Sulfa drugs are known to cause hemolysis in patients with G6PD.
Chloroquine	Induce production of RBC antibodies, which leads to hemolysis. This antimalarial drug is also known to cause hemolysis in patients with G6PD.
Phenytoin (Dilantin)	This anti-seizure medication interferes with folate metabolism, leading to megaloblastic anemia.
Chloramphenicol	This antibacterial drug inhibits formation of peptide bonds, thus temporarily causing bone marrow suppression (myelosuppression, neutropenia, and thrombocytopenia).

Source

Drug	Rationale
Chemotherapy agents	Anti-neoplastic drugs generally cause bone marrow suppression (chemotherapeutic agents preferentially target cells with fast mitotic activity, such as the bone marrow).
Zidovudine (AZT)	This reverse transcriptase inhibitor (used for the management of symptomatic and asymptomatic HIV infections) suppresses myeloid and erythroid progenitor cells.

MCCQE
USMLE

Iron Deficiency Anemia

The most common cause of anemia in North America, associated with the following symptoms and circumstances:
- Women of reproductive age due to menstrual blood loss.
- Children, pregnant, or breast-feeding women due to increased requirements.
- Asymptomatic chronic cases are often related to colon cancer.
- Often presents as fatigue, dyspnea on exertion, dizziness, and palpitations.
- Rarely, patients with iron deficiency anemia develop craving for ice or dirt (pica).

Diagnosis:
- Low iron
- Low ferritin level
- Increased total iron binding capacity (TIBC or transferrin)
- Low TIBC saturation
- In menstruating women, a presumptive diagnosis of menstrual blood loss can be made.
- In postnatal care, breast-fed babies do not require supplementation. Formula-fed babies should receive iron supplementation (most infant formulas and cereals contain iron, if not give separately) at 4-6 months of age (2 months of age for preemies).

Gonzales, 2009

Screening for Anemia

- Screen all pregnant and high risk infants ages 6-12 months via blood testing for hemaglobin and hematocrit%.
- In all patients more than 40 years of age (men and post menopausal women), rule out colon cancer as a cause of chronic, asymptomatic blood loss. A stool occult blood test (FOBT) should be performed (this test is also called Hemascreen in the RSNC). If the test returns a positive result or there is family history of colon cancer, seriously consider a colonoscopy.

Plummer-Vinson Syndrome

Plummer-Vinson syndrome is a triad of esophageal web (leading to dysphagia), iron deficiency anemia, and glossitis.
- Plummer-Vinson syndrome is of unknown etiology.

Source

NPLEX

Pizzorno, 2006

9. Guidelines for First-line Naturopathic Treatment of Iron Deficiency

Approach: The cause of any presenting anemia should always be explored first.

1. Dietary measures
- Encourage liberal consumption of green leafy vegetables and/or other dietary sources of iron.

2. Clinical nutrition
- Hydrolyzed (liquid) liver extract: 500-1500 mg t.i.d. before meals as a rich source of heme iron, as well as folic acid and vitamin B-12; or ingestion of 4-6 oz of calf liver q.d.
- Iron succinate (or iron fumarate): 30 mg b.i.d. between meals. If abdominal discomfort occurs, change posology to 30 mg t.i.d. with meals.
- Supplementing simultaneously with vitamin C may increase absorption of iron. Adequate stomach acid production is required for absorption (see GERD section in GI module).

- Follow these treatment protocols for 3 to 6 months to replete body iron stores.
- Monitor CBC monthly to determine when values normalize.

Differential DDx for Thalassemia and Iron Deficiency Anemia

- Iron levels are normal in thalassemia, whereas in iron deficiency anemia the iron levels are low.
- Both presentations should be differentiated because they both lead to microcytic hypochromic anemia. In thalassemia, hemoglobin A2 levels will also be elevated on hemoglobin electrophoresis.
- Remember that iron supplementation is contraindicated in thalassemia because it causes iron overload and subsequent hemochromatosis.

Langlois, 2008

Bastian, 2007

Screening: Current guidelines recommend offering screening to pregnant or conceiving women of high risk ethnic backgrounds (Mediterranean, Middle East, and southeast Asia) to identify carriers, and establish risk of trait inheritance (intrauterine death in α-thalassemia major with 4 Hb deletions, β-thalassemia - severe anemia and jaundice 3-6 months after birth).

Folate Deficiency

NPLEX
MCCQE
USMLE

Commonly seen in alcoholics and pregnant women. Since folate deficiency causes congenital neural tube defects, women of reproductive age should take folate-containing supplements.

Causes:
- Poor diet
- Malabsorption
- Chronic use of some medications, including Methotrexate, sulfa drugs (trimethoprim sulfamethox-azole "TMP"), and phenytoin.

Diagnostic Tests:
- The laboratory studies will show macrocytes and hyper-segmented neutrophils *without* neurologic signs (i.e., loss of sensation and position sense, paresthesia, ataxia, spasticity, hyperreflexia, positive Babinski sign, and dementia), which suggest B-12 deficiency.
- Confirm with serum or RBC folate assay.

Source

NPLEX

Guidelines for First-line Naturopathic Treatment of Folate Deficiency

1. Address the cause of the deficiency
- Stop or change medications.
- Correct deficient diet.

2. Clinical nutrition
- Hydrolyzed (liquid) liver extract: 500-1500 mg t.i.d. before meals as a rich source of heme iron, as well as folic acid and vitamin B-12; or ingestion of 4-6 oz of calf liver q.d.
- Folic acid: 800-1200 mcg t.i.d.
- Vitamin B-12: 1000 mcg q.d. orally. It is always necessary to complement vitamin B-12 with folic acid to prevent the folate from masking a B-12 deficiency.

- Follow this treatment protocol for 3 months.
- Monitor CBC monthly to determine when values normalize.

NPLEX
MCCQE
USMLE

Vitamin B-12 Deficiency Anemia

Vitamin B-12 deficiency anemia is subtype of megaloblastic anemias.

Pizzorno,
2006

Causes:
- Pernicious anemia (most common cause)
- Gastrectomy
- Terminal ileum resection
- Crohn's disease
- Strict vegan diet
- Chronic pancreatitis

Diagnostic Tests:
- The peripheral smear looks exactly the same as in folate deficiency (macrocytes, hypersegmented neutrophils), but patients will have neurologic deficiencies (e.g., loss of sensation and position sense, paresthesia, ataxia, spasticity, hyperreflexia, positive Babinski sign, and dementia).
- Achlorhydria is a diagnostic feature of pernicious anemia.
- Confirm diagnosis with serum B-12 assessment and/or the Schilling test.

NPLEX

Guidelines for First-line Naturopathic Treatment of Vitamin B-12 Deficiency Anemia

Clinical nutrition
- Hydrolyzed (liquid) liver extract: 500-1500 mg t.i.d. before meals as a rich source of heme iron, as well as folic acid and vitamin B-12; or ingestion of 4-6 oz of calf liver q.d.
- Oral vitamin B-12: 1000 mcg (sublingual methylcobalamin is preferred over cyanocobalamin) b.i.d. for 1 month followed by a maintenance dose of 1000 mcg q.d. Although it is popular to inject vitamin B-12, oral administration of an appropriate dose, even in the absence of intrinsic factor, is effective in achieving therapeutic elevation of serum B-12 levels.
- Alternative: Intramuscular vitamin B-12: 1000 mcg injection weekly for 8 weeks, followed by a maintenance dose of 1000 mcg once a month.
- Monitor CBC monthly until values normalize.

Source

Autoimmune Anemia

NPLEX
USMLE

Coombs test is positive in most cases of autoimmune anemia (e.g., secondary to SLE, lymphoma, leukemia, or long term of some prescription medications)

Lead Toxicity as a Cause of Anemia

NPLEX
USMLE

The human body can tolerate approximately 1 mg of lead per day without succumbing to deleterious side effects. In urban environments, the average intake of lead is about 2.5 mg per week. The World Health Organization estimates that 10% of ingested lead is absorbed by adults. However, recent research has demonstrated that children absorb and retain much higher amounts of lead than adults.

Acute (high-level exposure): Acute lead toxicity presents with vomiting, ataxia, colicky abdominal pains, irritability, aggression, behavioral regression, encephalopathy, cerebral edema, and/or seizures. Screen with serum lead assay.

Chronic (low-level exposure): Lead poisoning exhibits hypochromic microcytic anemia (CBC) and basophilic stippling (smear), as well as elevated free protoporphyrin. This presentation occurs almost always in children. Usually, lead toxicity is chronic and low-level with minimal nonspecific symptoms. Notwithstanding, chronic lead exposure has been linked to hyperactivity, attention deficit disorder (with or without hyperactivity), and behavioral disorders. Screen with CBC and blood, urine, or hair mineral analysis.

Risk Factors:
- Residence in old buildings that may have chipping or unstable lead-containing paint (building codes now prohibit lead based paints).
- Residence near lead-smelting or battery-recycling plants.
- Family members who work in lead-smelting or battery-recycling plants.
- Supplementation with oyster shell calcium, dolomite, and bone meal products (unless lead levels are stated on label).
- In underdeveloped countries still utilizing leaded fuels, living near highways or heavy traffic is a risk factor.
- In some underdeveloped countries, building codes do not prohibit lead pipes to be used in plumbing.

Screening: Routine screening of asymptomatic patients is not recommended. Assess risk factors for all infants (living in old building, eat paint chips, living near battery recycling plant, have a parent who works in battery recycling plant). In high risk children, test serum lead levels + CBC at 6 months of age and retest at 12 months. In low-risk children, screen at 12 months and retest at 24 months.

Gonzales,
2009

Source

NPLEX

Pizzorno,
2006

Guidelines for First-line Naturopathic Treatment of Lead Toxicity

Approach
- Find the cause (environmental, dietary, or lifestyle).
- Decrease exposure.
- Increase elimination (chelation).

1. First-line conservative chelation
- Vitamin C: 3 g q.d.
- Apple pectin
- Seaweed alginate
- Methionine
- Cysteine
- Cystine
- Encourage specific foods, such as beans, onions, and garlic

2. Second-line chelation
- For acute toxicity or in cases where laboratory evidence of improvement is not noted within 1 month of above treatment plan, consider the following lead-chelation measures:
  - Children: recommend Succimer (lead chelator). Add ethylenediamine tetracetic acid (EDTA) in severe cases.
  - Adults: recommend Dimercaprol (lead chelator). Add EDTA in severe cases.

NPLEX
MCCQE
USMLE

Anemia of Chronic Disease

Anemia of chronic disease can be either normocytic or microcytic.

Signs and Symptoms:
- Serum iron is low.
- Decreased total iron binding capacity (this is increased in iron deficiency anemia – an easy differential diagnosis).
- Serum ferritin will also be elevated.

Management:
- Treat the cause. Obviously, you should do your best to determine the disease that is causing this anemia (e.g., rheumatoid arthritis, SLE, cancer, or tuberculosis).
- Remember that chronic (often asymptomatic) renal disease causes normocytic anemia with reduced reticulocyte count due to decreased erythropoietin secretion.
- Refrain from prescribing iron supplementation.

Source

NPLEX
MCCQE
USMLE

Sickle Cell Disease

80% of African Americans are heterozygous for sickle cell trait.

Diagnosis:
- Diagnosis is established via peripheral blood smear exhibiting characteristic sickled erythrocytes; Howell-Jolly bodies in RBCs (nuclear remnants in erythrocytes); and elevated reticulocytes >8% to10%.
- Diagnosis is confirmed via hemoglobin electrophoresis (screening is done at birth in Canada and the United States).

Clinical manifestations:
- Acute chest syndrome (presents like pneumonia)
- Bone pain (due to microinfarcts which may lead to avascular necrosis of femoral head)
- Dactylitis (hand-foot syndrome in children)
- Priapism
- Tendency for strokes
- Patients are also susceptible to pigment cholelithiasis; *Pneumococcucs*, *Hemophilus*, and *Niesseria* infections; and aplastic crisis after parvovirus infection.

Management Guidelines:
- Folate supplementation
- Prophylaxis against infectious diseases
- Early and aggressive treatment of infections
- Proper hydration
- Severe presentations are termed "sickle cell crisis" and require hospitalization, oxygen administration, intravenous fluids, and analgesics (the pain is so severe that narcotic analgesics are the mainstay of pain management in hospitals).
- If all these measure fail in alleviating the sickle cell crisis, blood transfusion is considered.

Glucose-6-phosphatase Deficiency

NPLEX
MCCQE
USMLE

G6PD is an X-linked recessive disorder, affecting males. It is most common in African American and Mediterranean populations. These patients are susceptible to sudden hemolytic episodes after exposure to fava beans, certain drugs (e.g., antimalarials, salicylates, sulfa drugs, IV vitamin C), infections, or DKA (diabetic ketoacidosis).

Diagnosis: RBC enzyme assay. G6PD assay.

Treatment: Avoidance of inducers is the key to managing patients with G6PD.

Source

NPLEX
MCCQE
USMLE

BLEEDING DISORDERS

Conditions Prolonging and Differentiating Coagulation Tests

Condition	PT	PTT	BT	Platelets	RBCs	Facts
Hemophilia A or B (deficiency in factor VIII or IX, respectively)	Normal	High	Normal	Normal	Normal	Mostly men are affected since it is X-linked. Common. Look for positive family history.
von Willebrand factor deficiency	Normal	High	High	Normal	Normal	Autosomal dominant inheritance. Common. (vWF deficiency) Look for positive family history.
Liver failure	High	High	High	Low	Normal or low	Look for stigmata of liver disease.
Vitamin K deficiency	High	Normal	Normal or High	Normal	Normal	Seen in malabsorption, alcoholism and prolonged antibiotic use.
Vitamin C deficiency (scurvy)	Normal	Normal	Normal	Normal	Normal	Easy bleeding from fingernails and gums.
Idiopathic thrombocytopenic purpura (ITP)	Normal	Normal	High	Low	Normal	May follow upper respiratory tract infections.
Thrombotic thrombocytopenic purpura (TTP)	Normal	Normal	High	Low	Low	Characteristics of hemolysis is usually present in peripheral smear.
Disseminated intravascular coagulation	High	High	High	Low	Low	Diagnosed largely from the presenting history (see above).

Source

NPLEX
MCCQE
USMLE

Clotting Tests Measure

- Prothrombin Time (PT) = extrinsic clotting pathway; prolonged by Warfarin (Coumadin or dicumarol).
- Activated Partial Thromboplastin Time (PTT) = intrinsic clotting pathway; prolonged by Heparin.
- Bleeding Time (BT) = platelet function; prolonged by Aspirin.

NPLEX
MCCQE
USMLE

Disseminated Intravascular Coagulation (DIC)

A severe emergent condition, where thrombosis engages clotting factors, leading to their deficiency in circulating blood. DIC does not usually present to outpatient facilities. However, it should be suspected with bleeding disorders that prolong prothrombin time and partial thromboplastin time, as well as bleeding time.

Causes:
- Pregnancy and obstetric complications (50%)
- Malignancy (33%)
- Sepsis
- Trauma
- Prostate surgery
- Snake bites

Eosinophilia
Although it is not a bleeding disorder per se, eosinophilia is an increase in the amount of circulating eosinophils.

Common Causes:
- Atopic conditions (such as allergy, eczema, angioedema)
- Parasitic infections
- Autoimmune disease (e.g., SLE and rheumatoid arthritis)
- Drug reaction
- Adrenal insufficiency
- Blood dyscrasias (such as lymphoma)

NPLEX
MCCQE
USMLE

Thrombocytopenia

Bleeding from thrombocytopenia occurs as petechiae, nosebleeds, and easy bruising.

Common Causes of Low Platelet Count:
- Purpura (ITP or TTP)
- Hemolytic uremic syndrome (HUS)
- Disseminated intravascular necrosis (DIC)
- HIV
- Medications (especially heparin, quinidine, and sulfa drugs)
- Autoimmune disease
- Alcoholism

Source

NPLEX
MCCQE
USMLE

Petechiae in the Absence of Thrombocytopenia

Petechiae Causes:
- Vitamin C deficiency (from poor dietary habits) is the main factor that causes splinter and gum hemorrhages (due to connective tissue 'collagen' instability rather than thrombocytopenia), myalgia, arthralgia, and capillary fragility.
- Chronic steroid use also leads to capillary fragility due to poor collagen formation.
- Less common causes are uremia (chronic renal failure), inherited connective tissue disease (this will also manifest as weak joint capsules, joint hypermobility, hemorrhoids, and/or varicose veins), Marfan's syndrome, and osteogenesis imperfecta.

NPLEX
MCCQE
USMLE

Esonophilia and Infectious Mononucleosis

Affectionately called the kissing disease, mononucleosis is caused by the Epstein-Barr virus.

Signs and Symptoms:
- Low-grade fever
- Malaise
- Pharyngitis
- Lymphadenopathy

Diagnosis:
- Lymphocytosis is diagnostic for this infectious disease.
- Diagnosis is confirmed by the specific Monospot test.

Examination Board References

NPLEX (II): North American Board of Naturopathic Examiners
Naturopathic Physician Licensing Examination Part II (NPLEx II) Blueprint. Portland, OR: North American Board of Naturopathic Examiners (NABNE), 2010.

USMLE: National Board of Medical Examiners
Brochert A. Crush Step 3. The Ultimate USMLE Step 3 Review. 3rd ed. New York, NY: Saunders, Elsevier, 2008.

MCCQE: Medical Council of Canada
Dugani S, Lam D, eds. 2009. MCCQE Review Notes & Lecture Series. Medical Counsel of Canada Qualification Examination Review Notes. Toronto, ON: McGraw Hill Professional, Canadian edition, 2009.

Related References

Baustian GH, Djulbegovic B, Rao DS. Thalassemia. First Consult: Elsevier Inc., 2007. Online at www.mdconsult.com

Dawson J, Taylor M, Reide P. Crash Course Pharmacology. 2nd ed. Philadelphia, PA: Mosby Inc, 2002.

Gonzales, R., Kutner, J. Current Practice Guidelines in Primary Care 2009. Toronto (ON): McGraw Hill, 2009.

Langlois S, Ford JC, Chitayat D, Desilets VA, Farrell SA, Geraghty M, Nelson T, Nikkel SM, Shugar A, Skidmore D,

Allen VM, Audibert F, Blight C, Gagnon A, Johnson JA, Wilson RD, Wyatt P. Carrier screening for thalassemia and hemoglobinopathies in Canada. J Obstet Gynaecol Can. 2008;30(10):950-59.

Lederly F. Oral Cobalamin for pernicious anemia: Medicine's best kept secret. JAMA 1991;265:94-95.

Marz RB. Medical Nutrition from Marz. 2nd ed. Portland, OR: Omni-Press, 1999.

Murray M. Encyclopedia of Nutritional Supplements. New York, NY: Prima Publishing, Random House Inc., 1996.

Pizzorno JE, Murray MT. 2006. Textbook of Natural Medicine. 3rd ed. New York, NY: Churchill Livingstone, Elsevier, 2006.

IMMUNOLOGY AND GENETICS

HYPERSENSITIVITY

IMMUNODEFICIENCY DISORDERS

GENETIC DISORDERS

HYPERSENSITIVITY

Presentation

There are four types of hypersensitivity reactions:
1. Anaphylactic (type 1)
2. Cytotoxic (type II)
3. Immune complex-mediated (type III)
4. Cell-mediated/delayed (type IV)

Type I Hypersensitivity

True anaphylactic hypersensitivity is due to preformed immunoglobulin type E (IgE) that binds with its target, leading to the release of vasoactive amines (like histamine and leukotrienes) from mast cells and basophils. Symptoms of this type of hypersensitivity depend on the extent and tissue location of mast cells.

Signs and Symptoms:
- Anaphylaxis
- Atopy
- Hay fever
- Urticaria
- Allergic rhinitis
- Asthma
- True food allergies (e.g., peanut or shellfish)
- Bee sting allergy
- Medication allergy (e.g., penicillins and sulfa drugs)
- Rubber glove allergy (latex allergy)

Diagnosis:
- Eosinophilia
- Elevated IgE levels
- Positive family history of allergies, seasonal exacerbations
- Shiners (i.e., bilateral infraorbital edema)
- Bluish edematous nasal mucosa

Allergen Tests

- Allergens that react with preformed IgE are identified clinically by cutaneous scratch antigen test battery or intradermal antigen testing.
- Blood testing via radioallergosorbent test (RAST) quantify specific levels of preformed IgE as well as IgG.

Source

NPLEX
MCCQE
USMLE

Food Sensitivities

20% of food reactions exhibit IgE-mediated (type I) immediate allergy symptoms toward food antigens. However, the most common food reactions (food sensitivities) are IgG and IgG complex mediated (type III).

NPLEX
MCCQE
USMLE

Type II Hypersensitivity

Due to preformed IgG and IgM that bind to cell-bound antigens (or parts of a cell) leading to secondary inflammation. Examples include:

■ Hyperacute transplant rejection
■ Cytopenias caused by antibodies (e.g., idiopathic thrombocytopenic purpura)
■ Transfusion reactions
■ Erthythroblastosis fetalis (due to Rh incompatibility between parents)
■ Goodpasture's syndrome
■ Myasthenia gravis
■ Graves' disease
■ Pernicious anemia
■ Pemphigus
■ Autoimmune hemolytic anemia (e.g., due to exposure to methyldopa, penicillin, or sulfa)

Test for Hypersensitivity Induced Anemia

Coomb's test (usually direct Coomb's test).

NPLEX
MCCQE
USMLE

Type III Hypersensitivity

Immune-complex-mediated hypersensitivity is due to antigen-antibody complexes that are deposited in tissues and/or vascular endothelium leading to a delayed inflammatory response. Examples include:

■ Food sensitivities
■ Serum sickness
■ Lupus erythematosus
■ Rheumatoid arthritis
■ Glomerulonephritis (some types)
■ Polyarteritis nodosa

Pizzorno,
1999

NPLEX
MCCQE
USMLE

Type IV Hypersensitivity

Cell-mediated/delayed sensitivity is due to sensitized T-lymphocytes that release inflammatory mediators. Examples include:

■ Chronic transplant rejection
■ Granulomas (such as tuberculous Ghon's focus, syphilitic gumma, and sarcoidosis)
■ Contact dermatitis (poison ivy, nickel earrings, cosmetics, and medications)

IMMUNODEFICIENCY DISORDERS

IgA

IgA deficiency, which causes recurrent respiratory and gastrointestinal infections, is the most common primary immunodeficiency. IgA levels are always low (as well as IgG2).

HIV

HIV often initially presents to primary care providers as fever, malaise, pharyngitis, rash and/or lymphadenopathy. You need to distinguish HIV from a diagnosis of infectious mononucleosis.

HIV Diagnosis:
- Established with enzyme-linked immunosorbent assay (ELISA), which, if positive, is confirmed with retesting and Western blot test.
- Because it takes at least 1 month for HIV antibodies to develop, if a patient wants testing because of a recent unprotected sex encounter, the test should be repeated in 6 months if the initial test is negative.

Screening: Routine screening is recommended for pregnant women and adults in healthcare settings who are treated for TB or evaluated for STIs.

Hereditary Angioedema

A deficiency in C1 esterase inhibitor (complement enzyme) is the usual cause of hereditary angioedema. This term denotes some form of facial swelling.

Diagnosis:
- Patients exhibit diffuse swelling of the lips, eyelids, and possibly the airway, *unrelated* to allergen exposure.
- Look for positive family history because this disease is autosomal dominant.
- Laboratory investigations will show decreased levels of C4 complement levels.

Treatment: Acute treatment is the same as for anaphylaxis. Androgens are used for long-term management because they increase liver production of C1 esterase inhibitor.

Recurrent Neisseria Infections

Complement deficiencies of C5 through C9 predispose patient to recurrent *Neisseria* sp. infections. In practice, if you are presented with any patient with recurrent Neisseria infection, request a complement assay.

Source

NPLEX
MCCQE
USMLE

Chronic Mucocutaneous Candidiasis

A cellular immunodeficiency specific for candidal infection.

Diagnosis:
- Patients have oral thrush and other candidal infections of the scalp, skin, and nails.
- Skin testing will confirm if it displays no reaction toward *Candida* sp. This is a peculiar finding since everyone in Canada and the United States is exposed and should exhibit a positive result.
- Consider this condition if a patient exhibits susceptibility to candidal infections without any other immune function disorders (i.e., susceptibility to other types of infections).
- Often this condition is associated with hypothyroidism.

NPLEX

Guidelines for Naturopathic Immune Modulating and Stimulating Botanicals

- *Astragulus membranaceus*
- *Boswella serrata*
- *Echinacea spp.*
- *Ganoderma lucidum*
- *Lentinus edodes*
- *Ligustrum lucidum*
- *Thuja occidentali*
- *Withania somnifera*
- *Spilanthes acmella*
- *Uncaria tomentosa*

GENETIC DISORDERS

Patterns of Inheritance of Genetically Transmitted Disorders

Pattern of inheritance	Genetically Transmitted Disorders		
Autosomal Dominant (no generations are skipped)	Von Willebrand's hemophilia	Neurofibromatosis	Hereditary spherocytosis
	Achondroplasia (dwarfism)	Huntington's chorea	Marfan's syndrome
	Adult polycystic kidney disease	Familial hypercholesterolemia	Familial polyposis coli
	Myotonic dystrophy	Multiple endocrine neoplasia syndrome (MEN I/II)	
Autosomal Recessive (generations are skipped)	Glycogen storage diseases	Tay-Sachs sphingolipidosis	Cystic fibrosis
	Galactosemia	Amino acid disorders (e.g., phenylketonuria or PKU)	Sickle cell disease
	Children polycystic kidney disease	Wilson's disease	Hemochromatosis (usually)
	Ambiguous genitalia due to Androgenital Syndrome (e.g., 21-hydroxylase deficiency)		
X-Linked Recessive	Hemophilia	Glucose-6-phosphate-deficiency	Bruton's agammaglobulinemia
	Fragile X syndrome	Duchenne's muscular dystrophy	
Chromosomal	Down syndrome (trisomy 21)	Edward's syndrome (trisomy 18)	Patau's syndrome (trisomy 13)
	Turner's Syndrome (XO)		
Polygenic	Pyloric stenosis	Cleft lip/palate	Type II diabetes
	Obesity	Neural tube defects	Schizophrenia
	Bipolar disorder (I/II)	Ischemic heart disease	Alcoholism

Source

NPLEX
MCCQE
USMLE

Autosomal Dominant Transmission

What is the likelihood of a woman's autosomal dominant condition being passed to her child? Assuming that the father does not have the disease (a proper deduction since autosomal dominant conditions express themselves in carriers), the likelihood is 50%, unless the patient was told that she was homozygous for the gene defect, which is extremely rare.

NPLEX
MCCQE
USMLE

Autosomal Recessive Transmission

If both parents are carriers of an autosomal recessive condition, what are the odds that their child will develop the condition? The easy way to navigate autosomal genetic counseling questions is by applying binomial statistics (there are only two genes per parent). Thus, in this example you would multiply both parents' genetic factor ($0.5 \times 0.5 = 0.25$). Therefore, you can confidently answer this question by saying that the child has a 25% chance of developing the condition, a 50% chance of being a carrier, and a 25% chance of not inheriting the trait at all.

NPLEX
MCCQE
USMLE

X-linked Recessive Disorder (male)

If a father has an X-linked recessive disorder, what are the odds that his child will be affected if the mother is not a carrier? Obviously, if his child is male, there will be no chance of him inheriting the trait (as the father would have only contributed the Y chromosome to his son). If the child is female, the X chromosome will always be passed, but since this a recessive disorder, there will be no chance that his daughter will develop the condition (i.e., she will only be a carrier for the trait).

NPLEX
MCCQE
USMLE

X-linked Recessive Disorder (female)

If a mother is a carrier of an X-linked recessive disorder and the father is healthy, what are the odds that their son or daughter will develop the disease? There is a 50% chance for a son and no chance for a daughter to develop the disorder. However, there is a 50% chance that she will be a carrier.

NPLEX
MCCQE
USMLE

Down Syndrome

Occurrence of three genetic alleles (trisomy) on chromosome # 21 leads to Down syndrome, which is the most common cause of mental retardation in North America. At birth there is hypotonia, microgenia (small chin), round face, macroglossia (oversized or protruding tongue), upslanting palpebral fissures, shorter limbs, a single transverse palmar crease (instead of the normal double crease), poor muscle tone, and a larger than normal space between the big and second toes. Congenital cardiac defects, such as ventricular septal defect (VSD), increased risk of leukemia, duodenal atresia, recurrent otitis media, GERD, and early Alzheimer's disease are also common.

Sheets,
2011

Screening: Down syndrome can be diagnosed via amniocentesis during pregnancy or blood testing at any age. Early childhood intervention, enaging family environment, vocational training, and proper care will improve overall development and quality of life, despite the genetic limitations.

Signs and Symptoms:
- At birth there is hypotonia, transverse palmar crease, and characteristic facies.
- Congenital cardiac defects, such as ventricular septal defect (VSD), increased risk of leukemia, duodenal atresia, and early Alzheimer's disease are also common.

Risk Factors:
- Maternal age (1 in 1500 of 16-year-old mothers compared to 1 in 25 of 45-year-old mothers)
- Paternal age is a lesser factor when maternal age is above 35-years old.
- The rise in prevalence of Down syndrome in America and Canada is directly related to the increased number of births to parents over age 35, (more than doubled in the last 20 years).

Fragile X Syndrome

The second most common cause of inherited mental retardation after Down syndrome, this syndrome is X-linked recessive.
- Affected males often exhibit large testicles.

Patau's Syndrome

Another trisomy on chromosome # 13 (i.e., trisomy 13) that causes mental retardation.

Signs and Symptoms:
- Apnea
- Deafness
- Fusion of cerebral hemispheres (holoprosencephaly)
- Myelomeningocele
- Cardiovascular abnormalities

Turner's Syndrome

Occurs in females who exhibit XO instead of XX.

Signs and Symptoms:
- Short stature
- Webbed neck
- Widely spaced nipples
- Amenorrhea
- Lack of appropriate breast development (due to primary ovarian failure)
- Infertility
- Coarctation of the aorta
- Horse-shoe kidneys or cystic hygroma

Diagnosis: Established through karyotyping and absence of Barr bodies on a buccal smear.

Source

NPLEX
MCCQE
USMLE

Klinefelter's Syndrome

Occurs in males who exhibit XXY instead of XY.

Signs and Symptoms:
- Tall stature
- Small testicles
- Gynecomastia
- Infertility
- Slightly decreased IQ

NPLEX
MCCQE
USMLE

Marfan's Syndrome

An autosomal dominant connective tissue disorder.

Signs and Symptoms:
- Positive family history
- Tall stature
- Arachnodactyly (long, thin fingers)
- Hyperextensible joints
- Mitral valve prolapse
- Dislocation of the ocular lens
- High risk for thoracic aortic aneurysm (i.e., aortic dissection)

MCCQE
USMLE

Cri-du-Chat Syndrome

Appropriately named after the propensity of affected infants to emit a high-pitched cry, which sounds similar to a cat's cry.
- Caused by the deletion of the short arm of chromosome 5.
- Leads to severe mental retardation.

NPLEX
MCCQE
USMLE

Galactosemia

An autosomal recessive inherited disorder that manifests as elevated levels of galactose in the blood, congenital cataracts, and neonatal sepsis.
- These infants are born with a congenital inability to metabolize galactose and lactose. Affected infants should avoid all foods containing galactose or lactose.
- The affected newborn will consistently vomit after breast-feeding, leading to failure to thrive.

Examination Board References

NPLEX (II): North American Board of Naturopathic Examiners
Naturopathic Physician Licensing Examination Part II (NPLEx II) Blueprint. Portland, OR: North American Board of Naturopathic Examiners (NABNE), 2010.

USMLE: National Board of Medical Examiners
Brochert A. Crush Step 3. The Ultimate USMLE Step 3 Review. 3rd ed. New York, NY: Saunders, Elsevier, 2008.

MCCQE: Medical Council of Canada
Dugani S, Lam D, eds. 2009. MCCQE Review Notes & Lecture Series. Medical Counsel of Canada Qualification Examination Review Notes. Toronto, ON: McGraw Hill Professional, Canadian edition, 2009.

Related References

Dains J, Baumann L, Scheibel P. Advanced Health Assessment & Clinical Diagnosis in Primary Care. 2nd ed. City, St. Louis: Missouri: Mosby Inc, 2003.

Dains J, Baumann L, Scheibel P. Advanced Health Assessment & Clinical Diagnosis in Primary Care. 4th ed. St Louis, MO: Mosby C.V. Co. Ltd., 2011.

Gonzales R, Kutner J. Current Practice Guidelines in Primary Care 2009. Toronto, ON: McGraw Hill, 2009.

Pizzorno JE, Murray MT. Textbook of Natural Medicine, Vol. 1 and 2. 2nd ed. New York, NY: Churchill Livingstone, 1999.

Pizzorno JE, Murray MT, Joiner-Bey H. The Clinician's Handbook of Natural Medicine. New York, NY: Churchill Livingstone, 2002.

Pizzorno JE, Murray MT. Textbook of Natural Medicine, 3rd ed. New York, NY: Churchill Livingstone, Elsevier, 2006.

Sheets KB, Best RG, Brasington CK, Will MC. Balanced information about Down syndrome: What is essential? American Journal of Medical Genetic A. 2011;155(6): 1246-57.

INFECTIOUS DISEASES

Infectious Disease Reportng

Fever

Microbial Infections

INFECTIOUS DISEASE REPORTING

Public Health Reporting

The list of reportable diseases varies somewhat depending on provincial or state regulations. In the Province of Ontario, for example, the following infectious diseases are to be reported to the local medical officer of health according to Ontario Regulation 559/91 and amendments under the Health Protection and Promotion Act. For all other jurisdictions, contact your local medical officer of health.

- If you suspect one of these diagnoses but are unable to ascertain the etiology because of lack of experience and/or when confirmatory work-up is unavailable, report the condition as 'possible' and consult with another practitioner who can ascertain the diagnosis.

Infectious Disease Reporting:

Immediate reporting required

- Anthrax
- Botulism
- Brucellosis
- Cholera
- Clostridium difficile
- Cryptosporidiosis
- Cyclosporiasis
- Diphtheria
- Encephalitis
- Food poisoning (all causes)
- Gastroenteritis, institutional outbreaks
- Giardiasis, except asymptomatic cases
- Group A Streptococcal infections, invasive
- Haemophilus influenza B disease, invasive
- Hemorrhagic fevers (e.g., Ebola, Marbug, and other viral causes)
- Hepatitis A
- Lassa fever
- Legionellosis
- Listeriosis
- Measles
- Meningitis, acute (bacterial)
- Meningococcal disease, invasive

Reporting by next working day required

- Acquired Immunodeficiency Syndrome (AIDS)
- Amebiasis
- Campylobacter enteritis
- Chancroid
- Chickenpox (Varicella)
- Chlamydia trachomatis
- Cytomegalovirus, congenital (CMV)
- Gonorrhea
- Group B Streptococcal infections, neonatal
- Hepatitis B, C, D
- Herpes, neonatal
- Influenza
- Leprosy
- Lyme disease
- Malaria
- Mumps
- Meningitis, acute (viral, other)
- Ophthalmia neonatorum
- Pertussis (whooping cough)
- Psittacosis / Ornithosis
- Q fever
- Rubella, congenital syndrome
- Salmonellosis

Source	Immediate reporting required	Reporting by next working day required
	■ Paratyphoid fever ■ Plague ■ Poliomyelitis ■ Rabies ■ Rubella ■ Severe acute respiratory syndrome (SARS) ■ Shigellosis ■ Smallpox ■ Typhoid fever ■ Tularemia ■ Verotoxin-producing E. Coli, causing Hemolytic Uremic Syndrome (HUS) ■ West Nile Virus ■ Yellow fever	■ Syphilis ■ Tetanus ■ Transmissible spongiform encephalopathy ■ Trichinosis ■ Tuberculosis ■ Tularemia ■ Yersiniosis

FEVER

NPLEX
MCCQE
USMLE

Presentation

When patients present with FWS, take a complete history and conduct a physical exam.

Dains,
2011

Signs and Symptoms: Specifically inquire about the presence (or absence) of these symptoms during your evaluation of febrile presentations:
- Headache or sinus pain
- Purulent nasal discharge
- Ear pain
- Toothache
- Sore throat
- Chest pain
- Dyspnea
- Cough
- Breast tenderness
- Abdominal pain
- Flank pain
- Dysuria
- Pelvic pain
- Vaginal discharge
- Rectal pain
- Testicular pain
- Calf pain
- Neck stiffness
- Joint swelling or stiffness
- Localized pain or heat

Source

- Focal neurological deficits
- Body temperature greater than 41.1C (106F) almost always indicates central nervous system disease or heat illness (over bundling) with or without infectious etiology.
- Infectious diseases in neonates, immune-compromised patients, patients with chronic renal insufficiency, and elderly patients usually do not present as febrile conditions.

In Children:

- Fevers in infants under 2 months of age are *rare* and should be viewed as serious until proven otherwise.
- During early childhood, fevers up to 40C (104F) are common, even with minor infections.
- All febrile infants < 3 months of age are considered to have sepsis or meningitis until proven otherwise.
- Toxic appearing febrile infants < 3 months old have 17% chance of bacterial infections, 11% chance of bacteremia, and 4% chance of meningitis.
- Non-toxic appearing febrile infants < 3 months have 8.6% chance of bacterial infections, 2% chance of bacteremia, and 1% chance of meningitis.
- Febrile children between 3 and 36 months have a 4.3% chance of bacteremia.
- The risk for bacteremia is directly related to the age of patient and elevation of the WBC count (leucocytosis).

Serious Febrile Diseases

NPLEX
MCCQE
USMLE

Infectious diseases typically present as a febrile condition; however, in neonates, immune-compromised patients, patients with chronic renal insufficiency, and elderly patients, infectious diseases usually do not present as a febrile condition.

Serious Febrile Presentations:

- Progressive acute fever > 38.9C/102F (oral)
- Persistent fever for 3 weeks or longer
- Toxic appearance of patient (especially in pediatric presentations), altered consciousness, persistent vomiting, diarrhea with tenesmus, convulsions, lethargy, anorexia, or poor feeding, as well as the signs of sepsis (e.g., respiratory distress, temperature instability, jaundice, and apnea)
- Significant increases in WBC counts (e.g., leucocytosis, lymphocytosis)
- Infants:
  - Bulging or tightness of anterior fontanelle
  - Nuchal rigidity, Brudzinski's, or Kernig's signs

Normal Body Temperature

NPLEX

Bickley,
2003

Dains,
2011

Because body temperature follows a normal daily variation, instead of referring to the usually quoted 37C or 98.9F absolute as a measure of normal, practitioners need to be aware of the following normal ranges:
  1. Oral temperature: 35.8 to 37.3C (96.4 to 99.1F)
  2. Rectal temperature: 36.3 to 37.8C (97.2 to 99.9F)
  3. Tympanic temperature: 36.6 to 38.1C (97.7 to 100.4F)
  4. Axillary temperature: 34.8 to 36.3C (94.8 to 97.5F)

Source

Cause of Fever

Fever can be caused by three distinct pathophysiological processes:

1. Hypothalamic set point elevation: infections, collagen disease, vascular disease, and malignancy trigger the hypothalamus to reset core body temperature. Subsequently, there is elevation of T-lymphocytes and increased effectiveness of interferons.

Dains, 2011

2. Excessive heat production despite normal heat loss: hyperthyroidism, hyperthermia, and aspirin overdose usually lead to elevation of basal metabolic rate beyond the normal capacity of heat-loss mechanisms. Antipyretic agents are not effective in managing this type of fever.
3. Defective heat loss despite normal heat production: burns, heat stroke, overbundling a child, anticholinergic overdose, and ectodermal dysplasia often lead to decreased efficiency of heat-loss mechanisms. Again, antipyretic agents would not be effective in managing this type of fever.

Measurement Methods:

- In infants under 3 months of age, rectal temperatures are required. Pediatric clinical guidelines unanimously use rectal temperature ranges.
- Axillary and thermal-tape skin temperatures are not considered accurate enough for clinical management.
- Tympanic (auditory canal) and temporal artery temperature are gaining acceptance as quick and comfortable methods of recording body temperature for children and adolescents.
- Remember to follow the appropriate reference range of your method of choice.

NPLEX
MCCQE
USMLE

Fever Without Identifiable Source (FWS)

History:

- Onset, duration, and pattern of fever
- Alertness
- Hydration status
- Illness in other household members
- Immunizations, blood transfusions, HIV
- Exposure to animals
- Heat exposure
- Last Tylenol given
- History of febrile seizures
- Birth, family, and past medical history
- Child's social and home environment

Physical Exam:

- Vital signs
- Use standard evaluation scales, such as the Yale Observation Scale
- Nuchal rigidity (which is common in meningitis in infants under 3 months old)
- Check eyes for conjunctivitis (watch for bilateral injection in Kawasaki Disease)

Source

- Examine ears, nose, throat, and sinuses
- Check for lymphadenopathy
- Skin exam (watch for roseola between 6 and 36 months)
- Assess lungs and heart
- Assess for suprapubic and CVA tenderness
- Rule out UTI
- Rule out arthritis, osteomyelitis and meningitis

Guidelines for Naturopathic Antipyretic and Diaphoretic Botanical Remedies

NPLEX

Yarnell, 2000

Saunders, 2000

- *Achilia millefolium*
- *Eupatorium perfoliatum*
- *Filipendula ulmaria*
- *Pimpinella anisum*
- *Populus tremloides*
- *Salix alba/nigra*
- *Tilia europa*

MICROBIAL INFECTIONS

Principles of Antimicrobial Therapy

NPLEX
MCCQE
USMLE

Assessment of Benefit and Risk: Selection of antibiotics should be guided by comparing the potential harms from the presenting illness versus those of the pharmacological agent.
- Like most pharmacological agents, antimicrobials may have various side effects.
- The severity of the illness, immune status of the host, previous adverse reactions, allergies, pregnancy or breast-feeding status, and other medications the patient is taking must also be considered.
- Clinicians should identify the causative organism (through culture and sensitivity testing) of infectious presentations to improve the outcome of treatment.
- However, in outpatient settings, it may not be practical to wait for C&S results before implementing time-sensitive treatment. A prudent approach is to start addressing infectious diseases by using antimicrobial agents that are empirically recommended for particular conditions, and then refine the selection based on C&S results.

Antimicrobial Drugs for Treating Bacterial Pathogens

Condition	Usual Causative Organism(s)	Antimicrobial(s) of choice	Alternatives	Background Information
Typical Pneumonia	*Streptococcus pneumoniae*	Penicillin	Cephalosporin (1st or 3rd gen) Erythromycin Vancomycin	Some S. *pneumoniae* are penicillin resistant; 30% of H. *influenza* is aminopenicillin resistant. Erythromycin is only used in mild infections. Vancomycin is reserved for serious infections.
	Haemophilus influenzae	Ampicillin or Amoxicillin		
Atypical Pneumonia	*Mycoplasma Chlamydia pneumoniae trachomatis*	Erythromycin	Tetracycline Cephalosporin (3rd generation)	Although tetracycline is as effective as macrolides (erythromycin), the latter covers *Pneumococcus*, which mimics *Mycoplasma*.
AIDS Pneumonia	*Pneumocystis jiroveci (PCP)*	TMP-SMZ	Pentamidine	In AIDS (i.e., HIV +ve patient with CD4 < 200). PJP is the most common opportunistic infection.
	Cytomegalovirus (CMV)	Ganciclovir	Foscarnet	
Tuberculosis	*Mycobacterium tuberculosis*	Isoniazid + Rifampicin + Ethambutol	Streptomycin Flouroquinolone Cycloserine Clarithromycin Capreomycin	Isoniazid and rifampin should be given for 6-12 months duration. Add ethambutol in immune-compromised patients. Isoniazid is used for preventive therapy.
Bacterial Bronchitis	*Mycoplasma pneumoniae Haemophilus influenzae*	Amoxicillin or Erythromycin	Cephalosporin (3rd generation) Cholramphenicol	Although tetracycline is as effective as the macrolides (erythromycin), the latter covers *Pneumococcus*, which mimics *Mycoplasma*.

Condition	Usual Causative Organism(s)	Antimicrobial(s) of choice	Alternatives	Background Information
Urinary Tract Infection	*Escherichia coli*	TMP-SMZ (supersulfa) or Nitrofurantoin	Ciprofloxacin Gentamicin	Beta-lactam antibiotics (penicillins and cephalosporins) are less effective than TMP-SMZ, nitrofurantoin, and ciprofloxacin.
Osteomyelitis	*Staphylococcus aureus* *Salmonella sp.*	Antistaphylo-coccal penicillin (e.g., Methicillin)	Cephalosporin (1st generation) Vancomycin	Vancomycin is required for Methicillin-resistant *Staph. aureus* (MRSA).
Cellulitis	*Staphylococcus aureus* *Streptococcus pneumoniae*	Antistaphylo-coccal Penicillin	Cephalosporin (1st generation) Vancomycin	Antistaphylococcal penicillins, such as flucloxacillin, target both causative organisms.
Meningitis (in neonates)	*Streptococcus B* *Escherichia coli* *Listeria monocytogenes*	Ampicillin +Gentamicin	Vancomycin Cephalosporin (3rd generation)	Vancomycin is an alternative for ampicillin, but should still be combined with gentamicin.
Meningitis (children & adults)	*Streptococcus pneumoniae* *Neisseria meningitidis*	Amoxicillin+ Chloramphenicol	Penicillin Cephalosporin (3rd generation)	*Haemophilus influenzae* is the most likely cause of childhood meningitis, if there is no history of immunization.
Sepsis	*Enterococcus sp.* *Streptococci* *Staphylococci*	Penicillin or Ampicillin+ Streptomycin	Cephalosporin (3rd generation) + Gentamicin	There are some *Enterococci* sensitive to synergism with streptomycin, but not with gentamicin. Some strains are resistant to both types of aminoglycosides.
Septic arthritis	*Staphylococcus aureus* *Neisseria gonorrhea*	Antistaphylo-coccal Penicillin Cephalosporin (3rd generation)	Vancomycin (for MRSA) Ciprofloxacin	*Neisseria gonorrhea* should be suspected in any patient who is sexually promiscuous (especially younger adults).

Source

NPLEX
MCCQE
USMLE

Dains,
2011

Sputum Characteristics in Cough Presentations

Characteristics	Common Etiology
Malodorous sputum	Anaerobic infection of the lungs and sinuses
Brown or black	Smoking
Very thick, dark sputum that is hard to expectorate	Bronchiectasis
Cloudy thick sputum	Lower respiratory tract infection or sequelae of asthmatic process (i.e., due to manifesting esinophila)
Scanty mucopurulent sputum (less than 2 tbsp/day)	Viral or low grade bacterial bronchitis
Purulent sputum more than 2 tbsp/day	Bacterial bronchitis
Hemoptysis	Bacterial pneumonia, acute inflammatory bronchitis, cystic fibrosis, tumor, or foreign body.

NPLEX
MCCQE
USMLE

Classic Infections

Infection	Presentation	Probable Cause
Pneumonia	In a malnourished patient or in patients who exhibit silicosis. Also in immigrants or after recent ravel to a developing country.	*Mycobacterium tuberculosis*
	After recent travel to Southwest U.S.A. (Arizona, New Mexico, and southern California) and northern Mexico.	*Coccidioides immitis*
	In cave explorers (bird or bat droppings) or after recent travel to Midwest United States (Ohio and Mississippi River valleys)	*Histoplasma capsulatum*
	After exposure to parrots or exotic bird's droppings	*Chlamydia psittaci*
	After spending time in a low-budget centrally air-conditioned hotel	*Legionella pneumophila*

Infection	Presentation	Probable Cause
Acute Diarrhea	After hiking trips and drinking from streams	*Giardia lamblia*
	After travel to Mexico	Montezuma's revenge caused by *Escherichia coli*
	After antibiotics (especially clindamycin)	*Clostridium difficile*
	In young children	Norwalk virus
	Food poisoning after eating improperly stored meats or custard-filled pastries (profuse non-bloody diarrhea with cramping and vomiting)	*Staphylococcus aureus*
	Food poisoning after eating raw seafood	*Vibrio parahaemolyticus*
	Food poisoning after eating reheated rice	*Bacillus cereus*
	Food poisoning after ingestion of improperly preserved food, poultry or eggs (bloody diarrhea with cramping and vomiting)	*Salmonella sp.*
	Profuse painful & bloody diarrhea after ingesting contaminated water or food	*Entamoeba histolytica*
	Bloody diarrhea after anal sex (fecal-oral transmission)	*Shigella sp.*
	Bloody diarrhea in day care settings	*Shigella sp.*
	Profuse watery diarrhea that is painless; Rice-water diarrhea that occurs after ingestion of contaminated water or seafood.	*Vibrio cholera*
	Hemolytic uremic syndrome	*Escherichia coli* 0157:H7
Hemoptysis	After 'resolved' tuberculosis Cavitary lesion on CXR	*Aspergillus sp.*
Abscess	After getting stuck with a thorn	*Sporothrix schenckii*
Vesicular genital lesions	Without recent sexual activity (umbilicated)	*Molluscum contagiosum*

Source	Infection	Presentation	Probable Cause
	Cellulitis	After cat or dog bite	*Pasteurella multocida*
	Pregnant woman	Lives with cats	*Toxoplasma gondii*
	Aplastic crisis	In a patient with sickle cell disease	Parvovirus B19
	Burn site infection	Purulent with blue/green color	*Pseudomonas arginosa*
	Burn site infection	Purulent with yellow color	*Staphylococcus aureus*
	UTI	With green urine	*Pseudomonas arginosa*
	UTI	Without green urine	*Escherichia coli*
	Reiter's Syndrome and Lympho-granuloma venereum		*Chlamydia trachomatis*

Guidelines for Naturopathic Botanical Antimicrobials

NPLEX

Yarnell,
2000
Saunders,
2000

Antibacterial	Antiviral	Antiparasitic	Antifungal
Allium sativum	*Allium sativum*	*Allium sativum*	*Berberis aquifolium*
Arctostaphylos uva ursi	*Astragalus membranaceus*	*Artemisia absinthium*	*Calendula officinalis*
Baptisia tinctoria	*Echinacea spp.*	*Artemisia annua*	*Chilopsis linearis*
Berberis aquifolium	*Glycyrrhiza glabra*	*Berberis aquifolium*	*Commiphora molmol*
Capsicum spp.	*Hypericum perforatum*	*Chenopodium ambrosoides*	*Melaleuca alternifolia*
Commiphora molmol	*Larrea tridentate*	*Cucurbita pepo*	*Tabebuia avellanedae*
Coptis chinensis	*Lentinus edodes*	*Dryopteris filix-mas*	*Thymus vulgaris*
Echinacea spp.	*Ligusticum porterii*	*Hydrastis canadensis*	*Usnea barbata*
Grapefruit seed extract	*Lomatium dissectum*	*Juglans nigra*	
Hydrastis canadensis	*Melissa officinalis*	*Picrasma excelsa*	
Ligusticum porterii	*Phyllanthus spp.*	*Ricinus communis*	
Ligustrum lucidum	*Populus candicans*	*Tanacetum vulgare*	

Antibacterial	Antiviral	Antiparasitic	Antifungal	Source
Lomatium dissectum	Salvia officinalis	Verbena spp.		
Rosmarinus officinalis	Silybum marianum	Zingiber officinalis		
Salvia officinalis	Tabebuia avellanedae			
Tabebuia avellanedae	Uncaria tomentosa			
Tussilago farfara	Zingiber officinalis			
Thymus vulgaris				
Uncaria guyanensis				
Usnea barbata				

Guidelines for Naturopathic Botanical Anti-inflammatories

NPLEX

Saunders, 2000

Yarnell, 2000

Phytotherapeutic Agent	Background Information
Achillia millefolium	Gentle anti-inflammatory and antipyretic. Clinical trial showed that combination of 100 mg Filipendula + 90 mg Populus + 60 mg Achillia had the same efficacy as 400 mg Ibuprofen on severe OA (reported to have fewer S/E). Used in febrile condition and diarrheal presentations.
Boswellia serrata	Inhibits 5- but not 12-lipoxygenase/cycloxygenase. Used in arthritis and ulcerative colitis.
Calendula officinalis	Anti-inflammatory and vulnerary. Used in proctitis, colitis, anal fistulas (with Echinacea and Commiphora), PUD, URI, and wound dressing.
Camellia sinensis	Antioxidant, stimulates B-cell regeneration. Used in atherosclerosis, hyperlipidemia, elevated liver enzymes, and dental caries.
Curcuma longa	Inhibits 5- and 12-lipoxygenase/cycloxygenase. Used primarily for musculoskeletal inflammation.
Filipendula ulmaria	Similar to Salix nigra. Used in febrile conditions, rheumatic disease, hyperchlorhydria, GERD, and diarrheal presentations.
Glycyrrhiza glabra	Anti-inflammatory, inhibits T-suppressor lymphocytes, inhibits endogenous cortisol degradation; bactericidal towards H. Pylori, and is an antioxidant. Used in inflammatory conditions in the GI, respiratory, or GU tract.

Source	*Phytotherapeutic Agent*	*Background Information*
	Larrea tridentata	Antimicrobial, anti-inflammatory. Used for skin injuries, PMS, rheumatic disease, and autoimmune diseases.
	Matricaria recutita	Antispasmodic, anti-inflammatory, anxiolytic, and carminative. Used in oral mucositis, chronic GI inflammation (e.g., esophagitis, PUD, and IBD), stasis ulcers (with plantago lanceolata), wounds, and atopic dermatitis.
	Salix alba/nigra	Antipyretic, analgesic. Used in febrile conditions, OA, RA, prostatitis, urethritis and cystitis.

Morrison, 1998

Homeopathic Remedies for Infectious Diseases

Presentation	Remedy of Choice and Background Information
Pharyngitis and Tonsillitis	
Rapid onset of inflammation and burning sensation. Bright red swollen mucosa; with visible aphthae; strawberry tongue; high fever; flushed face; cold extremities.	*Belladonna:* the most commonly used remedy for acute tonsillitis with rapid onset. Also considered a remedy for peritonsillar abscess. Mainly right sided complaints.
Exquisite sharp throat pain, commonly described as splinters in the throat. There may be ulceration on the throat; pain radiates to ears on swallowing.	*Hepar Sulphur:* used for more advanced pharyngitis and suppurative tonsillitis. One of the main remedies for peritonsillar abscess.
Tonsils are swollen, mucosa is deep red or purple; uvula is swollen; advanced cases exhibit ulceration, excoriation, and bleeding. Sensation of a lump or constriction in the throat. Mainly left-sided.	*Lachesis:* used for mild sore throats as well as serious inflammation and peritonsillar abscess. Mainly left-sided complaints.
Suppurative pharyngitis with offensive halitosis 'sick breath'; sensation of something lodged in the throat; metallic taste in the mouth; night sweats, and cervical lymphadenopathy.	*Mercurius Vivus:* used for suppurative pharyngitis, acute or recurring pharyngitis, or tonsillitis of any severity.
Urinary Tract Infections	
Intense burning with urination; each drop feels like scalding acid as it passes. The patient feels that emptying the bladder will bring relief.	*Cantharis:* used for mild or moderate urethritis and cystitis. This remedy is prescribed when pain is the main symptom.
Constant urging and full sensation, but only small, non-satisfying amounts are passed.	*Nux Vomica:* used in renal colic, cystitis, and pyelonephritis. This remedy is prescribed when frequent urging is the main symptom.

Presentation	Remedy of Choice and Background Information
Intense itching or tingling deep in the urethra; sudden intense urges to urinate; pain if the patient cannot void immediately.	*Petroselinum:* prescribed when urethral itching or irritation is the main symptom.
Sudden urges to void with no capacity to hold back the urine. Involuntary urination; pain increases every moment voiding is resisted.	*Pulsatilla:* prescribed when the pain is irregular, paroxysmal, or with spurting. Indicated when urine is copious, bloody, and mucousy.
Copious urination with marked burning pain at the end of micturition; pain occurs only with the last few drops.	*Sarsparilla:* prescribed when the main symptom is pain at the end of voiding.

Impetigo

Sores become crusted, cracked, and eventually thickened. Oozing of thin, smelly, or sometimes honey-like discharge.	*Antimonium Crudum:* the most commonly prescribed remedy for acute and recurring cases of impetigo. Location – face, corners of mouth, or nose.
Thick crusts, characteristic honey-like discharge, itching, and prompt suppuration.	*Graphites:* Location – intertriginous areas, mouth, or behind ears.
Moist eruptions or pustules over an erythematous base.	*Mercurius:* Location – scalp or face.
Moist eruptions (as opposed to the above dry and crusty variety), large coalescing pustules, surrounded by erythema, seen in neglected wounds or poor hygiene.	*Sulphur:* may be indicated in skin infections where the eruption itches or burns.

Fungal Infections

Patches of scaly dry skin that are somewhat itchy; tinea versicolor.	*Sepia:* the most commonly prescribed remedy for skin conditions exhibiting scaly round patches.
Ringworm on the scalp; tinea corporis	*Calcarea Carbonica, Dulcamara,* or *Radium bromatum*
Fungal infections of toenails; thick, hard, yellow, friable nails. Also a remedy for tinea pedis.	*Graphites:* used for moist, crusty eruption with thick borders.
Tinea pedis or cruris with excessive exudate. Burning athlete's foot infections.	*Sulphur:* used for markedly itchy tinea cruris, especially when intertriginous areas are erythematous.

Source

Presentation	Remedy of Choice and Background Information
Abscesses	
Abscess continues to discharge for weeks after opening; creamy yellow discharge; fistula formation.	*Calacarea sulphurica:* recommended for chronic abscess formation and hydradenitis suppurativa.
Crops of slowly developing abscesses and indurated boils. Also used in bartholinitis; paronychia; and nape carbuncles.	*Silica:* indicated for abscesses developing around retained foreign bodies.
Recurring boils in patients with poor hygiene; yellow offensive discharge.	*Sulphur:* indicated for recurring boils anywhere in the body.
Painful abscess that is exquisitely sensitive to touch; recurring crops of abscesses with offensive discharge 'old cheese'.	*Hepar Sulphur:* the main remedy for paronychia and also recommended for hydradenitis.
Infectious Conjunctivitis	*Pulsatilla, Argenticum nitricum, Euphrasia,* or *Graphitus*
Acute Otitis Media	*Chamomilia, Belladonna, Ferrum phosphoricum, Hepar,* or *Mercurius*
Chronic Otitis Media	*Pulsatilla, Mercurius, Graphites, Calcarea carbonica,* or *Lycopodium*

NPLEX

Probiotic Therapy

Dains, 2003

Non-pathogenic symbiotic flora, known as probiotics, are touted for their protective effect on the tissues they colonize (e.g., GI, bladder, and vagina). Probiotics generally exhibit a dose-response relationship, where the observed effect depends of the dose administered (2.5-20 billion organisms per day) and is somewhat reversible. The bulk of published evidence suggests that the use of probiotics in management of infectious or inflammatory presentations is safe at any age and can be synergistically combined with herbal or pharmaceutical antimicrobial therapy.

Types of Probiotics: Several types of probiotics have been the subject of rigorous studies over the past few years:
- *Lactobacillus acidophilus*
- *L. sporogenes*
- *L. Casei, L. rhamnosus*
- *Bifidobacterium bifidus*
- *Saccharomyces boulardii*

Yarnell, 2000

Mechanism of Action: The actual mechanism of action appears to be a complex interplay between the following functions:
1. Spatial competition with pathogenic strains for adherence sites (crowding)

2. Resource competition with pathogenic strains for food (competitive inhibition)
3. Secretion of antimicrobial mediators (such as bacteriocins)
4. Gut-associated lymphoid tissue modulation (systemic immune response modification)
5. Inducing mucus secretion
6. Support intestinal integrity and permeability

Conditions for Probiotic Therapy:

Condition	Published Evidence
Antibiotic-induced diarrhea	*Saccharomyces boulardii* was effective for treatment and prevention.
Pseudomembranous colitis	*Saccharomyces boulardii* was effective in prevention treatment of chronic and recurrent *Clostridium difficile* colitis. *Saccharomyces boulardii and Lactobacillus spp* better the outcome of treatment when combined with antibiotics.
Infectious diarrhea	*Lactobaccilus casei* was effective in viral (rotavirus) and vaccination-induced diarrhea. Positive evidence also exists for vancomycin-resistant *Enterococcus faecalis* infection, GI *Staphylococcal* infection, *Shigella*, Salmonella, pathogenic *Escherichia coli*, and *Campylobacter jejuni*.
Traveler's diarrhea	Mixed evidence; positive studies prevail.
Inflammatory bowel disease (IBD)	*Saccharomyces boulardii* was helpful in relieving chronic diarrhea in patients with Crohn's disease. Various other probiotics have induced and maintained remission in ulcerative colitis patients (e.g., non-pathiogenic *E. coli*).
Irritable bowel syndrome (IBS)	Mixed evidence; negative studies prevail.
Lactose intolerance	Negative studies with lactic acid bacteria (theoretical hypothesis).
Increase intestinal permeability	Probiotics have a normalizing effect on enterocyte permeability.
Aphthous ulcers	*Lactobacillus acidophilus* is promising.
Infectious vaginitis	Oral and topical probiotics have shown efficacy in treatment and prevention of bacterial vaginosis.
Hyperlipidemia	*Lactobacillus sporogenes, Enterococcus faecum,* and *Streptococcus thermophilus* may play a future role in LDL reduction.
Atopic dermatitis	Probiotics have reduced severity in infants.
Food allergy	Trials suggest that probiotics may decrease food allergies.

Condition	Published Evidence
Bladder cancer	Two studies suggest that *Lactobaccilus casei* can reduce the rate of recurrence of urinary bladder cancer.
Cystic fibrosis	Probiotics have reduced the incidence of pulmonary infection in one trial

- Probiotic efficacy and effective dosing appear to be condition-specific. Consult a protocol manual or review publications for appropriate use.
- Please note that some severely immune compromised patients have developed probiotic sepsis.

Examination Board References

NPLEX (II): North American Board of Naturopathic Examiners
Naturopathic Physician Licensing Examination Part II (NPLEx II) Blueprint. Portland, OR: North American Board of Naturopathic Examiners (NABNE), 2010.

USMLE: National Board of Medical Examiners
Brochert A. Crush Step 3. The Ultimate USMLE Step 3 Review. 3rd ed. New York, NY: Saunders, Elsevier, 2008.

MCCQE: Medical Council of Canada
Dugani S, Lam D, eds. 2009. MCCQE Review Notes & Lecture Series. Medical Counsel of Canada Qualification Examination Review Notes. Toronto, ON: McGraw Hill Professional, Canadian edition, 2009.

Related References

Bickley LS, Szilagyi PG. Bates' Guide to Physical Examination & History Taking. Philadelphia, PA: Lippincott, Williams & Wilkins, 2003.

Canadian Pharmaceutical Association. Compendium of Pharmaceuticals & Specialties (CPS). Toronto, ON: Canadian Pharmaceutical Association, 2004.

Dains J, Baumann L, Scheibel P. 2003. Advanced Health Assessment & Clinical Diagnosis in Primary Care. 2nd ed. St. Louis, MI: Mosby C.V. Co. Ltd., 2003.

Dains J, Baumann L, Scheibel P. Advanced Health Assessment & Clinical Diagnosis in Primary Care. 4th ed. St Louis, MO: Mosby C.V. Co. Ltd., 2011.

Dawson JS. Pharmacology. Crash Course Series. Philadelphia, PA. Mosby/Elsevier Science Ltd, 2002.

Morrison R. Desktop Companion to Physical Pathology. Nevada City, CA: Hahnemann Clinic Publishing, 1998.

Ontario Health Protection and Promotion Act. Regulation 559/91 and amendments.

Pizzorno JE, Murray MT. 1999. Textbook of Natural Medicine. Vol. 1and 2. 2nd ed. New York, NY: Churchill Livingstone, 1999.

Pizzorno JE, Murray MT. Textbook of Natural Medicine. 3rd ed. New York, NY: Churchill Livingstone, Elsevier, 2006.

Saunders, PR. Herbal Remedies for Canadians. Toronto, ON: Prentice Hall-Pearson Canada Inc., 2000.

Yarnell E. Naturopathic Gastroenterology. Scottsdale, AZ: Naturopathic Medical Press, 2000.

NEPHROLOGY

RENAL FAILURE

NEPHROTIC SYNDROME

GLOMERULONEPHRITIS

PYELONEPHRITIS

NEPHROLITHIASIS

RHABDOMYLOSIS

RENAL FAILURE

Presentation

Loss of kidney function due to any number of reasons. Renal failure can be acute or chronic and is classified as prerenal, renal/intrarenal, or postrenal. Azotemia, which is defined as excess blood urea (BUN) or nitrogenous waste (creatinine), is the hallmark of loss of kidney function.

Acute Renal Failure

Rapid and progressive elevation of blood urea (BUN) with or without oliguria (oliguria =daily excretion of < 500 ml of urine). This condition is fatal in 40% of cases.

Signs and Symptoms:
- Edema, HTN, CHF
- Urine output may be completely arrested (anuria) or diminished (oliguria) or normal

Laboratory findings that warrant referral to emergency care:
1. Progressive rise in serum creatinine
2. Urinalysis: RBCs, WBCs, proteinuria, and casts
3. CBC: normochromic normocytic anemia

Prerenal Failure

- Prerenal implies that the kidney is not adequately perfused. This may be secondary to hypovolemia (dehydration or hemorrhage), sepsis, heart failure, liver failure, or renal artery stenosis.
- BUN: Creatinine ratio will be >15-20.
- There will also be systemic signs of hypovolemia = tachycardia, weak pulse, loss of skin turgor (tenting), and depressed fontanelle in infants.

Treatment: Address the cause:
- Rehydrate (IV fluids)
- Treat CHF
- Support the liver
- Balloon dilation of stenotic renal arteries if present (PCD review: renal artery bruit)

Postrenal Failure

Urinary excretion is somehow blocked at the ureters, prostate, or urethra (i.e., distal to the kidneys).

Cause: Most common cause is benign prostatic hypertrophy (BPH). Nephrolithiasis will not produce postrenal failure unless stones exist bilaterally (rare).

Source

Signs and Symptoms:
- Patient is male >50 years of age with hesitancy, frequency, and dribbling on urination.
- In men and women, diagnostic ultrasound will reveal bilateral hydronephrosis.

Treatment:
- Acute treatment involves catheterization to prevent further renal damage.
- Then, a more permanent solution needs to be sought (such as transurethral prostatic resection or naturopathic treatment).

Intrarenal Failure

NPLEX
USMLE

Causes:
- Failure lies within the kidney.
- Basically, anything that causes tubular necrosis will lead to intrarenal failure.

Medications that Commonly Cause Renal Insufficiency or Failure

NPLEX
MCCQE
USMLE

Cohen,
2010

- Chronic use of NSAIDs may cause papillary necrosis and thus chronic renal failure.
- Women are 3 to 5 times more likely to develop this side effect.
- Cyclosporine and Methotrexate (immune suppressants used in psoriasis, rheumatoid arthritis, SLE, organ transplantation)
- Aminoglycosides (antibiotics known for their nephrotoxicity, such as gentanicin, neomycin, streptomycin).
- Cisplatin (chemotherapeutic agent used in small cell carcinoma, lymphoma, and germ cell tumors)
- Amphotericin (antifungal agent used intravenously for systemic infections)
- Radiocontrast media
- Furosemide (diuretic)
- Proton Pump Inhibitors (PPIs), e.g., omeprazole (Losec, Prilosec), lansoprazole (Prevacid), esomeprazole (Nexium)

Goodpasture's Syndrome

NPLEX
MCCQE
USMLE

Signs and Symptoms: A young man with hemoptysis, dyspnea, and hematuria (possibly renal failure, too).

Cause: Anti-glomerular basement membrane antibody. This antibody cross-reacts with lung and kidney parenchyma.

Treatment: Since the cause of this serious autoimmune condition is unknown, the recommended conventional treatment is cyclophosphamide + steroids.

Source

NPLEX
MCCQE
USMLE

Chronic Renal Failure (CRF)

Chronic Renal Failure Symptoms:

Early
- Nocturia, lassitude, fatigue, and decreased mental activity

Intermediate
- Bad taste in mouth
- Nausea and vomiting
- Stomatitis and diarrhea
- Muscle twitches and cramps
- Peripheral neuropathies
- Anorexia

Advanced
- GI ulcers and bleeding
- Yellow/brown skin
- Generalized tissue wasting
- Uremic frost on skin with pruritus
- HTN, CHF, acidosis, and anemia

Labs
- Azotemia
- Metabolic acidosis
- Hyperkalemia
- Waxy casts
- Anemia (due to lack of erythropoietin)
- Hypocalcemia and hyperphosphatemia (due to impaired vitamin D production, which in turn leads to bone demineralization)

Causes: Any cause of acute renal failure may lead to chronic failure if the insult is severe or prolonged. The following are the main causes of CRF worldwide:
- 40%: Glomerulonephritis (you will see RBC casts in urinalysis)
- 10% to 16%: Chronic pyelonephritis (you will see WBC casts in urinalysis)
- 14%: Hypertension and coronary artery disease
- 7% to 8%: Polycystic kidney disease
- 7%: Diabetes
- In developed countries, the etiology of CRF shifts toward diabetes and then hypertension. Polycystic kidney disease contribution to CRF remains unchanged.
- Polycystic kidney disease (= hypertension, hematuria, palpable renal masses, multiple cysts in the kidneys, berry aneurysms in the circle of Willis, and cysts in the liver), an autosomal recessive disease, is almost always diagnosed in children.

Risk Assessment

NFK, 2000

National Kidney Foundation (NKF), 2000, recommends assessing risk of CRF in all patients, but testing for markers of kidney damage and GFR only in individuals at increased risk.

Source

Gonzales,
2009

Risk Factors for CRF:
- Diabetes
- HTN
- Autoimmune dz
- Systemic infxn
- UTI
- Uurinary stones
- Uurinary obstruction
- FHx of CRF
- PHMx of acute RF
- Medications (see above)
- Old age

NPLEX

Chronic Renal Failure Treatment

Dugani,
2009
Csiky, 2010
Fatouris,
2010
Seherli,
2008
Kang,
2009

Regardless of the cause, the recommended treatment for CRF is as follows. This comprehensive and demanding regimen is usually adopted until kidney transplantation can be arranged.
1. Regular hemodialysis 3X per week
2. Water-soluble vitamin supplements (because they are lost in dialysis)
3. Phosphate restriction
4. Calcium supplementation
5. Erythropoietin administration
6. Hypertension treatment

First-line Naturopathic Treatment of Chronic Renal Failure

- L-carnitine: 500-1000 mg t.i.d. improves exercise capacity, enhances antioxidant status and may prevent cardiovascular complications associated with CRF.
- Alpha-lipoic acid: 200 mg t.i.d. May improve renal function by reducing inflammation and oxidative damage.
- *Ginkgo biloba* and *Withania somnifera*: shown to improve renal function in experimental models of renal failure. This is likely due to their antioxidant properties.

NEPHROTIC & NEPHRITIC SYNDROMES

NPLEX
MCCQE
USMLE

Nazarenko,
2003
Naidu,
2000
Jeyanthi,
2009

Presentation: Nephrotic Syndrome

A descriptive term meaning: proteinuria >3.5gm/day + central edema + hypo-albuminemia + hyper-lipidemia + lipiduria. It is a manifestation of glomerular disease, which may be immune mediated or metabolic. Establish diagnoses by measuring 24-hour urine protein.

Source

Causes:
- In children, it is usually due to minimal change disease secondary to an infection.
- In adults, it is most commonly due to membranous nephropathy (idiopathic or secondary to hepatitis B or SLE), diabetes, and amyloidosis, or as a side effect of medications (e.g., penicillamine, captopril, or gold).

Presentation: Nephritic Syndrome

NPLEX
MCCQE
USMLE

A descriptive term meaning: oliguria + azotemia + hematuria + hypertension. It may be accompanied with proteinuria, but not in the nephrotic range (see above). It is a manifestation of glomerulonephritis that is severe enough to obstruct glomerular capillaries, leading to renal hypoperfusion.

Causes:

Sisson,
2007

- In children, it is usually due to acute post-streptococcal-glomerulonephritis (Note that treatment of strep reduces prevalence of secondary rheumatic complications but it does not seem to alter prevalence of nephritic syndrome).
- In adults, the causes are:
  - Goodpasture's syndrome (see above)
  - Wegener's granulomatosis (vasculitis that affects kidneys, nose, and lungs)
  - IgA nephropathy (see below)
  - SLE (refer to Rheumatology module)
  - Idiopathic

Treatment depends on the cause:
- Treat all presenting infections, recommend (penicillin, erythromycin) for strep infections
- Manage hypertension according to guidines
- Manage autoimmune disease and consider immune suppression in progressive cases

GLOMERULONEPHRITIS

Acute Glomerulonephritis

NPLEX
MCCQE
USMLE

Signs and Symptoms: Typically patients are children with a history of upper respiratory tract infection 1 to 3 weeks before.
- Edema
- Hypervolemia
- Hypertension
- Hematuria
- Oliguria
- Microscopic urinalysis will show pathognomonic red blood cell casts.

IgA Nephropathy

NPLEX
MCCQE
USMLE

IgA nephropathy disease, also known as Berger disease, is the most commonly diagnosed glomerular disease worldwide. It is due to deposition of IgA around renal mesangial cells (no one knows why

Source

yet). This disease occurs most often in children and young adults. It is typically preceded by a mild respiratory, urinary, or gastrointestinal infection.

Signs and Symptoms: Clinical presentation is mild hematuria and proteinuria without systemic symptoms. However, despite this innocuous initial presentation, the disease is progressive, and approximately 50% of cases will ultimately develop end-stage kidney disease. Diagnosis is confirmed via kidney biopsy.

PYELONEPHRITIS

NPLEX
MCCQE
USMLE

Presentation

Occurs as an ascending UTI caused by *E. coli* in >80% of the time.

Signs and Symptoms:
- High fever
- Shaking chills
- Flank pain
- With or without UTI symptoms

Diagnosis:
- Positive costovertebral angle tenderness (CVA tenderness) and urinalysis.
- Confirm diagnosis with urine and blood cultures.
- In life-threatening conditions, such as this one, empiric treatment should be started while waiting for culture results.
- Look for WBC casts in urinalysis – these are pathognomonic for pyelonephritis.

Kim, 2010

Risk Factors:
- Impaired immune function (e.g., HIV, diabetes).
- Urine flow obstruction (pregnancy, BPH, polycystic kidney, dz, catheters, Vesicoureteral reflux.
- 30% of women with symptomatic bacterium develop pyelonephritis.
- Associated with preterm birth.

NEPHROLITHIASIS

NPLEX
MCCQE
USMLE

Presentation

Signs and Symptoms:
- Severe, intermittent, loin-to-groin unilateral flank pain.
- Most stones (calcium salts type) will be visible on a KUB image (kidney and urinary bladder x-ray), if not, request a renal ultrasound.

Tests: All passed stones should be collected and analyzed by the lab to determine the type and possible prophylactic measures.

Causes of Kidney Stones

For the majority of cases, no single etiology may be found. However, some individuals (stone-formers) appear to be more susceptible than others. The following is a list of underlying disorders that may lead to nephrolithiasis:

- Hypercalcemia: This may be due to hyperparathyroidism or malignancy.
- *Proteus sp.* Infection: *Proteus sp.* are ammonia producing microorganisms associated with stag-horn calculi that fill the renal pelvis (also known on NPLEX boards as struvite stones).
- Hyperuricemia: This may be due to gout or leukemia chemotherapy.
- Cystinuria/aminoaciduria: This condition needs to be considered in stone-formers (recurrent nephrolithiasis). Diagnose by laboratory assessment of urine as well as any passed stones.

Guidelines for First-line Naturopathic Treatment of Kidney Stones

Approach: Naturopathic treatment is effective, but varies according to stone type. Three distinct treatment guidelines exist for calcium, uric acid, or struvite (struvite is magnesium-ammonium-phosphate) stones. In refractory cases, lithotripsy, ultrasonic resonance dissolution, or endoscopic stone removal is recommended.

Lifestyle
In 85% of cases the risk of stone recurrence could be reduced through lifestyle changes:

- Hydration (adequate for prevention, aggressive for treatment)
- Diet: increase potassium, magnesium, vitamin K intake (fruits + vegetables), reduce animal protein and refined carbohydrates (vegetarians have reduced risk of stone formation)
- Maintain normal BMI
- Physical activity

Calcium Stones
1. Dietary measures
- Reduce urinary calcium and oxalate; increase magnesium.
- Increase consumption of green leafy vegetables.
- Increase high Mg:Ca foods, such as bran, buckwheat, rye, soy, brown rice, avocado, coconut, and lima beans.
- If calcium oxalate is depositing, then it is prudent to also restrict consumption of oxalates (black tea, spinach, cranberry, or nuts).

2. Clinical nutrition
- Vitamin B-6: 25 mg q.d. Reduce production and increase excretion of oxalates.
- Magnesium: 600 mg q.d. Magnesium significantly increases solubility of calcium phosphate and oxalate.
- Calcium: 300-1000 mg q.d. With oxalate stones, calcium supplementation is preventive.

3. Botanical medicine: Empirical approach involves combination therapy using *Hydrangea arborescens, Eupatorium purpurium, Parietaria diffusia,* and *Aphanes arvensis.* It important to note that the anthraquinones in *Rubia tinctura, Rumex crispus,* and *Aloe vera,* in oral doses lower than laxative, bind calcium and act as a urinary crystal inhibiting factor.

Source

Uric Acid Stones

1. Dietary measures

- Restrict consumption of red meat, fish, poultry, and yeast.
- Encourage more complex carbohydrates and green leafy vegetables.

2. Clinical nutrition

- Alkalinize urine using citrate or bicarbonate salts.

3. Botanical Medicine: Empirical approach involves combination therapy using *Hydrangea arborescens*, *Eupatorium purpurium*, *Parietaria diffusia*, and *Aphanes arvensis*.

Struvite Stones

- The critical factor in eliminating these stones is controlling the presenting infection by appropriate identification and tailored treatment. Follow-up assessment is required to ensure eradication.
- Empirically, clinicians recommend acidifying urine with ammonium (or potassium) chloride 100-200 mg t.i.d. and dietary approaches.

RHABDOMYLOSIS

NPLEX
MCCQE
USMLE

Presentation

Due to strenuous exercise (also occurs in burn victims, crush accident victims, and heat stroke), this acute condition produces cellular debris in the blood that plugs the renal filtration system.

Diagnostic Tests: Myoglobinuria (which is detected as hemoglobin in urinalysis) and elevated creatine phosphokinase (CPK) will establish diagnosis.

Treatment: IV hydration (watch the acid-base and electrolytes) and diuretics.

Examination Board References

NPLEX (II): North American Board of Naturopathic Examiners
Naturopathic Physician Licensing Examination Part II (NPLEx II) Blueprint. Portland, OR: North American Board of Naturopathic Examiners (NABNE), 2010.

USMLE: National Board of Medical Examiners
Brochert A. Crush Step 3. The Ultimate USMLE Step 3 Review. 3rd ed. New York, NY: Saunders, Elsevier, 2008.

MCCQE: Medical Council of Canada
Dugani S, Lam D, eds. 2009. MCCQE Review Notes & Lecture Series. Medical Counsel of Canada Qualification Examination Review Notes. Toronto, ON: McGraw Hill Professional, Canadian edition, 2009.

Related References

Cohen D. Acute kidney injury. First Consult Elsevier Inc., 2010. Online at www.mdconsult.com

Csiky B, Nyul Z, Toth G, et al. L-carnitine supplementation and adipokines in patients with end-stage renal disease on regular hemodialysis. Exp Clin Endocrinology Diabetes. 2010;118(10): 735-40.

Cutler P. Problem Solving in Clinical Medicine: From Data to Diagnosis. 3rd ed. Baltimore, MD: Lippincott, Williams & Wilkins Press, 1998

Dains J, Baumann L, Scheibel P. Advanced Health Assessment and Clinical Diagnosis in Primary Care. 2nd ed. St. Louis, MI: Mosby C.V. Co. Ltd, 2003.

Dains J, Baumann L, Scheibel P. Advanced Health Assessment & Clinical Diagnosis in Primary Care. 4th ed. Mosby C.V. Co. Ltd., 2011.

Damjanov I, Conran PB, Goldblatt PJ. Pathology: Rypins' Intensive Reviews. Philadelphia, PA: Lippincott-Raven, 1998.

Hoffmann D. The Complete Illustrated Holistic Herbal. Boston, MA: Elements Books, 1996.

Jeyanthi T, Subramanian P. Nephroprotective effect of Withania somnifera: a dose-dependent study. Renal Failure. 2009;31(9): 814-21.

Kang KP, Kim DH, Jung YJ, et al. Alpha-lipoic acid attenuates cisplatin-induced acute kidney injury in mice by suppressing renal inflammation. Nephrol Dial Transplant. 2009; 24(10):3012-20.

Kim A, Goldberg M, Gulati A, Junes, RC. yelonephritis. First Consult Elsevier Inc., 2010. Online at www.mdconsult.com

Monga M. Nephrolithiasis. First Consult Elsevier Inc, 2009. Online at. www.mdconsult.com

Moore R. Hematology Laboratory Diagnosis. Guelph, ON: McMaster University Press, 2001.

Naidu MU, Shifow AA, Kumar KV, Ratnakar KS. Gingko biloba extract ameliorates gentamicin-induced nephrotoxicity in rats. Phytomedicine. 2000;7(3):191-97.

Nazarenko, ME., Shtygol'Slu, Slobodin, VB. Nephroprotective effect of bilobil in experimental acute kidney failure. Eksp Klin Farmakol. 2003;66(6): 29-31.

Pizzorno JE, Murray MT, Joiner-Bey H.The Clinician's Handbook of Natural Medicine. New York, NY: Churchill Livingstone, 2002.
Pizzorno JE, Murray MT. Textbook of Natural Medicine. 3rd ed. New York, NY: Churchill Livingstone, Elsevier, 2006.

Sehirli O, Sener E, Cetinel S, et al. Alpha-lipoic acid protects against renal ischaemia-reperfusion injury in rats. Clin Exp Pharmacol Physiology. 2008;35(3): 249-55.

Sisson SD, Saver DF, Baustian GH, et al. Nephritic Syndrome. First Consult Elsevier Inc, 2007 Online at www.mdconsult.com

Straub M, Hautmann RE. Developments in stone prevention. Current Opinion in Urology. 2005; 15(2):119-26.

Teichert J, Tuemmers T, Achenback H, et al. Pharmacokinetics of alpha-lipoic acid in subjects with severe kidney damage and end-stage renal disease. Journal of Clinical Pharmacology. 2005;45(3): 313-28.

NEUROLOGY

MOTOR NEURON DISORDERS

HEADACHE

SYNCOPE AND SEIZURES

DEMENTIA

ALZHEIMER DISORDER

PARKINSON'S DISORDER

STROKE & TRANSIENT ISCHEMIC ATTACKS

MOTOR NEURON DISORDERS

Motor Neuron Lesions

Type	Lower MNL	Upper MNL
Causes	Peripheral motor neurons (corticospinal tract) are interrupted beyond the level of decussation	Due an interruption of the same corticospinal tract, but above the level of decussation (brain or cord lesion).
Presentation	Flaccid paralysis; decreased or no reflexes; fasciculations; and muscle atrophy.	Spastic paralysis; hyperreflexia; and clonus.
Babinski's sign	Negative	Positive

- Electromyography (EMG) exhibits fasciculations or fibrillation in LMNL. In contrast, intrinsic muscle diseases exhibit no muscle activity at rest on EMG with decreased amplitude upon stimulation.

Primary Neurological Deficit in Common Neurological Conditions

Loss of motor functions

Amyotrophic Lateral Sclerosis

Botulism – descending paralysis

Huntington's Chorea

Parkinson's Disease

Polymyositis

Tick paralysis – ascending paralysis

Loss of motor and sensory functions

Guillain-Barré syndrome

Multiple Sclerosis

Acute Poliomyelitis

Stroke

Peripheral Neuropathies

Multiple Sclerosis (MS)

An autoimmune demyelinating disease of the CNS.

Signs and Symptoms:
- Symmetric muscle weakness (legs > arms) and clumsiness (GAIT disturbances + trips a lot)
- Paresthesias
- Sudden radiating pain (especially after exposure to heat – showers and baths)
- Visual disturbances (diplopia, blurring, and scotomas)

Source

- More common in white females 20-40 years of age
- Course exhibits characteristic exacerbations, followed by periods of remission
- Other manifestations: emotional lability, scanning speech, and a positive Babinski's sign

Diagnosis:

- Positive diagnosis is suspected when magnetic resonance imaging shows demyelination plaques (MRI is sensitive, but not specific to MS).
- Confirm with CSF analysis (if it shows high levels oligoclonal IgG levels, lymphocytes, and possibly myelin basic protein).

Treatment: Conventional treatment is not considered highly effective. These may include corticosteroids and interferons.

NPLEX

Guideline for First line Naturopathic Treatment of MS

Smolders, 2011
Yadav, 2005
Zhu, 2011

Goal is to reduce relapse and prolong remission. The following therapies are gaining acceptance in the scientific literature.

Clinical Nutrition:

- Vitamin D: $\geq$ 4,000 IU and $\leq$ 40,000 IU q.d.
- Alpha-lipoic acid: 600 mg b.i.d. or 1200 mg qd.
- Other cited therapies are: fish oil, Swank or low-fat diet, green tea extract, and vitamin B-12.

NPLEX
MCCQE
USMLE

Common Neurological Symptoms and Diagnosis

Gradual and Progressive	Sudden or Insidious	Waxes and Wanes	Regressive
Amyotrophic Lateral Sclerosis	Guillain-Barré syndrome	Multiple Sclerosis	Guillain-Barré syndrome
Huntington's Chorea	Multiple Sclerosis Poliomyelitis Polymyositis Stroke Tick paralysis Meniere's disease	Myasthenia Gravis	Poliomyelitis

NPLEX
MCCQE
USMLE

Gullain-Barré Syndrome (GBS)

Presentation:

- Usually presents as symmetric distal weakness or paralysis of the feet and legs (along with paresthesia) with loss of deep tendon reflexes.
- Ascending loss of motor function without significant sensory impairment, which usually occurs 1 week after mild respiratory infections (other infections are also implicated) or immunization.
- Although demyelination is ultimately observed (note that GBS and MS exhibit demyelination), the pathophysiology of this condition remains elusive.

Diagnosis:

- Taking a thorough history and performing a complete neurological assessment usually establishes this diagnosis.
- Confirmatory tests include evoked nerve potential testing (nerve conduction velocity will be slowed) and CSF analysis (markedly increased protein).
- Be on the lookout for respiratory impairment (assess via spirometry), which may require intubation and assisted respiration.

Treatment:

- Plasmapheresis is of value in reducing the severity and overall duration of this self-limiting neurological syndrome.
- It is important to note that steroidal anti-inflammatory agents are contraindicated as they may exacerbate this condition.

Myasthenia Gravis (MG)

Signs and Symptoms:

- Loss of motor function (general muscle fatigability after steady or continued use, ptosis, and diplopia) without any loss of sensory function. The progressive motor impairment is due to autoimmune antibodies that destroy postsynaptic acetylcholine receptors.
- Incidence rates in women (between the ages of 20 and 40 years) are higher than in men (in their 50s).
- Symptoms in women often exacerbate prior to menses and during prenatal or postpartum periods.

Diagnosis:

- Tensilon test (administration of edrophonium, a short acting anticholinesterase inhibitor) establishes diagnosis if it improves the presenting muscle weakness.
- Nerve stimulation tests are also of value in confirming this diagnosis.
- MG patients are prone to developing thymomas and most improve after removal of the thymus, which is considered part of standard conventional treatment (along with long acting acetylcholinesterase inhibitors, such as neostigmine and pyridostigmine).

Amyotrophic Lateral Sclerosis (ALS)

An idiopathic degenerative disease of anterior horn cells. Previously called Lou Gehrig's disease.

Signs and Symptoms:

- ALS = LMNL + UMNL. In other words, you will see spasticity and hyperreflexia (which are characteristic of UMNL) in addition to fasciculations and muscle atrophy (features of LMNL).
- Whenever you are faced with both upper and lower motor neuron lesion signs and symptoms, think of ALS.
- More common in men (in their mid-50s).

Prognosis: The prognosis is poor because the course is progressive and, ultimately, leads to loss of all motor function without dementia or sensory deficits (50% of ALS patients die within 3 years of onset).

Source

Izumi,
2007
Zoccolella,
2010
Graf, 2005
Weighaupt,
2006
Piquet,
2006
Desport,
2000

NPLEX
MCCQE
USMLE

Management Plan

- Pharmacotherapy with Riluzole may slow down progression, but only by about 3-5 months (SE nausea and fatigue).
- Vitamin B-12 in high doses of(50 mg q.d. IM 2x/wk) has been shown to prolong survival time. This may be due to methylcobalamin's ability to reduce homocysteine, shown to be elevated in ALS.
- Vitamin E, melatonin, and vitamin
- Preventing malnutrition (affecting 16-50% of ALS patients) may prolong survival as well

Vitamin Deficiencies

Deficiency	Manifestations
Vitamin B-12	Peripheral neuropathy; loss of vibration sense; loss of position sense; spasticity; ataxia; hyperreflexia; positive Babinski's sign; and dementia.
Vitamin B-6	Peripheral sensory neuropathy (often secondary to the use of isoniazid in anti-tuberculosis therapy).
Thiamine	Confusion; delirium; dementia; peripheral neuropathy; ophthalmoplegia; ataxia; and nystagmus ('dry' beriberi often seen in alcoholics).
Vitamin E	Loss of proprioception; loss of vibration sense; areflexia; ataxia; and gaze palsy.
Vitamin A	Vision loss (night blindness).

NPLEX
MCCQE
USMLE

Botulism

Sudden onset bilateral descending paralysis, common in infants who ingest raw honey or adults who consume home-canned foods. This condition is caused by the neurotoxin of *Clostridium botulinum* bacteria, which flourishes under anaerobic conditions.

Signs and Symptoms:
- In infants, the main presentation of botulism is that of a 'floppy' or 'flaccid' baby.
- In adults, there is usually a prodromal state (N&V, abdominal pain, diarrhea, diplopia, and dysphagia) that precedes frank paralysis.

Diagnosis: Confirmed by identifying *C. botulinum* or its toxin in the stool.

Hoffman,
1996

Treatment: This is an emergency condition that requires inpatient monitoring (for respiratory function) and often involves intubation and assisted respiration (otherwise patients die from respiratory muscle paralysis). This is a self-limiting condition that usually resolves within 1 week of onset with supportive care.

Source
NPLEX
MCCQE
USMLE

Tick Paralysis

A paralytic syndrome caused by toxins from tick bites. History is the key to solving this condition. This presentation is most common in children who play in tick-infested areas.

Signs and Symptoms:
- Flaccid paralysis that progress from proximal to distal
- Areflexia
- Incoordination
- Anorexia
- Without sensory deficits

Treatment: This is a self-limiting condition that subsides approximately 2 days after removal of tick.

HEADACHE

Presentation

NPLEX
MCCQE
USMLE

Serious Headache Signs and Symptoms:
- New onset headache
- Patient describes it as the 'worst headache ever'
- Different and more severe than ever experienced
- Sudden onset of maximal intensity
- Fever, nausea, and vomiting
- Altered level of consciousness
- Focal neurological symptoms
- Recent head injury
- Optic disc edema
- Signs of meningeal irritation
- Progressively worsening headache (crescendo headache)

Types of Headaches: The majority of headaches are classified as benign or primary (i.e., migraine, tension, and cluster). Serious or secondary headaches are manifestations of underlying pathology (i.e., meningitis, temporal arteritis, increased intracranial pressure, tumor, or abscess).

Diagnosis: A systematic approach that involves a thorough history, followed by complaint-oriented physical examination, is paramount to differentiate among the types as well as causes of headaches. Rule out serious and potentially fatal pathologies that may manifest in headaches.

Source	Red Flags in Headache	Clinical Response
	■ Headaches that occur daily with nausea and projectile vomiting, mental status changes, and papilledema.	Beware: these are the signs of intracranial hypertension → Request a CT/MR scan promptly.
	■ Headaches with fever, positive Brudzinski's and/or Kernig's sign	Be concerned: these are the signs of meningeal irritation. → Request lumbar tap (for CSF analysis).
	■ The worst headaches in a patient's life with sudden onset of maximal intensity and/or history of trauma	STAT: these are typical manifestations of subarachnoid hemorrhage. → Request a CT/MR scan and lumbar tap.
	■ Severe temporal headaches with palpatory tenderness over temple and scalp and sudden painless loss of vision	Suspect temporal arteritis (Giant cell arteritis): this is more common in women with history of polymyalgia rheumatica (PMR). If untreated, it leads to blindness in 20% to 25% of cases. → Request ESR, CRP, and temporal artery biopsy.

Migraine, Cluster, and Tension Headache

Migraine
- Classic migraine headaches are associated with an aura (peculiar sensation – noise, smell, or flash of light) that announces to the patient that a migraine is coming.
- Presentation: photophobia, nausea, vomiting, and positive family history. Age of onset is usually between 10 and 30 years of age.

Cluster
- These unilateral excruciating headaches occur in clusters (i.e., few frequent episodes for a week and then none for couple of months).
- Presentation: no prodrome, flushing, diaphoresis, or lacrimation.

Tension
- These 'garden-variety' (most common) headaches usually manifest as bilateral frontal or occipital tenderness.
- Presentation: long history of headaches and stress; feeling of tightness or stiffness; better with stress reduction activities.

Tension Headaches

Causes:
- Eye pain due to optic neuritis; eye strain; refractive errors; glaucoma; and iritis.
- Middle ear pain due to otitis media or mastoiditis
- Sinus pain due to sinusitis or allergic rhinitis
- Herpes zoster infection affecting cranial nerves
- Toothache or oral cavity pain
- Illness or general malaise from any cause
- Food sensitivities: caffeine withdrawal; tyramine; nitrites; MSG; red wine.
- Stress
- Fasting
- Menstruation
- Ovulation

SYNCOPE AND SEIZURES

Source

NPLEX
MCCQE
USMLE

Presentation: Syncope

The most common cause of 'passing-out' is Vasovagal syncope, which usually follows situations of stress or fear. Be concerned if you suspect other more serious causes:

■ If you suspect cardiac arrhythmias or other cardiac pathology (check ECG).
■ If you suspect transient ischemic attacks or carotid stenosis (refer for carotid ultrasound/duplex scan).
■ If you suspect neurological disorders especially seizures or intracranial lesion (request an electroencephalogram 'EEG' and/or CT/MR scan).

Miller,
2005

When dealing with a case of reported syncope without above suspicions it is prudent to get a base-line blood pressure measurement (upright and supine) and a resting ECG.

NPLEX
MCCQE
USMLE

Presentation: Seizures

General Type	Characteristics and Management
Simple partial	■ Most commonly occur in older children and adults. ■ Consciousness is never impaired. ■ Paroxysmal functional disturbances of sensory, motor, or autonomic systems. ■ Motor or 'Jacksonian seizure' is most common. ■ Hallucinations, cognitive, and affective variants exist. *Treatment:* ■ Rule out focal neurological disease (EEG + CT/MR scan). ■ Conventional treatment = phenytoin, valproate, or carbamazepine.
Complex partial 'Focal Cortical'	■ Similar to simple partial characteristics, but is followed by loss of consciousness ■ Patients often perform purposeless movements (e.g., staring, chewing movements, smacking, and unintelligible noises) and may become aggressive if restrained. *Treatment:* ■ Recommended first-line therapy is carbamazepine.
Absence seizure 'Petit Mal'	■ Patients are always younger than 20 years of age. ■ Main manifestation is loss of awareness (but not consciousness) for 10 to 30 seconds with eye or muscle fluttering. ■ The 'petit' child usually stares into the void for a while and then resumes prior activity (looks like abrupt daydreaming). This scenario can occur up to 100X per day. *Treatment:* ■ Recommended first-line therapy is ethosuximide.

Source

General Type	Characteristics and Management
Tonic-clonic seizure 'Grand Mal'	■ Primary epilepsy of adulthood, where tonic muscle contraction is followed by clonic contractions. ■ Lasts 2 to 3 minutes with loss of consciousness. ■ Sometimes there is an aura; incontinence; and tongue lacerations. ■ This is followed by a postictal state, during which patient feels headachy, drowsy, confused and sore. *Treatment:* ■ Conventional treatment = phenytoin, valproate, or carbamazepine.
Febrile seizure	■ Infants and children (<6 years of age) may get seizures during febrile conditions. ■ Assume organic cause until proven otherwise (i.e., rule out meningitis, tumors, or other serious causes of seizures). *Treatment:* ■ These children do not have epilepsy, and as such should not receive antiepileptics. ■ Treat the cause of the fever and provide supportive measures.
Secondary seizure	■ Occur secondary to organic causes (e.g., tumor, meningitis, encephalitis, toxoplasmosis, cysticercosis, hemorrhage, hypoglycemia, PKU, hyponatremia, lead/cocaine/carbon monoxide poisoning, substance withdrawal, severe hypertension, pheochromocytoma, eclampsia, trauma, and stroke). *Treatment:* ■ A full work-up is essential in determining the best course of action.

DEMENTIA

NPLEX
MCCQE
USMLE

Presentation

Memory loss with impairment of at least one of the following cognitive capacities:
1. Language ability
2. Orientation
3. Attention or ability to concentrate
4. Frontal executive function (like judgment and problem solving)
5. Apraxia (inability to perform acquired motor skills)
6. Activity of daily living

Diagnosis: To qualify for the diagnosis, the impairment must be at a level that interferes with social or occupational functioning. Major depression can present similarly, but due to lack of motivation (to recall or learn) rather than ability. This is termed pseudodementia. Delirium, psychiatric disorders, mental retardation, and mild cognitive impairment can also be mistaken for dementia.

Source

Causes:

- Alzheimer's disease (leading cause)
- Severe depression
- Cerebrovascular disease (multi-infarct dementia)
- Parkinson's disease
- Hypothyroidism
- Multiple medications
- Substance abuse
- Carbon monoxide, organophosphates, solvent inhalation
- Vitamin B-12 deficiency
- Brain tumor
- Liver or kidney failure

Screening for Dementia

NPLEX
MCCQE
USMLE

AAN
Gonzales,
2009

- American Academy of Neurology (AAN 2004) cites insufficient evidence for screening asymptomatic adults for dementia, though patients already diagnosed should be re-evaluated on regular basis for progression.
- Short test of Mental Status (STMS) is more effective than Mini Mental State Examination (MMSE) in differentiating between cognitively healthy and those with cognitive impairment.

Delirium and Dementia Characteristics

Delirium

Delirium is state of confusion that occurs abruptly and is usually associated with precipitating causes, such infections, acid/base imbalance, electrolyte imbalance, and cardiac events (in fact it, can be viewed as a marker for them).

Decreased attention span is a presenting feature.

Waxing and waning in the level of consciousness.

Waxing and waning in the level of arousal.

Dementia

Dementia is a slower progressive decline of cognitive function that may be exacerbated by social stressors, such as bereavement, unfamiliar environment, and high stress social functions.

Decreased attention span is a late feature.

Level of consciousness is usually not affected.

Level of arousal is normal.

Source

NPLEX

Foster,
2011
Teixeira,
2011
Cole, 2009
Hermann,
2011
Selhub,
2010
Gray, 2007

Guidelines for First-line Naturopathic Treatment of Dementia

Naturopathic Prevention and Treatment

Approach
- Identify modifiable risk factors
- Reduce disease burden
- Delay progression of condition
- Provide symptom relief

Clinical Nutrition
- Diet high in antioxidants, mono and polyunsaturated fatty acids, and proteins may prevent artherosclerosis and plaque formation
- Omega-3 fatty acids (especially DHA) have been shown to reduce risk of dementia
- B-vitamins (especially B-6 and B-12) may prevent rise in homocysteine, an emerging biomarker of neurodegenerative diseases

Physical Exercise
- Daily physical activity promotes circulation and vascular health, increases cognitive plasticity, delays neurodegeneration and enhances neurogenesis

Cognitive Exercises
- Solving puzzles, playing challenging games, and reading have been shown to delay cognitive decline

Safety
- Remove environmental hazards
- Counsel against driving

Source

ALZHEIMER DISEASE

Presentation

NPLEX
MCCQE
USMLE

Alzheimer disease is a progressive neurodegenerative disorder characterized by the development of β-amyloid plaques and neurofibrillary tangles in frontal, temporal, and parietal cortex.

Signs and Symptoms:

Dugani,
2009

- Anterograde amnesia (can't learn new things)
- One of following:
  - Aphasia (trouble with speech production and comprehension)
  - Apraxia (motor difficulties)
  - Agnosia (can't recognize objects)
  - Disruption of executive functions (planning, organizing, sequencing, abstracting)

Risk Factors

NPLEX
MCCQE
USMLE

Dugani,
2009
Gray, 2009

- FHx of AD
- Previous head injury
- Low education level
- Smoking
- Aluminum
- Elevated homocysteine
- Down syndrome.

Conventional Therapy: Involves cholinesterase inhibitors (donepezil, rivastigmine, galantamine) and NMDA receptor antagonists (memantine).

Guidelines for First-line Naturopathic Treatment of Alzheimer Disease

NPLEX

Alt Med
Rev, 2010
Di Stefano
2010
He, 2011
Mandell,
2011
Janssen,
2010

Approach
General guidelines as per Dementia above, in addition to:

Clinical Nutrition
- Acetyl-L-carnitine: 1-3g q.d. Improves long term memory, attention, and learning while delaying behavioral deterioration
- Alpha-lipoic acid: 200 mg t.i.d. Reduces inflammation and may protect against neurodegeneration as a potent antioxidant
- Green tea extract (better effect when taken with fish oils) may slow down progression of AD via its antioxidant and metal chelating abilities.

Botanical Medicine
- *Ginkgo biloba*: 240 mg q.d. Improves quality of daily living and cognitive symptoms

Source

NPLEX
MCCQE
USMLE

Dugani,
2010

PARKINSON'S DISEASE

Presentation

Parkinson's disease (PD) is a neurodegenerative motor disorder affecting 2% of the North American population over 60 years of age. The degeneration occurs within the basal ganglia; specifically the dopaminergic neurons of substantia nigra undergo apoptosis. These neurons project to the striatum and are very important in motor control. The motor symptoms of PD develop when 80% of the neurons are affected.

- Motor symptoms
- Resting tremor, "pill rolling"
- Muscle rigidity, flexed posture
- Bradykinesia, shuffling gait, facial hypomimia
- Postural instability, freezing (increased risk of falls)
- Autonomic symptoms: constipation, inadequate bladder emptying, sleep disturbances, anosmia

Diagnosis:
- PD is diagnosed based on clinical symptoms and neurological exam.
- While there is no test that will clearly identify the disease, the clinician needs to exclude secondary Parkinson's, drug and metabolism induced Wilson's disease, multiple systematrophies, benign essential tremor, Corticobasilar degeneration.
- Motor symptoms

USMLE

Conventional Treatment

Dugani,
2010

Class/ Function	Name	Side Effects
Dopamine precursor	Carbidopa-levodopa	Painful cramps, dyskinesias
Dopamine agonist	Bromocriptine, pergokide, pramipexole, ropinirole	Orthostatic hypotension, hallucinations
Dopamine releaser	Amantadine (Early PD)	Dizziness, constipation
MAO B Inhibitor	Selegeline (Early PD)	Muscle pain, insomnia

Deep Brain Stimulation: (thalamic, pallidal, subthalamic) - implant sends electrical impulses on behalf of the under-functioning substantia nigra.

Embryonic Dopaminergic Transplantation: may offer clinical benefits in younger patients with PD, as replacement of the dead dopaminergic neurons.

Source

NPLEX

Ransmayer, 2011
Filippin, 2010
Kim, 2004
Vankampen, 2003

Guidelines for First-line Naturopathic Treatment of Parkinson's Disorder

Lifestyle
- Exercise: treadmill walking improves motor and non-motor symptoms. Balance training may reduce risk of falls.

Clinical Nutrition
- Coenzyme Q10: 300-1000 mg q.d. Potent antioxidant has been shown to slow down PD progression
- Alpha-lipoic acid: 200-300 mg t.i.d. Antioxidant shown to improve blood-brain-barrier, which has been shown to be compromised in neurodegenerative conditions
- Magnesium: 100 - 200 mg t.i.d. symptomatic relief of painful cramps (s/e of medication) and constipation

Botanical Medicine
- *Ginkgo biloba*: 120 mg b.i.d.: Offers neuroprotection via its antiapoptotic and antioxidant properties and may reduce neurotoxicity of levodopa
- Green tea extract (EGCG): Has both antioxidant and metal chelating properties, which may delay neurogeneration.
- Panax ginseng: May offer neuroprotection to the dopaminergic neurons according to animal models of PD

STROKE & TRANSIENT ISCHEMIC ATTACKS

NPLEX

Dugani, 2009
Billar, 2010
Prabhakaran, 2010

Presentation and Definition

TIA is a transient obstruction of blood flow to cerebral arteries. The symptoms of obstruction resolve completely within minutes, but can last up to 24 hours ($\geq$ 24 hours $\neq$ TIA). Within the next 3 months following a TIA, 10-15% will develop a stroke.

Symptoms:
- Sudden loss of consciousness (more typical of stroke than TIA)
- Severe and sudden headache
- Rapid onset nausea and vomiting
- Sensory or motor changes (hemaparesis, hemaplegia, facial weakness, unilateral weakness)
- Aphasia, apraxia
- Dizziness, vertigo, loss of balance or coordination
- Monocular blindness, visual field deficit, diplopia

Source

NPLEX
MCCQE
USMLE

Dugani,
2009
Prab-
hakaran,
2010
Billar, 2011

Risk Factors

Age	Obesity	Dyslipidemia
Hypertension	Diabetes mellitus	Carotid stenosis
Smoking	Drugs (BCP, cocaine)	Physical inactivity
Myocardial infarction	FHx stroke (<65 yo)	Sickle cell disease
Mitral stenosis	Migraines (esp with aura)	Sleep apnea
Atrial fibrillation	Hyperhomocysteinemia (m/c cause of stroke in young adults)	

NPLEX
MCCQE
USMLE

Billar, 2011
Dugani,
2009

Sequelae of stroke

- Long-term complications: The long-term or permanent changes that result may include depression, memory loss, communication deficits, pain, motor difficulties (paralysis), emotional liability, confusion and apathy. Rehabilitation and secondary prevention are important, and may be impeded by depression (typical after stroke).
- Serious complications: DVT/PE, seizures, cerebral edema (onset 2-3 days after stroke - worsening of symptoms) and pressure sores (d/t immobility)
- Rate of recurence: 25-45% in the next 5 years

USPSTF

Gonzales,
2009

Screening

United States Preventive Services Task Force (USPSTF) 2007 does not recommend screening asymptomatic adults for internal carotid artery stenosis (ICAS) via duplex ultrasound. The prevalence of ICAS is highest in ≥ 54 yo, diastolic BP ≤ 83mmHg (stenosis over carotid body causes reflex hypotension) and those with peripheral artery disease patients. Carotid duplex ultrasound is 94% sensitive and 92% specific for detecting carotid artery stenosis $\geq 60\%$ (endarterectomy or stenting is advised with $\geq 70\%$ stenosis).

NPLEX
MCCQE
USMLE

Management Plan

Tests:
- CBC, electrolytes, creatinine, PT, PTT, glucose, lipids
- CT head (or MRI)
- ECG, echocardiogram
- DDX: Migraine, intracranial hemorrhage, seizure, hypoglycemia

Dugani,
2009
Prab-
hakaran,
2010
Billar, 2011

Therapy:
1. Acutely ischemic strokes are circumvented by thrombolysis (Alteplase) if administered within 4 hours of onset
2. Antiplatelet agents (aspirin, clopidogrel)
3. Statins (regardless of lipid status)
4. Warfarin (in the case of atrial fibrillation)

Source

NPLEX

Guidelines for First-line Naturopathic Treatment Post-stroke

Lifestyle
- Physical activity: treadmill walking and physiotherapy improve circulation, prevent muscle atrophy, and improve function (likely to benefit mood)
- Diet: Reduce or eliminate saturated fats, hydrogenated oils, cholesterol, fried foods, simple carbohydrates, and food sensitivities. Increase consumption of fiber, apples, onions, garlic, vegetables, and cold-water fish.

Clinical Nutrition
- Alpha-lipoic acid: 200 mg t.i.d.
- Taurine: 500-2000 mg t.i.d.
- Folic acid 2 mg + Vitamin B-6 25 mg + Vitamin B-12 500 mcg
- Vitamin C: 500 mg t.i.d.
- L-carnitine: 500 - 1000 mg t.i.d.
- Coenzyme Q10: 100 - 300 mg t.i.d.
- Melatonin: 3 - 10 mg qd

Botanical medicine
- *Ginkgo biloba*: 120 mg b.i.d. Increases cerebrovascular perfusion, but must be used with caution as it may potentiate the effects of anticoagulation therapy (monitor INR).
- Panax ginseng: May improve neurological deficits after ischemic stroke; anti-apoptotic, may stimulate CNS regeneration

Yamori, 2010
Almeida, 2010
Lin, 2009

Zheng, 2011
Li, 2010

Examination Board References

NPLEX (II): North American Board of Naturopathic Examiners
Naturopathic Physician Licensing Examination Part II (NPLEx II) Blueprint. Portland, OR: North American Board of Naturopathic Examiners (NABNE), 2010.

USMLE: National Board of Medical Examiners
Brochert A. Crush Step 3. The Ultimate USMLE Step 3 Review. 3rd ed. New York, NY: Saunders, Elsevier, 2008.

MCCQE: Medical Council of Canada
Dugani S, Lam D, eds. 2009. MCCQE Review Notes & Lecture Series. Medical Counsel of Canada Qualification Examination Review Notes. Toronto, ON: McGraw Hill Professional, Canadian edition, 2009.

Related References

Almeida, OP., Marsh, K., Alfonso, H., et al. B-vitamins reduce the long-term risk of depression after stroke: the VITATOPS-DEP trial. Ann Neurology. 2010;68(4):503-10.

Alternative Med Review. Acetyl-L-carnitine Monograph. Alternative Medicine Review. 2010;15(1): 76-83.

Billar J, Wijdicks EFM, Misulis KE, Ferri FF. Stroke - ischemic. First Consult Elsevier Inc. 2011. Online at www.mdconsult.com

Cao F, Sun S, Tong ET. Experimental study on inhibition of neuronal toxical effect of levodopa by gingko biloba extract on Parkinson disease in rats. J Huazhong Univ Sci Technolog Med Sci. 2003;23(2):151-53.

Cole GM, Ma QL, Frautschy SA. Omega-3 fatty acids and dementia. Prostaglandins Leukot Essential Fatty Acids. 2009;81(2-3): 213-21.

Dains J, Baumann L, Scheibel P. Advanced Health Assessment & Clinical Diagnosis in Primary Care. 2nd ed. St. Louis, MO: Mosby C.V. Co. Ltd., 2003.

Desport JC, Preux PM, Truong CT, Courat L, Vallat, JM., Couratier, P) Nutritional assessment and survival in ALS patients. Amyotrophic Lateral Sclerosis Other Motor Neuron Disorders, 2000;1(2): 91-96.

Di Stefano A, Sozio P, Cerasa S, Iannitelli A, et al. Ibuprofen and lipoic acid diamide as co-drug with neuroprotective activity: pharmacological properties and effects in beta-amyloid (1-40) infused Alzheimer's disease rat model. Int J Immunopathol Pharmacology. 2010;23(2):589-99.

Filippin ND, Da Costa PH, Mattioli R. Effects of treadmill-walking training with additional body load on quality of life in subjects with Parkinson's disease. Rev Bras Fisioter 2010;14(4): 344-50.

Foster PP, Rosenblatt KP, Kuljis RO. Exercise-induced cognitive plasticity, implications for mild cognitive impairment and Alzheimer's disease. Frontiers in Neurology. 2011;2(28).

Gonzales R, Kutner J. Current Practice Guidelines in Primary Care 2009. Toronto (ON): McGraw Hill, 2009.

Graf M, Ecker D, Horowski R, et al.High dose vitamin E therapy in amyotrophic lateral sclerosis as add-on therapy to riluzole: results of a placebo-controlled double blind study. Journal of Neural Transmission. 2005;112(5):649-60.

Gray J. Therapeutic Choices. 5th ed. Ottawa, ON: Canadian Pharmacists Association, 2004.

He Y, Cui J, Lee JC, et al. Prolonged exposure of cortical neurons to oligomeric amyloid-beta impairs NMDA receptor function via NADPH oxidase-mediated ROS production: protective effect of green tea (-)-epigallocathin-3-gallate. ASN Neuro, 2011.

Hermann W, Obeid R. Homocysteine: a biomarker in neurodegenerative diseases. Clin Chem Lab Med. 2011;49(3): 435-41.

Izumi Y, Kaji R. Clinical trials of ultra-high-dose methylcobalamin in ALS. Brain Nerve, 2011;59(10): 1141-47.

Janssen IM, Sturtz S, Skipka, G, et al. Gingko biloba in Alzheimer's disease: a systematic review. Wien Med Wochenschr. 2010;160(21-22):539-46.

Kim MS, Lee JL, Lee WY, Kim, SE. Neuroprotective effect of Gingko biloba L. extract in a rat model of Parkinson's disease. Phytotherapy Research, 2004;18(8): 663-66.

Li Y, Tang J, Khatibi NH, et al. Ginsenoside Rbeta1 reduces neurologic damage, is anti-apoptotic, and down-regulates p53 and BAX in subarachnoid hemorrhage. Current Neurovascular Research, 2010;7(2):85-94.

Lin HW, Lee EJ.009). Effects of melatonin in experimental stroke models in acute, subacute, and chronic stages. Neuropsychiatr Dis Treat. 2009;5:157-62.

Mandel SA, Amit T, Weinreb O, Youdim, MBUnderstanding the broad spectrum neuroprotective action profile of green tea ppolyphenols in aging and neurodegenerative diseases. Journal of Alzheimer's Disorder, 2011.

Mandel S, Maor G, Youdim, MBH.004). Iron and alpha-synuclein in the substantia nigra of MPTP-treated mice. Journal of Molecular Neuroscience. 2004; 24: 401-416.

Miller TH, Kruse JE. Evaluation of syncope. American Family Physician.2005;72(8): 1492-1500.

Piquet MA. Nutritional approach for patients with amyotrophic lateral sclerosis. Rev Neurol. 2006; 162 Spec No 2: 4S117-4S187.

Pizzorno JE, Murray MT. Textbook of Natural Medicine. Vol. 1 and 2. 2nd ed. New York, NY: Churchill Livingstone, 1999.

Pizzorno JE, Murray MT, Joiner-Bey H. The Clinician's Handbook of Natural Medicine. New York, NY: Churchill Livingstone, 2002.

Pizzorno JE, Murray MT. Textbook of Natural Medicine, 3rd ed. New York, NY: Churchill Livingstone, Elsevier, 2006.

Prabhakaran S, Wijdicks EFM, Misulis KE, Ferri F. Transient Ischemic Attack. First Consult Elsevier Inc., 2010. Online at www.mdconsult.com.

Ransmayr G. Physical, occupational, speech and swallowing therapies and physical exercise in Parkinson's disease. Journal of Neural Transmission. 2011;118(5):773-81.

Selhub, J., Troen, A., Rosenberg, IH. B vitamins and the aging brain. Nutr Rev. 2010;68 Suppl 2:S112-18

Smolders J. Vitamin D and Multiple sclerosis: correlation, causality and controversy. Autoimmune Disease: 2007;629538.

Teixeira CV, Gobbi LT, Corazza DI, et al. Non-pharmacological interventions on cognitive functions in older people with mild cognitive impairment (MCI). Arch Gerontol Geriatr. 2011.

Weishaupt JH, Bartels C, Polking E, et al. oxidative damage in ALS by high-dose enteral melatonin treatment. Journal of Pineal Res. 2006;41(4): 313-23.

Van Kampen J, Robertson H, Hagg T, Drobitch R. (2003). Neuroprotective actions of the ginseng extract G115 in two rodent models of Parkinson's disease. Exp Neurology, 2003;184(1): 521-29.

Yadav V, Marracci G, Lovera J, et al. Lipoic acid in multiple sclerosis: a pilot study. Multiple Sclerosis. 2005;11(2):159-65.

Yamori Y, Taguchi T, Hamada A, et al. Taurine in health and disease: consistent evidence from experimental and epidemiological studies. Journal of Biomedical Science, 2010,17 Suppl 1: S6.

Zheng GQ, Cheng W, Wang Y, et al. Ginseng total saponins enhance neurogenesis after focal cerebral ischemia. Journal of Ethonopharmacology.2011;133(2):724-28.

Zhu Y, He ZY, Liu HN. Meta-analysis of the relationship between homocysteine, vitamin B(12), folate, and multiple sclerosis. Journal of Clinical Neuroscience. 2011.

Zoccolella S, Bendotti C, Beghi E, Loqroscino G. Homocysteine levels and amyotrophic lateral sclerosis: a possible link. Amyotrophic Lateral Sclerosis. 2010;11(1-2):140-7.

OPHTHALMOLOGY

Contributing author: Martin Downorowicz

OPHTHALMOLOGY

NPLEX
MCCQE
USMLE

Presentation

Common Complaints:
- In practice, red eyes are the most common complaint, which can result from chemical irritation, physical irritation (contact lenses), acute glaucoma, keratitis, uveal tract or scleral inflammation, vascular or retinal disease, and conjunctivitis.
- Sensory innervation of the eyelids, cornea, conjunctivae, and uveal tract. Note that sinus and orbit diseases can have referred pain to the eye.
- Gradual loss of vision; cataracts, diabetes, glaucoma, tumor infiltration, toxic degeneration, and refractive error.
- Acute loss of vision; vitreous hemorrhage, cortical blindness, optic neuropathy, central retinal vein/artery occlusion, MS, acute glaucoma, acute iritis, and retinal detachment.

Eye Examinations

NPLEX
MCCQE
USMLE

Gonzales,
2009
AAO, 2007
AAFP, 2007
USPSTF,
2005

Always start any vision test with corrected vision (i.e., with corrective eye wear). Recommendations for routine eye and vision examinations range between 2-10 years for patients 6 years old and older , with more frequent screening in elderly and pediatric patients and those with risk factors. Infants should be screened at birth, 3 months, and at 3, 4, and 5 years old. Annual examinations are advised for patients with diabetes, hypertension, FHx ocular dz, hazardous or visual-straining occupations, contact lens users, or use of eye-damaging medications.

Visual acuity test: performed on left, right, and both eyes using Snellen Eye chart.
Snellen Fraction = testing distance (6 meters or 20 feet)
Smallest line patient can read on the chart

Visual field test: examines any loss in the visual fields and is done by confrontation of all visual quadrants. Pupils should be examined relative to each other in shape, size, equality, and reactivity to light in both direct and consensual.
Flashlight test: can be performed for relative afferent pupilary defect
Near flex test: for lens accommodation, eye convergence, and pupil constriction.

H Pattern: the six muscles of the eye are tested using the "H" pattern movement noting for diplopia and nystagmus.

General external inspection: should include primary position of the eyes, possible strabismus, irregular lateral or vertical jitter of eyes.

Hirschberg test: examines corneal light reflex and should be symmetric and near center of each cornea.

External eye exam: includes lids, lashes, lacrimal apparatus and lymph nodes.

Slit lamp: using slit-lamp the iris, lens, cornea, anterior chamber, conjunctiva, and sclera can be examined.

Ophthalmoscopic test: allows for the examination of the anterior segment (cataract, corneal opacity, red reflex) and posterior segment (macula, retina, vitreous, optic disc).

Source

NPLEX
MCCQE
USMLE

Differential Diagnosis of Red Eyes

	Pain	Discharge	Photophobia	Pupil	Vision
Conjunctivitis	No	Virus – serous Bacterial – pus Allergy – mucous	No	Normal	Normal
Acute Iritis	Yes	No	Yes, severe	Smaller	Reduced
Acute Glaucoma	Yes, severe	No	Yes	Fixed – mid dilation	Reduced
Acute Closure Keratitis	Yes, with blinking	Profuse tearing	Yes	Normal or smaller	Varies, depending on site of lesion

NPLEX
MCCQE
USMLE

Ocular Emergencies

Trauma, lacerations and foreign bodies	Orbital cellulitis
Acute angle closure glaucoma	Chemical burns
Gonococcal conjunctivitis	Giant cell arteritis
Central retinal artery occlusion	Retinal detachment
Corneal ulcer	Endophthalmitis

NPLEX
MCCQE
USMLE

Van Rooij,
1999

Uveitis

- The uveal tract is composed of the iris, ciliary body, and choroids. In the case of uveitis, the uveal tract is inflamed with common manifestations, such as photophobia and injection.
- A number of systemic diseases also are associated with uveitis, including ankylosing spondylitis, Reiter's syndrome, lupus erythematosus, rheumatoid arthritis, sarcoidosis, juvenile rheumatoid arthritis, and inflammatory bowel disease. Infectious cases, such as cytomegalovirus, varicella zoster, herpes simplex, syphilis, and Lyme disease, can also be associated with uveitis.
- Common treatment for uveitis includes topical cycloplegics to systemic steroids. With this treatment an adjunct of vitamin C (500 mg twice daily) and vitamin E (100 mg twice daily) can improve the condition by way of antioxidant scavenging mechanism.

Source

Conjunctivitis

- Conjunctivitis is inflammation or infection of the conjunctiva. The conjunctiva is a membrane that covers the eye and lines the inner surface of the eyelid.
- Symptoms include red, watery eyes, inflamed inner eyelids, sensitivity to light, scratchy feeling in eyes, pus or watery discharge, and swelling of eyelids. The most common causes are viral upper respiratory infection, bacterial infection, allergic reaction, and chemical irritation.

NPLEX

Guidelines for First-line Naturopathic Treatment of Conjunctivitis

Hagen, 2003

Approach:
- Address inflammation or infection.
- Provide symptom relief.

1. Compresses: A warm compress should be applied to the affected eye or eyes. In an allergic conjunctivitis a cool compress will be more soothing.

2. Hygeine: Remember to keep area around affected eye or eyes clean and keep hands away to prevent any further spread to other people. Infectious conjunctivitis is easily and quickly spread, thus infection control measures should be stressed.

3. Irrigation: the following are eye irrigation formulas that can be used to treat conjunctivitis. Note that some compounding pharmacies provide sterile ocular preparations (which should be used if available):
1. Echinacea: Euphrasia: Hydrasis equal parts tea, apply q.i.d.
2. Calendula: Berberis: Foeniculum equal parts tea, apply q.i.d.
3. Sambucus canadensis flowers or white walnut applied p.r.n.

MCCQE NPLEX

Keratitis

The corneal epithelium can be infected by a variety of viral agents. The most common agents are herpes simplex and herpes zoster.

Herpes Simplex Signs and Symptoms
- Pain, tearing, foreign body sensation, redness
- May have visual acuity loss
- Occasional cold sore on lip
- Corneal hypoesthesia
- Dendritic lesion seen in corneal epithelium with fluorescein staining and cobalt blue illumination

Herpes Zoster Signs and Symptoms
- Ocular tearing, pain and photophobia
- Neuralgia-type pain
- Corneal hypoesthesia
- Hutchinson's sign

Source

NPLEX
PCS

NPLEX

Hagen,
2003
Zolfaghari,
2001
Bowie,
2000

NPLEX

USPSTF,
2005
Gonzales,
2009

Causes of Sensation of a Foreign Body in the Eye

- Trichiasis
- Corneal or conjunctival abrasion
- Corneal or conjunctival foreign body
- Punctate epitheliopathy caused by chemical irritation or dryness

Sty and Chalazion

Presentation:
- A sty typically presents as acutely painful and suppurative due to a bacterial infection.
- A chalazion is due to chronic sterile granuloma of a meibomian gland and is painless.

Management Plan:
Compresses: typical management for chalazion is a warm compress and the chalazion usually subsides. A sty can be treated similarly by applying a warm compress four times a day for 10 minutes at a time to relieve the pain and help the sty come to a point sooner. The sty should be allowed to open on its own and the area to be washed thoroughly.

Alternative: black tea bags and hot Epsom salt packs can be used for treatment of a sty or chalazion, t.i.d. x20min.

Vitamin C and A: a number of studies suggest using vitamin C (4 g q.d. with bioflavanoids) and vitamin A (50,000 IU q.d.) as a treatment partly due to their anti-inflammatory properties.

Glaucoma

Presentation:
Glaucoma is a progressive optic neuropathy involving characteristic structural changes to the optic nerve head, which in turn produce visual field changes. Glaucoma commonly presents with increased intraocular pressure. Given that the United States Preventive Services Task Force 2005 reports insufficient evidence to recommend for or against screening adults for glaucoma, the primary care physician should refer for evaluation only those patients who present with the following symptoms.

Primary Open-angle Glaucoma
(most common, about 55% of all cases)
- Caused by the obstruction to aqueous drainage within the trabecular meshwork and its drainage into the canal of Schlemm. Symptoms include coloured halos around lights, possible hemorrhage at disk margin, and bilateral eyes affected. The condition is asymptomatic until severe visual field or central loss occurs.

Primary Closed-angle Glaucoma
(about 12% of all cases)
- Caused by peripheral iris bowing forward in a susceptible eye with shallow anterior chamber causing an obstruction of the aqueous access to the trabecular meshwork. Symptoms include red, painful eye, unilateral, halo around lights, decreased visual acuity, abdominal pain, nausea and vomiting.

Source

Secondary Open-angle Glaucoma

- There are numerous reasons for secondary open angle glaucoma, such as increased ocular pressure secondary to ocular or systemic disorder that blocks the trabecular meshwork, traumatic glaucoma, steroid-induced glaucoma, neovascular glaucoma, pseudoexfolation syndrome, and pigmentary dispersion syndrome.

Secondary Closed-angle Glaucoma

- Caused by an inflammation of the iris, which in turn adheres to the lens.

Congenital Glaucoma

- Caused by improper development of the filtering mechanism of the anterior chamber angle. In this case, signs and symptoms include photophobia, buphthalmos, blepharospasm, tearing, cloudy cornea, and increased ocular pressure.

Conventional Medications for Treating Glaucoma

MCCQE
USMLE

The drug classes used in the management of glaucoma inhibit aqueous humor production by the ciliary body or increase drainage via the trabecular meshwork. To minimize their systemic effects, most drugs used in eye disease are administered topically. Avoid corticosteroids or other medication that increases intraocular pressure unless medically necessary.

Open-angle Glaucoma

Yanoff,
2008

- Prostaglandin analogues increase acqueous fluid outflow by relaxing the cilary muscles. They can be used simultaneosly with other treatments. This class of topical agents may cause permanent increase in pigmentation of the iris, eyelids, and eyelashes. Contraindicated in hypersensitivity to PG analogues and pregnancy.
- Beta-adrenoceptor antagonists (Beta blockers), such as Timolol and Betaxolol, block beta-2 receptors on the ciliary body leading to vasoconstriction. This class of topical drugs sometimes leads to transient dry eyes and allergic blepharoconjunctivitis. Remember that all beta blockers are C/I in asthma, bradycardia, heart block, and CHF.
- Adrenoceptor agonists (sympathomimetics), such as Adrenaline, Dipivefrine, and Brimonidine stimulate alpha receptors on the ciliary body leading to vasoconstriction. This class of topical agents may cause eye pain and redness. C/I are closed-angle glaucoma, hypertension, and heart disease.

Prum,
2010

- Carbonic anhydrase inhibitors, such as Acetazolamide and Dorzolamide, lead to ciliary body deprivation of bicarbonate (bicarbonate is required in aqueous humor production). These drugs can be given orally, topically, and intravenously. The side effect profile includes eye irritation, nausea, vomiting, diarrhea, and diuresis. C/I are renal impairment, hypokalemia, and hyponatremia.
- Muscarinic agonists (e.g., Pilocarpine) will increase the drainage of aqueous humor by stimulating the constrictor pupillae muscle (which produces miosis). The side effect profile includes eye irritation, headache, blurred vision, and hypersalivation. C/I are acute iritis and anterior uveitis.

Closed-angle Glaucoma

- The drugs used in closed-angle galaucoma lower intraocular pressure (IOP). Pilocarpine and carbonic anhydrase inhibitors are used topically as first-line agents, while mannitol and glycerol (osmotic agents) are used systemically in resistant or more serious cases.
- Yttrium-aluminum-garnet (YAG) laser iridotomy is used to permanently increase the flow of aqueous humor.

Source

NPLEX

Pizzorno,
1999

Boyd, 1995
Gaspat,
1995

MCCQE
NPLEX

USMLE
NPLEX

Pizzorno,
2006

Blades,
2001

Guidelines for First-line Naturopathic Treatment of Glaucoma

Approach:
- Early diagnosis essential
- Support conventional medical and surgical recommendation
- Delay progression of condition
- Improve condition

1. Dietary measures
- Eliminate food allergies
- Increase fresh fruits and vegetables, especially those high in vitamin C and flavanoids tomatoes, broccoli, strawberries, red peppers, spinach and especially berries.
- Increase consumption of cold-water fish. These fish are high in omega-3 fatty acids, which have been shown to lower intra ocular pressure.
- Avoid caffeine.

2. Clinical nutrition
- Flaxseed oil: 1 tbsp q.d.
- Vitamin C: 2000 mg q.d.
- Bioflavonoids (especially anthocyanosides): 1000 mg q.d.
- Chromium: 200-400 mcg q.d.
- Magnesium: 200-600 mg q.d.

3. Botanical medicine
- Ginkgo biloba extract (24% ginkgo flavonglycosides) 40-80 mg t.i.d.
- Vaccinium myrtillus extract (25% anthocyanidin): 80 mg t.i.d.

Ischemic injury

Presentation:
- The appearance of cotton wool spots in the fundus indicates ischemic injury to the superficial nerve layer of the retina. These spots are caused by an obstruction or poor blood flow through the capillaries.
- The appearance of these spots can be commonly seen in diabetic patients who develop diabetic retinopathy.
- Other cases where these spots can be seen are in patients with anemia, endocarditis, AIDS, leukemia, collagen vascular disease, and severe hypertension.

Dry-eye Syndrome

Presentation:
Patients with keratoconjunctivitis sicca (dry eye syndrome) often experience blurring vision, a burning sensation, and foreign body sensation. Numerous reasons underlie the dry eye syndrome, such as normal aging process, lid abnormality (ectropion), decreased blinking (CN VII palsy), post-cataract surgery, systemic diseases (Sjogren's syndrome, leukemia, lymphoma), and medications (diuretics, anticholinergics, antihistamines).

Conventional Treatments:
Lubricating agents: Mild to moderate forms may not display any obvious signs of redness or discomfort to the patient. The most common treatment methods are over-the-counter lubricating agents

that can be applied by the patient. Success of this treatment is determined by patient's adherence to the protocol (frequency and duration of application).

Vitamin A: Evaluate the patient's vitamin A status, especially if malnourishment is suspected and assign an appropriate dose (e.g., 5,000-50,000 IU q.d. but for short-term only as this dose may cause hypervitaminosis A when used for longer periods).

Other Supplements: Other antioxidants to consider are vitamin C, E, and bioflavonoids, due to their ability to improve tear stability and conjunctival health.

Cataract

NPLEX
MCCQE
USMLE

Patients with cataract present with a gradual, painless, and progressive loss of vision produced by the increased opacity of the lens. The opacity distorts with a gradual light refraction, resulting in patients reporting seeing haloes around lights at night, dimness, and glare. It also reduces the red reflux and may interfere with fundoscopy.

Causes:
- Age (90% of all cataracts)
- Metabolic (diabetes, hypocalcemia)
- Trauma (UV radiation, toxin, mechanical)
- Congenital (Down syndrome, maternal rubella exposure)

Treatment:
- Surgery option is dependent on the degree of visual impairment and impact on quality of life
- Smoking cessation can slow down progression
- Glucose control in patients with diabetes
- Antioxidants may help reduce cataract formation in patients at high risk of oxidation damage
- UV protective sunglasses may delay development and slow down progression

AAO, 2006
AREDS,
2001
Fernandez,
2008

Examination Board References

NPLEX (II): North American Board of Naturopathic Examiners
Naturopathic Physician Licensing Examination Part II (NPLEx II) Blueprint. Portland, OR: North American Board of Naturopathic Examiners (NABNE), 2010.

USMLE: National Board of Medical Examiners
Brochert A. Crush Step 3. The Ultimate USMLE Step 3 Review. 3rd ed. New York, NY: Saunders, Elsevier, 2008.

MCCQE: Medical Council of Canada
Dugani S, Lam D, eds. 2009. MCCQE Review Notes & Lecture Series. Medical Counsel of Canada Qualification Examination Review Notes. Toronto, ON: McGraw Hill Professional, Canadian edition, 2009.

Related References

Blades K, Patel S, Aidoo K, Original communication oral antioxidant therapy for marginal dry eye. *British Journal of Clinical Nutrition* 2001:55:589-97.

Bowie A, O'Neill L. Vitamin C inhibits NF-kappa B activation by TNF via the activation of p38 mitogen-activated protein kinase. *J. Immunol.* 2000;12(165):7180-18.

Boyd HH. Eye pressure lowering effect of vitamin C. *J. Orthomolecular Med.* 1995;10:165-68.

Dains J, Baumann L, Scheibel P. Advanced Health Assessment & Clinical Diagnosis in Primary Care. 2nd ed. St Louis, MO: Mosby C.V. Co. Ltd., 2003.

Gaspar AZ. Gasser P, Flammer J. The influence of magnesium on visual field and peripheral vasospasm in glaucoma. *Ophthalmologica.* 1995;209:11-13.

Dawson J, Taylor M, Reide P. Crash Course in Pharmacology. 2nd ed. St Louis, MO: Mosby, Elsevier Science Ltd, 2002.

Hagen, P. Mayo Clinic Guide to Self-Care, Answers to Everyday Health Problems. 4th ed. Rochester, MN: Mayo Clinic Health Information, 2003.

Mladenovic J. Primary Care Secrets. 3rd ed. Philadelphia, PA: Hanley & Belfus, 2004.

Pizzorno JE, Murray MT. Textbook of Natural Medicine. Vol. 1& 2. 2nd ed. New York, NY: Churchill Livingstone, 1999.

Van Rooij J, Schwartzenberg SGWS, Mulder PGH, et al. Oral vitamins C and E as additional treatment in patients with acute anterior uveitis: a randomised double masked study in 145 patients. Br J Ophthalmol. 1999;83:1277-1282.

Zolfaghari R, et al. Fatty acid delta desaturasc mRNA is regulated by dietary vitamin A and exogenous retinoic acid in liver of adult rats. Archives of Biochemistry and Biophysics. 2001;39(1):8-15.

ORTHOPEDICS

MUSCULOSKELETAL PAIN

DISK HERNIATION

HIP DISORDERS

MUSCULOSKELETAL PAIN

Presentation

Nothing beats good history taking skills in managing musculoskeletal pain conditions. In fact, it has been argued that a good history will indicate an accurate diagnosis without resorting to batteries of diagnostic tests in approximately 70% of primary care musculoskeletal presentations.

Musculoskeletal Pain Diagnostic Characteristics

Musculoskeletal pain differentials	Etiology or contributing factors	Musculoskeletal pain differentials	Etiology or contributing factors
Dull and aching with diminished passive ROM	Joint capsule	Cramping, dull, and aching	Muscle pain
Sharp, shooting	Nerve root	Sharp, non-shooting	Peripheral nerve
Sharp, intolerable, and always present	Fracture	Deep, nagging, dull,	Bone pain
Throbbing, diffuse	Vascular compromise	Burning, aching, pressure-like, or stinging	Sympathetic nerve irritation
Pain that improves with activity	Chronic inflammation causing edema	Pain that worsens with activity	Vascular insufficiency; muscular or articular pathology
Pain that is not affected by activity	Bone pain, tumors, and visceral referral	Pain that worsens at night	Peripheral nerve entrapment; thoracic outlet syndrome
Intermittent claudications	Vascular insufficiency or spinal stenosis	Severe pain at night	Serious organic pathology (tumor)
Pain that worsens by sitting or bending	Inter-vertebral disc	Pain that improves by sitting or bending	Lumbar facet joint inflammation

Source

NPLEX
MCCQE

Orthopedic Tests

Test	Performance	Interpretation
Cervical spine compression	Push down on seated patient's head – repeat with bilateral bending	Pain = inter-vertebral nerve root compression
Cervical spine distraction	Traction head upwards via occiput	Relief = nerve root impingement Pain = ligament or joint capsule pathology
Adson's	Take radial pulse with arms internally rotated and abducted 45 degrees – ask patient to rotate and extend neck to each side	Disappearance of pulse indicates thoracic outlet syndrome, cervical rib syndrome, or tight anterior scalene
Drop arm test	Patient seated with arms at the side – slowly abduct arm and hold at maximal abduction	Arm drop = rotator cuff tear
Apprehension test	Place hand of affected arm on opposite shoulder – push posteriorly on the elbow of the affected arm	Pain in shoulder = anterior dislocation of shoulder
Lippmann's test	Forearm is flexed to 90 degrees – palpate biceps tendon 2.5 inches distal to shoulder	Sharp pain = bicipital tendonitis
Allen's test	Compress both arteries of the wrist – ask patient to flex and extend digits until palm turns pale – release one side (repeat, but release the other)	Non patent radial or ulnar artery
Phalen's test	Place dorsae of hands together – press both wrists into significant flexion for 30 to 60 seconds.	Pain during test or upon release = carpal tunnel syndrome
Tinel's test	Tap over middle of flexor wrist retinaculum.	Pain over the distribution of the median nerve = carpal tunnel syndrome
Straight leg raise	Patient is supine – passively raise leg to tolerable range of hip motion	Shooting pain at 35 degrees = disc herniation Pain at 70 degrees = SI pathology
Kemp's test	Rotate and extend torso to both sides, then press anteriorly on lumbar spinal processes	DDx facet joint irritation, lumbar strain, and disc herniation

Test	Performance	Interpretation
Valsalva	Patient is seated – patient takes deep breath and blows out with a pursed mouth	Pain in the back or neck = space occupying lesion (disc herniation) anywhere along the spinal canal
Ely's test	Patient is prone – flex patient knee to maximum tolerance	Ipsilateral hip flexion = tight rectus femoris
Gaenslen's test	Patient is supine – bring knee of affected side (of lumbar pain) to chest	Pain in the sacroiliac area = SI pathology or nerve root lesion
Ober's test	Patient is lying on their side – abduct supported limb – extend hip slightly then lower the limb in a supported fall	Leg remains abducted and doesn't fall below table level = iliotibial tract syndrome (tightness)
FABER (Patrick's) test	Patient is supine – flex, abduct, and externally rotate hip – then extend the hip	Hip pain = bursitis, arthritis, ligament strain, or tight capsule in the hip joint
Thomas' test	Patient is supine – bring knee to chest	Contralateral limb comes off the table = tight iliopsoas
Pelvic rock	Patient is supine – compress iliac crests bilaterally toward midline	Pain = SI lesion
McMurray's test	Patient is supine – flex hip and knee – then externally and internally rotate knee (change angle of knee flexion and repeat)	Snap or click sound = meniscus tear in knee joint
Patellar bulge	Patient is seated – milk medial side of patella superiorly – keep medial pressure – then milk inferiorly on the lateral side	Fluid wave = minor knee joint effusion, and patellofemoral syndrome
Patellar ballottement	Patient is supine – compress patella into patellofemoral groove then rapidly release	Click = major patellar effusion, and patellofemoral syndrome
Kernig's test	Patient is supine – flex knee and hip to 90 degrees – then attempt to extend knee while keeping the hip in flexion	Attempt to extend knee is significantly resisted = meningeal irritation (meningitis, herniated disc, cauda equina syndrome)
Brudzinski's test	Patient is supine – examiner passively flexes the neck	Involuntary hip flexion = ominous sign of meningitis

Source

NPLEX
MCCQE
USMLE

Compartment Syndrome

Since the deep fascia that surrounds muscular compartments is non-elastic, any condition that causes swelling inside a muscle compartment will cause some degree of nerve compression. This manifestation is seen in the extremities when edema or hemorrhage cases swelling inside the affected muscle compartment (e.g., anterior compartment syndrome of the leg or shin splints). This mechanism is considered to be protective since it invariably leads to the cessation of the offending activity (e.g., running), but sometimes the pain is tolerated (or the patient resorts to potent analgesics) so that compartmental pressure progressively rises, causing more severe nerve dysfunction (it can even lead to permanent nerve damage).

Signs and Symptoms:
- Severe pain (even on passive movement)
- Firm-feeling muscle compartment
- Signs of nerve compression: decreased sensation; decreased two-point discrimination; paresthesia; formications; numbness; or hypesthesia
- Decreased distal pulse amplitude (since arterial supply is also compressed)
- Cyanosis or pallor
- Paralysis and absence of peripheral pulses (late, ominous signs)

Exercise-induced Compartment Syndrome:
- Mild presentations that are caused by excessive (often novel sports activity that the patient is not used to) muscular exercise can be addressed with rest, massage, hydrotherapy, and supportive physical therapy.

Non-exercise Induced Compartment Syndrome:
- Fractures (mid-shaft tibial fractures in adults and supracondylar humeral fractures in children)
- Burns (especially electrical burns of sufficient magnitude leading to soft tissue edema)
- Vascular compromise (this offsets the balance of interstitial fluid formation and drainage → edema)

Emergency Care:
- Surgical intervention is warranted for severe non-remitting presentations to avoid any permanent neurological damage.
- A compartment syndrome presentation of such magnitude is an emergency that requires prompt fasciotomy.

NPLEX
MCCQE

Motor and Sensory Functions of the Cardinal Peripheral Nerves

Nerve	Motor	Sensory
Radial	Wrist extension Palsy manifests in 'wrist drop'	Back of forearm and hand (first three digits)
Ulnar	Finger abduction. Palsy manifests in 'claw hand deformity'	Front and back of last two digits

Nerve	Motor	Sensory	Source
Median	Forearm pronation and thumb opposition. Usually affected in carpal tunnel syndrome	Palmar surface of hand and front of the first three digits	
Axillary	Abduction and lateral rotation of arm (football throwing stance)	Lateral shoulder	
Fibular (Peroneal)	Dorsiflexion and eversion of foot Palsy manifests in foot drop	Lateral aspect of leg and dorsum of foot	

Cruciate Ligaments of the Knee Joint

NPLEX
USMLE

Anterior and posterior drawer tests are specific orthopedic tests that assess the anterior and posterior cruciate ligament, respectively.

Scaphoid Bone Fracture

NPLEX
USMLE

Presents clinically as palpatory tenderness in the anatomical snuff-box along with other signs of wrist fracture.

DISK HERNIATION

Presentation

NPLEX
MCCQE

Lumbar disk herniation is a common and often correctable cause of low back pain.

L5-S1 Disk Herniation Signs and Symptoms: The most likely location of herniation is the L5-S1 disc, which leads to nerve compression of the S1 nerve root. Features of this presentation include:
- History of lumbar trauma or strain
- Sciatica with positive straight leg raise (SLR) finding
- Decreased ankle jerk
- Weakness of plantar flexors of the foot
- Cauda equina syndrome (see below) with cerntal disk herniation

L4-L5 Disk Herniation Signs and Symptoms: The second most common location for herniation is L4-L5 disc, which leads to nerve compression of the L5 nerve root. Features of this presentation include:
- Pain in the hip or groin
- Decreased biceps femoris reflex
- Weakness of the extensors of the foot

Cauda equina syndrome: Leg weakness, rectal pain, perineal numbness, loss of bowel/bladder control

Source

ACP
APS, 2007
Chou,
2007

C6-C7 Disk Herniation Signs and Symptoms: Although less common, the third most common site of herniation is the C6-C7 disc, which affects the C7 nerve root. Features of this presentation include:

- Neck pain
- Decreased biceps and triceps reflexes
- Weakness of forearm extension

Diagnosis: Definitive diagnosis is established via computed tomography (CT) or magnetic resonance imaging (MRI). According to the American College of Physicians (ACP) and American Pain Society (APS) 2007 guidelines, CTs and MRIs should only be requested in cases where surgery or epidural steroid injections are being considered.

Treatment: Treatment of these conditions should always start as a conservative approach – bed rest and pain management. If such approach fails in reducing the symptoms, surgical intervention may be considered.

Septic Arthritis

Redness + pain + swelling + joint dysfunction

Causes: Most commonly caused by *Staphylococcus aureus* (gram negative cocci). In patients who exhibit high-risk sexual activity, *Neisseria gonorrhea* should also be ruled out.

Diagnosis: Definitive diagnosis and treatment require CBC + differential white cell count + joint fluid culture and gram stain.

Most Common Type of Bone Tumors

The most common bone tumors are metastatic from:
- Breast cancer
- Prostate cancer
- Lung neoplasia

HIP DISORDERS

Presentation

Disorder	Onset	Epidemiology	Presentation	Treatment
Developmental Dysplasia of the Hip (DDH)	At birth	Female, first born, breech delivery	Positive Ortolani's and Barlow's signs	Harness
Legg Calve-Perthes Disease	4-10 years	Short male with delayed bone age	Knee, thigh, and groin pain + limp	Orthoses
Slipped Capital Femoral Epiphysis	9-13 year	Overweight male adolescent	Knee, thigh, and groin pain + limp	Surgery

Screening for DDH

America Academy of Family Physicians (AAFP 2008) and United States Preventive Services Task Force (USPSTF 2006) do not recommend screening for DDH given that >90% of identified cases will resolve spontaneously without intervention and that the potential harms of associated treatment both surgical and non-surgical are not warranted.

Osgood-Schlatter Disease

Results from osteochondritis of the tibial tubercle. It usually occurs bilaterally in boys 10 to 15 years of age. The patient will exhibit knee pain (referred – no palpatory tenderness or knee swelling), as well as pain and swelling of the tibial tubercles.

Treatment: Since most cases resolve spontaneously, the treatment of this condition always starts as conservative:
■ Rest
■ Activity restriction (no jumping down stairs)
■ Anti-inflammatory approaches

Functional and Structural Scoliosis

The most reliable assessment of scoliosis is having the patient bend forward while the doctor evaluates the alignment of the vertebral column:
■ Functional scoliosis (listing) will exist in the upright position, but disappear in the bent forward position (this is not true for structural).
■ Structural scoliosis is idiopathic and disproportionately affects pre-pubertal girls.
■ Leg length discrepancy.
■ Patients with congenital scoliosis are at higher risk for cardiac and urinary tract abnormalities. For pediatric patients, screen for scoliosis annually.

Treatment:
- Functional scoliosis is treated by addressing the causes for listing (knee or foot problems).
- Structural scoliosis is usually correctable via vertebral column braces. Surgery is reserved for severe presentations.

Examination Board References

NPLEX (II): North American Board of Naturopathic Examiners
Naturopathic Physician Licensing Examination Part II (NPLEx II) Blueprint. Portland, OR: North American Board of Naturopathic Examiners (NABNE), 2010.

USMLE: National Board of Medical Examiners
Brochert A. Crush Step 3. The Ultimate USMLE Step 3 Review. 3rd ed. New York, NY: Saunders, Elsevier, 2008.

MCCQE: Medical Council of Canada
Dugani S, Lam D, eds. 2009. MCCQE Review Notes & Lecture Series. Medical Counsel of Canada Qualification Examination Review Notes. Toronto, ON: McGraw Hill Professional, Canadian edition, 2009.

Related References

Chou R, Qaseem A, Snow V, et al. Clinical Efficacy Assessment Subcommittee of the American College of Physicians, American College of Physicians, American Pain Society Low Back Pain Guidelines Panel. (2007). Diagnosis and treatment of low back pain: a joint clinical practice guideline from the American College of Physicians and the American Pain Society. Ann Internal Medicine, 147(7): 478-91.

Dains J, Baumann L, Scheibel P. Advanced Health Assessment & Clinical Diagnosis in Primary Care. 4th ed. St Louis, MO. Mosby C.V. Co. Ltd., 2011.

Damjanov I, Conran PB, Goldblatt PJ. Pathology: Rypins' Intensive Reviews. Philadelphia, PA: Lippincott-Raven, 1998.

Driscoll, C. The family practice desk reference 3rd ed. St Louis, MO: Mosby, 1996.

Gonzales R, Kutner J. (2009). Current Practice Guidelines in Primary Care 2009. Toronto, ON: McGraw Hill, 2009.

Mercier LR. Ferri: Ferri's Clinical Advisor 2011 1st ed: Scoliosis. St Louis, MO: Mosby, 2010.

Pizzorno JE, Murray MT. Textbook of Natural Medicine. Vol. 1 and 2. 2nd ed. New York, NY: Churchill Livingstone, 1999.

Pizzorno JE, Murray MT. Textbook of Natural Medicine. 3rd ed. New York, NY: Churchill Livingstone, Elsevier, 2006.

PEDIATRICS

Contributing author: Jared Skowron, ND

BIRTH CONDITIONS

GROWTH AND DEVELOPMENT

SCREENING

FEVER

ACUTE OTITIS MEDIA

STREP THROAT

URINARY CONDITIONS

SKIN CONDITIONS

PUBERTY

CHILD ABUSE

GI CONDITIONS

PULMONARY CONDITIONS

PSYCHIATRIC CONDITIONS

BIRTH CONDITIONS

Normal Pediatric Vital Signs

- Heart rates >100 are normal.
- Respiratory rates >20 are normal.
- Consult developmental charts for age-specific vital sign parameters.

Changes that Occur in Circulation at Birth

1. First breaths inflate the lungs → decreased pulmonary resistance → enables blood flow to pulmonary arteries (instead of the monopoly that the ductus arteriosus had thus far).
2. Clamping of the umbilical cord → increases left ventricular pressure → functional closure of foramen ovale.
3. The resulting increased oxygenation of the blood → inhibits prostaglandin production in the ductus arteriosus → gradual atresia of the ductus arteriosus.

Pediatric Vital Sign Parameters

Children have lower blood pressures and higher heart rates than adults. Most PCPs check appropriate VS tables to help them gain an objective appreciation of when to refer. The following table lists normal vital sign ranges for various age groups. Refer your patient to a hospital, if one or more parameter is consistently outside the normal range listed:

Age	Heart Rate (beats/min)	Blood Pressure (mm Hg)	Respiratory Rate (breaths/min)
Premature	120-170	55-75/ 35-45	40-70
0-3 mo	100-150	65-85/ 45-55	35-55
3-6 mo	90-120	70-90/ 50-65	30-45
6-12 mo	80-120	80-100/ 55-65	25-40
1-3 yr	70-110	90-105/ 55-70	20-30
3-6 yr	65-110	95-110/ 60-75	20-25
6-12 yr	60-95	100-120/ 60-75	14-22
12yr - adult	55-85	110-135/ 65-85	12-18

- Remember that children also have different laboratory reference ranges (for example, a normal infant hemoglobin/hematocrit level will be considered abnormal or anemic if adult reference ranges are used). In short, age adjusted laboratory reference ranges are always available, especially on board examinations.

Source

NPLEX
MCCQE
USMLE

Common Congenital Heart Defects

Defect	Characteristics
Ventricular septal defect (VSD)	Most common heart defect. Pan-systolic murmurs are heard around the left middle border of the sternum. Most cases will resolve without intervention. Associated with Down syndrome, fetal alcohol syndrome, and maternal toxoplasma, rubella, cytomegalovirus, or herpes infections.
Tetralogy of Fallot	Most common cyanotic heart defect. Tetra=four: VSD, RVH, pulmonary stenosis, and overriding aorta. It is important to note that children with this condition often squat after exertion. This habitual squatting is termed tet spells.
Patent ductus arteriosus	Constant 'machine-like' murmur in upper left sternal border. Dyspnea and possible CHF. The defect needs to be closed – indomethacin (sclerosing agent) and/or surgery are recommended. Associated with maternal rubella infection.
Atrial septal defect	Asymptomatic until adulthood. Fixed split S2 and palpitations. Most atrial defects do not require surgical correction.
Coarctation of the aorta	Upper extremity hypertension only. Systolic bruit over upper/ mid back. Associated with Turner's syndrome.

NPLEX
MCCQE
USMLE

Cavernous Hemangiomas

Cavernous hemangiomas are common benign vascular tumors noticed a few days after birth. They usually increase in size but they tend to resolve spontaneously without a trace within the first 2 years of life. Reassure parents by educating them about this common mystery.

NPLEX
MCCQE
USMLE

Caput Succedaneum and Cephalhematoma

Both conditions are traumatic sequelae of vaginal delivery that you need to be able to distinguish:
- Caput succedaneum is diffuse edema of the scalp that presents as a swelling that crosses the midline, it is considered benign.
- Cephalhematoma is subperiosteal hemorrhage that presents as a swelling that is sharply defined by sutures and cannot cross the midline.
- Both conditions usually resolve on their own; however, in rare cases, a cephalhematoma may indicate an underlying skull fracture. In practice if you suspect a skull fracture, request radiography to confirm.

Source

NPLEX
MCCQE
USMLE

Anterior Fontanel

The anterior fontanel closes (via ossification) around the age of 18 months. In practice, when you are presented with case of a delayed closure of fontanels, suspect the classic causes:

- Hypothyroidism
- Vitamin-D deficiency
- Rickets
- Hydrocephalus
- Intrauterine growth delay

NPLEX
MCCQE
USMLE

Vaginal Discharge

Milky-white vaginal discharge is a physiologic neonatal response to maternal estrogen. Blood-tinged discharge is also considered normal consequence of withdrawal from maternal progesterone.

GI Congenital Malformations in Children

Condition	Age of Onset	Vomit Description	Findings
Pyloric stenosis	0-2 months	Projectile nonbilious	Incidence in males > females; palpable olive shaped mass in epigastrium; low serum Cl and K; metabolic alkalosis.
Intestinal atresia	0-1 week	Bilious	Common in Down syndrome.
Tracheoesophageal fistula	0-2 weeks	Food regurgitation	Respiratory distress during feedings; aspiration pneumonia; and gastric distention with air.
Hirschsprung's disease	0-2 years	Feculent	Abdominal distension; and obstipation. Males > females.
Anal atresia	0-1 week	Late and feculent	Detected on initial nursing examination after delivery; males > females.
Choanal atresia	0-1 week	None	There is cyanosis with feeding relieved by crying. These infants cannot breath simultaneously while feeding due to nasal obstruction.

- Surgical repair is the treatment of choice for all of the above conditions.

Common Pediatric GI Conditions

Condition	Age of Onset	Vomit Description	Findings
Intussusception	4 months-2 years	Bilious	Currant-jelly stools (blood and mucus mixed with stool); palpable sausage-shaped mass. Barium enema is diagnostic and commonly therapeutic.
Volvulus	0-2 years	Bilious	Sudden onset of pain; distention, rectal bleeding, peritonitis. Emergency surgical intervention is the only treatment for this condition.
Necrotizing enterocolitis	0-2 months	Bilious	Common in premature infants; fever; rectal bleeding. Refer to children's hospital for NGT, IV fluids, and antimicrobials.
Meconium ileus	0-2 weeks	Late & feculent	This is a manifestation of cystic fibrosis along with rectal prolapse.
Meckel's diverticulum	0-2 years	Varies	2% of population is affected; a 2-inch-long remnant of omphalomesenteric duct at the ileocolic junction. This condition may lead to intussusception, obstruction, or volvulus.
Strangulated hernia	Any age	Bilious	Palpation reveals intestinal loops in an inguinal hernia; there is also fever, distress and borborygmi.

Diarrhea in Children

- Viral gastroenteritis (e.g., Norwalk virus) is usually the culprit. It presents as fever, vomiting, diarrhea (check if other children in the daycare or school have similar symptoms).
- Diarrhea may be a sign of systemic illness.

IBS in Children

Irritable bowel syndrome is possible in children with these presentations:
- Separation anxiety (e.g., not wanting to go to school)
- Depression
- Child abuse
- Other psychiatric presentations

Source

Jaundice Assessment

NPLEX
MCCQE
USMLE

- Work-up of neonatal jaundice is to figure out whether it is physiologic or pathologic.
- Measure total, direct, indirect bilirubin, and microalbumin.
- There may be a concern that this infant will develop kernicterus (encephalopathy secondary to high levels of unconjugated bilirubin with seizures, flaccidity, opisthotonos, and irregular breathing).

Physiologic Neonatal Jaundice

NPLEX
MCCQE
USMLE

Causes:
- Approximately 50% of normal infants will have physiologic jaundice. It is caused by degradation of fetal hemoglobin (and its replacement by adult hemoglobin).
- In addition, the liver functions aren't developed yet. That is why bilirubin will be mostly unconjugated.

Bilirubin Levels:
- In full-term infants, physiologic bilirubin rise is <12 mg/dl and returns to normal by 2 weeks of age.
- In premature babies, physiologic bilirubin rise is <15 mg/dl and returns to normal by 3 weeks of age.

Pathologic Pediatric Jaundice

NPLEX
MCCQE
USMLE

- Jaundice presents at birth and/or bilirubin levels are above the levels mentioned above. In this case, send the patient to the emergency ward at a specialized children's hospital.
- Breast-milk jaundice: Occurs in breast fed infants with peak bilirubin level of 10-20 mg/dl at 2-3 weeks of age. Recommend temporary cessation of breast-feeding until jaundice resolves.
- Biliary atresia: Clay- or gray-colored stools and high levels of conjugated bilirubin. Refer for surgical intervention.
- Medication induced: SULFA drugs displace bilirubin from albumin.
- Illness: Infection or sepsis, hypothyroidism, liver disease, and cystic fibrosis may prolong physiologic jaundice, as well as lower the threshold for developing kernicterus.
- Metabolic disorders: Examples include Crigler's-Najjar disease (severe unconjugated hyperbilirubinemia); Gilbert's disease (mild unconjugated hyperbilirubinemia); and Dubin-Johnson disease (conjugated hyperbilirubinemia).

Pathologic Jaundice Treatments:
- Primary treatment is phototherapy to convert unconjugated bilirubin into a water-soluble form.
- If the unconjugated hyperbilirubinemia is >20 mg/dl, exchange transfusion may be performed to prevent kernicterus.

GROWTH AND DEVELOPMENT

Milestones

Growth and development should be charted at each visit. The age listed in this chart is the upper limit of the appearance of the milestone (National Center of Birth Defects and Developmental Disabilities, CDC 2010). Slight delay occurs and is considered normal. However, consistent and pervasive delay in more than one area is not normal and should be investigated. For premature infants, subtract duration of prematurity from date of birth to arrive at actual developmental age.

Age	Development Achievement	Age	Development Achievement
2 mo	Social smile	12 mo	Imitates others' sounds First words
4 mo	Lifts head up while prone Cooing	13 mo	Walks without help
5 mo	Voluntary grasp without release Rolls front to back	15 mo	Understand 1 step verbal command Separation anxiety
7 mo	Sits with no support	18 mo	Good use of cup and spoon
9 mo	Pulls to stand Stranger anxiety	2 yr	Builds tower of 6 cubes high Runs well
10 mo	Pat-a-cake, Voluntary grasp with release, Waves bye-bye	5 yr	Ties shoelaces

SCREENING

Source

Screening Tests for Metabolic and Congenital Disorders

NPLEX
MCCQE
USMLE

All jurisdictions screen for:
- Hypothyroidism
- Phenylketonuria
- Galactosemia
- Sickle cell disease

In some jurisdictions, such as the Province of Ontario, the newborn screening program covers additional disorders of metabolism, endocrine system, blood, and cystic fibrosis (Ontario Government, MHLTC, Newborn Screening Program, 2011). Early identification of neonates with one of these disorders is beneficial because early diagnosis and treatment can prevent serious consequences, such as recurrent illnesses, developmental disabilities, and/or death. Screening is done by pricking the heel of the neonate. The blood is transferred to a special paper card and sent to the laboratory. Acceptable samples can be taken between one day (24 hours) and seven days after birth.

The Ontario newborn screening program tests for the following disorders:

Amino Acid Disorders (AADs)

NPLEX
MCCQE
USMLE

Inherited metabolic conditions that occur when certain amino acids either cannot be broken down or produced by the body. These conditions lead to toxic accumulation of some substances and the deficiency of others.

- Argininosuccinic Acidemia (ASA)
- Citrullinemia (CIT)
- Homocystinuria (HCY)
- Maple Syrup Urine Disease (MSUD)
- Phenylketonuria (PKU)
- Tyrosinemia (TYR)
- Biotinidase deficiency (BIOT)
- Galactosemia (GALT)

Clinical Features:
- Lethargy
- Vomiting
- Eczema
- Hair loss
- Developmental disorders
- Clotting disorders
- Coma
- Liver disease
- Failure to thrive

Source

- Speech problems
- Abnormalities of motor function
- Premature ovarian failure
- Death

Treatment: Involves a low protein diet and/or a diet low in specific amino acids. Specific medications and/or vitamins may also be prescribed, depending on the disorder. It is also important for affected individuals to avoid fasting.

NPLEX
MCCQE
USMLE

Organic Acid Disorders (Organic Acidemias)

Inherited metabolic conditions that occur when certain components of proteins cannot be broken down by the body. These conditions lead to toxic accumulation of organic acids in the blood:

- Isovaleric Acidemia (IVA)
- Glutaric Acidemia type 1 (GA1)
- HMG-CoA lyase deficiency (HMG)
- Multiple Carboxylase Deficiency (MCD)
- Methylmalonic Acidemia (also known as mutase "MUT" deficiency)
- 3-Methylcrotonyl-CoA carboxylase (MCC) deficiency
- Propionic Academia (PROP)
- ß-Ketothiolase (BKT) deficiency

Clinical features:
- Acute Encephalopathy
- Vomiting
- Metabolic acidosis
- Ketosis
- Dehydration
- Coma
- Hyperammonemia
- Lactic acidosis
- Hypoglycemia
- Failure to Thrive
- Hypotonia
- Global Developmental Delay
- Sepsis
- Hematological disorders
- Death

Newborns with OAs are perfectly healthy at birth, but may become quite ill within the first few days of life.

Treatment: Involves a low protein diet and/or a diet low in specific amino acids. Specific medications and/or vitamins may also be prescribed, depending on the disorder. It is important for affected individuals to avoid fasting.

Fatty Acid Oxidation Defects (FAOD)

Occur when fatty acids cannot be broken down in the mitochondria. These defects hinder the ability of the body to produce energy in the fasting state (or illness), and lead to accumulation of fatty acids, hypoketotic hypoglycemia and tissue damage, especially in the liver, muscle, and heart tissue.

- Carnitine Uptake Defect (CUD)
- Trifunctional Protein (TFP) Deficiency
- Light Chain Acyl-Co-A dehydrogenase (LCHAD) Deficiency
- Medium Chain Acyl-Co-A dehydrogenase (MCAD) Deficiency
- Very Long Chain Acyl-Co-A dehydrogenase (VLCAD) Deficiency

Clinical Features:
- Lethargy
- Seizures
- Coma
- Sudden Infant Death Syndrome (SIDS).

Dietary supplementation with carnitine and/or cornstarch may also be part of the treatment for FAODs. It is very important for affected individuals to avoid fasting.

Hemoglobinopathies

Occur when genes coding for hemoglobin produce hemoglobin variants that are not physiologically capable of carrying oxygen and/or cause morphological disabilities of the red blood corpuscle. Examples include Sickle Cell Disease (HbSS, HbSC or HbS/ß-Thalassemia).

Clinical features of hemoglobinopathies include blockage of blood vessels leading to painful crises, increased susceptibility to infection, hemolysis, and anemia.

Treatment can involve blood transfusions and subsequent iron chelation therapy. Certain vitamins and medications, such as folic acid and hydroxyurea, may also be prescribed.

Endocrine Disorders

Congenital Hypothyroidism (CH) can cause developmental disabilities and failure to thrive if not recognized and treated. It is a relatively common condition and is the result of a thyroid hormone deficiency. Thyroid hormone replacement is a very effective treatment.

Congenital Adrenal Hyperplasia (CAH) is an inherited defect in which the adrenal gland cannot make cortisol and will over produce male hormones. Without cortisol, infants are unable to regulate salt and fluids. Some newborns with CAH can be symptomatic at birth with virilisation of females. Replacement of deficient hormones is an effective means of preventing a salt-wasting crisis and preventing long-term complications.

Source

NPLEX
MCCQE
USMLE

Cystic Fibrosis (CF)

Occurs when a protein called the Cystic Fibrosis Transmembrane Conductance Regulator (CFTR) is impaired. CFTR is a chloride channel that allows chloride (salt) and water to move out of certain cells of the body. Newborns with CF often develop respiratory problems and infections because the lungs are clogged with mucus. The mucus also obstructs the pancreas, preventing digestive enzymes from being released into the stomach and resulting in malabsorption and malnutrition. The sweat glands are also affected in CF; individuals with the disease will have sweat with higher chloride concentrations, a phenomenon which forms the basis for diagnostic sweat chloride testing. Individuals with CF (especially males) may have reduced fertility. Some infants will be identified as CF carriers by the screening and diagnosis process.

NPLEX
MCCQE
USMLE

Anticipatory Guidance

Anticipatory guidance is an umbrella term referring to when primary care providers educate parents about the following:
- Keep the water heater thermostat less than 43-49C (110-120F) to avoid accidental scalding of a neonate
- Using seatbelts, rear-facing child seats, placing child seat in back seat of care
- Put infant to sleep on their side or back to help prevent Sudden Infant Death Syndrome (SIDS), the most common cause of death in children less than 12 months of age
- Do not use infant walkers (cause injuries, can topple over, fall off stairs, etc)
- Watch out for small objects, which may be aspirated (choking hazards)
- Do not introduce cow`s milk before 1 year of age
- Introduce solid foods gradually, starting at 6 months
- Never leave an infant unattended in a bathtub, splash pool or swimming pool

NPLEX
MCCQE
USMLE

Growth Curves

- Height and weight measurements are routine until adulthood. Head circumference (HC) should be measured at every visit in the first 2 years. Abnormal values may suggest disease.
- The pattern of growth (plotted on growth curve) tells you more than any single measurement. Growth curve percentile refers to the percentage of children in the reference population who are shorter or weigh less than the patient; for example if your patient is plotted to be in the 50th percentile weight, this means that 50% of all infants of the same age in the population weight less than your patient. If an infant or child is consistently in the low or high percentiles, the growth pattern is considered normal. In practice , watch out if a child goes from being plotted on a high or normal percentile, to a low or below 5th percentile; this pattern is definitely abnormal and more worrisome.
- Increased HC may mean hydrocephalus or tumour; decreased HC may mean microcephaly due to intrauterine or perinatal infections with TORCH (Toxoplasmosis, Rubella, other congenital factors or viruses, Cytomegalovirus, Herpes simplex virus), HIV or other congenital anomaly. The pattern is more important that any single measurement.
- Failure to thrive is HC, height or weight less than the 5th percentile for age. It is usually due to psychological or functional problems. Common causes are neglect, child abuse, post partum depression, and inability for parents to cope with stress. Organic causes usually have specific clues (observe carefully, examine carefully, and obtain a thorough history).

Source

Hearing and Vision Screens

NPLEX
MCCQE
USMLE

Hearing and vision should be measured objectively (by a threshold audiometer or screening autore-fractor) at least once by 4 years of age. After initial screening, it is recommended to measure every few years until adulthood. Similar to in-office electrocardiography, threshold audiometers and screening autorefractors are gaining acceptance as part of primary care provision. In most practice settings, however, these screening services can be provided by public health or school nurses, optometrists, and audiologists. Other clinical grounds for screening are:
- Patient, parent, care provider, teacher concern
- After measles or mumps
- Chronic middle ear effusions or chronic recurrent otitis media
- After a bout of serious viral infection (meningitis)
- Congenital TORCH (see above)

Strabismus

MCCQE
USMLE

Strabismus or occasional ocular misalignment is normal until 3 months of age. Refer to an ophthal-mologist any infant above 3 months old with strabismus to prevent adaptive blindness (suppression of vision in the affected eye).

Anemia

NPLEX
MCCQE
USMLE

Routine screening for anemia is controversial and evidence is not supportive. However, if any iron deficiency risk factors exist (prematurity, low birth weight, ingestion of cow`s milk prior to 1 year of age, low growth curve percentile, low socioeconomic status) do not hesitate to order a complete blood count, hemoglobin, and hematocrit.

Prophylactic Iron Supplements

NPLEX
MCCQE
USMLE

Exclusively breast-fed babies definitely do not require supplementation. Formula fed babies should receive iron supplementation (most infant formulas and cereals contain iron, if not give separately) at 4-6 months of age (2months of age for preemies).

Lead Exposure

NPLEX
MCCQE
USMLE

In high-risk children (living in old building, eat paint chips, living near battery recycling plant, have a parent who works in battery recycling plant), test serum lead levels at 6 months of age and retest at 12 months. In low-risk children, screen at 12 months and retest at 24 months. If the lead value is high, closer follow-up and intervention (stopping exposure to lead is first-line, and lead chelation therapy can be tried).

Fluoride Supplementation

NPLEX
MCCQE
USMLE

Most domestic water sources are fluoridated. If, however, the child is fed exclusively from premixed ready-to-eat formulas, or the domestic source of water is not floridated (e.g., well water, distilled water, or reverse osmosis water), fluoride supplements are recommended. Remember to advise parents not to give too much fluoride because it will discolor teeth and cause bones to be brittle. This the main reason fluoride toothpaste is not recommended in early childhood.

Source

NPLEX
MCCQE
USMLE

Vitamin D Supplementation

Most pediatric guidelines now recommend vitamin D supplementation only for high-risk children who are exclusively breast fed beyond 6 months with inadequate maternal intake of vitamin D, little sunlight exposure, or dark skin.

NPLEX
MCCQE
USMLE

Tuberculosis

Universal screening for children with no risk factors (HIV infection, juvenile incarceration, living in a high risk area) is not recommended. If the only risk factor is socioeconomic (living in a high risk area) screen once at 4-6 years and another at 11-16 years.

NPLEX
MCCQE
USMLE

Routine Urinalysis

There is no evidence that supports this practice. However, you should screen for renal disease after repeated urinary tract infections in children less than 6 years old via a voiding cystourethrogram and renal ultrasound.

PEDIATRIC FEVER

NPLEX
MCCQE
USMLE

Presentation

Fever is defined as physiologic elevation of body temperature set-point above 38C (rectal or rectal equivalent) aimed at enhancing host defense mechanism. Once this set-point elevation is initiated, the body establishes a new balance of heat loss and production to maintain homeostasis. Fever in itself is not harmful. The febrile response rarely exceeds 41-42C. The most common cause of pediatric fever is infection, however it may also occur in malignancy, rheumatologic, or immunologic diseases.

Infants under 3 months of age (neonate): Pyrexia in neonates is considered rare and should be viewed as serious until proven otherwise. Remember that infectious diseases in neonates usually do not present as febrile conditions. Rectal temperatures are required because pediatric clinical guidelines unanimously use rectal temperature ranges.
- Toxic appearing infants < 3 months old have 17% chance of bacterial infections, 11% chance of bacteremia, and 4% chance of meningitis.
- Non-toxic appearing infants < 3 months have 8.6% chance of bacterial infections, 2% chance of bacteremia, and 1% chance of meningitis.

Infants between 3 and 36 months: Pyrexia is more common in this age group than in neonates. In general, the risk for bacteremia and SBI is directly related to the age of patient and elevation of the WBC count.

Children above 36 months (early childhood): Fevers up to 40C (104F) are common in this age group, even with minor infections.
- Body temperature greater than 41.1C (106F) almost always indicate central nervous system disease or heat illness (over bundling) with or without infectious etiology.

- In children and adolescents, tympanic (auditory canal) and temporal artery temperature are gaining acceptance as quick and comfortable methods of screening body temperature. Remember to follow the appropriate reference range of your method of choice.
- Axillary and thermal-tape skin temperatures, while valuable for parents to use for screening at home, they are not considered accurate enough for clinical management.

Primary Care versus Specialist Care: Infectious disease experts generally tend to emphasize their experience with the occasional child who does poorly, whereas primary care physicians emphasize their experience with the hundreds of children who do well. Both perspectives are equally important; however considering the dire consequences of "missing" the child with occult bacteremia, the prudent approach of the primary care ND needs to be centered on understanding the evidence behind current guidelines so that the patient with Serious Bacterial Infection (SBI - refers to bacteremia, bacterial gastroenteritis, cellulitis, meningitis, osteomyelitis, pneumonia, septic arthritis, and urinary tract infections), which is often difficult to rule out clinically, is appropriately identified and managed, no matter how rarely this scenario occurs.

Case Management

When pediatric patients present with fever, start by taking a focused history and conduct a thorough physical exam:

History
- Onset, evolution
- Alertness
- Hydration status
- Last Tylenol given (or other medications)
- Heat exposure (over bundling)
- Birth, family, and past medical history
- Illness in other household members
- Recent Immunizations
- Blood transfusions
- HIV
- Exposure to animals
- History of febrile seizures
- Child's social and home environment

Physical Exam
- Vital signs
- Use standard observation scales, such as the Yale Observation Scale
- Nuchal rigidity (which is common in meningitis in infants under 3 months old)
- Check eyes for conjunctivitis (bilateral injection with Kawasaki Disease)
- Examine ears, nose, throat, and sinuses
- Check for lymphadenopathy
- Skin exam (Roseola between 6 and 36 months)
- Assess lungs and heart
- Assess for suprapubic and CVA tenderness
- Rule out UTI
- Rule out arthritis, osteomyelitis and meningitis

Fever Without Source

- Even with a thorough history and a complete physical examination, 1 in 5 acutely ill, nontoxic-appearing children will prove to have Fever Without identifiable Source (FWS). Evidence also indicates that viral infection is the most common cause of FWS.
- Recent studies demonstrate that 1 in 60 (1.6-1.8%) of all febrile children have occult bacteremia and serious bacterial infection (SBI), which is in contrast to the 1 in 10 (7-13%) range that studies from the 1980s and 1990s previously indicated.

Evidence-based Management of Pediatric Fevers

Refer the child to a hospital for urgent or emergency care with the following presentations:

Presentation	Evidence-Based Action Required
Fever in a neonate younger than 29 days old	Pyrexia in a neonate < 29 days old is rare and is not within primary care scope. Refer to hospital for a complete sepsis work-up and observation until culture results are obtained or the source of the fever is ascertained.
*Toxic appearing febrile child, signs of sepsis, or ominous signs regardless of age	Refer to hospital for a complete sepsis work-up and observation until culture results are obtained or the source of the fever is ascertained.
Nontoxic-appearing febrile child 29 to 90 days of age	Order screening laboratory analysis (including a complete blood cell count with differential and a urinalysis), child can be sent home with a follow-up in 24 hours and detailed return precautions. This child can either be given no antibiotics at all or one dose of ceftriaxone (third generation penicillin "Rocephin") 50 mg per kg intramuscularly (presumptive treatment).
Nontoxic-appearing infant three to 36 months of age who have a fever higher than 39°C (102.2°F)	Option 1: Observe only & reevaluate in 24 to 48 hours, OR, Option 2: Order CBC count with differential, UA with culture, discharge home with follow-up in 24 to 48 hours. Notice that presumptive antibiotics are not recommended for this presentation.
Nontoxic-appearing infant three to 36 months of age who have a fever of 39°C (102.2°F) or less	Observe only with close follow-up. Child can be discharged without laboratory testing or antibiotics, and should have a follow-up visit if symptoms worsen or fever persists for longer than 48 hours.

* Toxic appearance = altered consciousness, persistent vomiting, diarrhea with tenesmus, convulsions, lethargy, anorexia or poor feeding
Signs of sepsis = respiratory distress, temperature instability, jaundice or apnea
Ominous signs = bulging or tightness of anterior fontanelle, nuchal rigidity, Brudzinski's or Kernig's signs

Physical Methods for Reducing Pyrexia

There are numerous commonly used physical methods of heat reduction (convection, evaporation, or conduction) that are often used by parents to counteract the body's attempt to maintain a higher temperature set-point. However, evidence indicates that the body will aggressively oppose physical cooling by attempting to re-establish the previously intended temperature set-point by shivering and vasoconstriction.

Source

Langley, 2007

- In instances where core temperature exceeds 41C or where the metabolic demands of fever are a consideration, unbundling or sponging with tepid water are recommended options.
- More aggressive physical methods such as sponging with cold water, bathing in ice -cold water, ice packs, and cooling blankets (hypothermia blankets), are uncomfortable, potentially dangerous and are never recommended because they invariably lead to rebound hyperthermia (with serious or life threatening sequelae)

Pharmacologic Antipyretic Therapy

NPLEX
MCCQE
USMLE

- There is little evidence that pharmacologic antipyretic therapy is beneficial to the child. In particular, it does not seem to prevent febrile seizure, alter the natural history of the underlying cause of the fever, or shorten illness duration.

- Acetaminophen and ibuprophen are the only therapeutic choices approved for managing fever in children. Both agents have antipyretic and analgesic properties, but ibuprophen has additional anti-inflammatory effects.
- Because acetaminophen has a larger body of safety data it is generally preferred as first-line therapy over ibuprophen, which is reserved for second line. However, safer does not mean safe; remember that acetaminophen is the most common cause of analgesic overdose in children under 6 years old.
- There is insufficient evidence to support the practice of alternating acetaminophen with ibuprofen. This is a mistaken belief often perpetrated by members of the healthcare workers citing anecdotal evidence.
- Educate parents that if using acetaminophen or ibuprophen to use doses based on child weight not age (this is in contrast to the dosing criteria on boxes of commonly sold OTC products such as Tempra or Children's Motrin). Therapeutic dose and maximum dose per day should be specified.
- **Para-aminophenol derivatives** (Acetomenophen, Paracetamol, Atasol, Tempra, Tylenol) Rx - 10-15 mg/kg Q4-6h PRN. MAX Rx 75 mg/kg q.d. or 4000 mg q.d., whichever is less.
  - Side effects: Rarely, hypersensitivity, agranulocytosis, anemia. Chronic use and overdose associated with hepatotoxicity and/or nephropathy. Potential for toxicity enhanced with concurrent dehydration, prolonged fasting, diabetes, obesity, viral infection, or family history.
- **NSAIDs** (Ibuprophen, Advil, Motrin Children's, Motrin IB) Rx 5-10 mg/kg Q6-8h PRN. MAX Rx 40 mg/kg q.d. or 2400 mg q.d., whichever is less.
  - Side effects: GI intolerance, GI bleeding, allergic reactions, tinnitus, visual disturbances, nephropathy. Potential for renal toxicity enhanced with concurrent dehydration.

Aspirin Caution:
- Reye's syndrome is rare but possible side effect of aspirin when used on children for influenza or varicella (a viral etiology). Remember that the only approved pharmacologic analgesics and antipyretics in general pediatrics are acetaminophen and ibuprophen
- Kawasaki syndrome, a rare disease that affects children younger than 5 years, is an exception to the ban on aspirin for pediatric use. Diagnostic criteria include fever for more than 5 days, bilateral conjunctival injection, strawberry tongue, changes in extremities (erythema, edema, desquamation), truncal rash, and cervical lymphadenopathy. The most feared complication of Kawasaki's syndrome involves the heart (coronary artery aneurysms, heart failure, arrhythmias, myocardial infarction). The treatment of choice is aspirin + IV immune globulin (together they prevent cardiac and coronary damage).

Source

NPLEX

Saunders,
2010

Guidelines for First-line Naturopathic Botanical Antipyretics and Diaphoretics

Approach: In general terms, the goals of management of pediatric pyrexia are:
1. Identify source of fever and treat it where possible
2. Provide patient comfort
3. Relieve parental anxiety
4. Avoid potentially harmful side effects in those with cardiac or pulmonary disorders

Antipyretic and Diaphoretic Botanicals:
- Achillea millefolium
- Eupatorium perfoliatum
- Filipendula ulmaria
- Pimpinella anisum
- Populus tremloides
- Salix alba/nigra
- Tilia europa

Immune modulating and stimulating botanicals:
- Astragulus membranaceus
- Boswella serrata
- Echinacea spp.
- Ganoderma lucidum
- Lentinus edodes
- Ligustrum lucidum
- Thuja occidentali
- Withania somnifera
- Spilanthes acmella
- Uncaria tomentosa

OTITIS MEDIA

Source

Presentation

NPLEX
MCCQE
USMLE

An inflammation of the middle ear, OM is extremely common in pediatric patients; in fact, it is the most common reason for pediatric (up to 15 years of age) primary care visits. This is largely due to the anatomy of the pediatric eustachian tube. Studies have found no bacterial etiology in approximately 60% of OM cases. However, the remaining of OM patients exhibit bacterial pathogens (*Haemophilus influenza, Streptococcus pneumonia & Brahnamella catarrhalis*).

Signs and Symptoms:
- Earache
- Fever, nausea, and vomiting
- Erythematous and bulging tympanic membrane
- No pain on manipulation of the auricle (this is a feature of otitis externa)
- Children who cannot talk may 'tell' you that their ear hurts by tugging on the ear.

Pizzorno,
2006

Prognosis:
Prognosis is excellent with the following common factors present:
- Well appearance of child
- Mild pain
- Mild or no fever
- Unilateral inflammation
- Little or no bulge in tympanic membrane
- Little or no erythema of tympanic membrane
- No perforation of tympanic membrane
- Presence of some movement of tympanic membrane with insufflation

Shapiro,
2002

Complications of Bacterial Otitis Media

NPLEX
MCCQE
USMLE

- Tympanic membrane rupture (from impeded drainage of fluid)
- Mastoiditis
- Meningitis
- Labyrinthitis
- Cranial nerve palsies
- Cerebral abscess
- Lateral sinus thrombosis
- Chronic otitis media
- Regardless of the cause, recurrent OM (> 4 episodes per year) is also reason for concern because it can cause hearing loss, which, in a child, leads to developmental problems in speech and cognition.

Periodic audiological screening should be done with children with recurring otitis media. However, the efficacy of universal screening on long-term language outcomes remains unclear.

Gonzales,
2009

Source

Mastoiditis

Although the most feared complication of OM, mastoiditis (which can lead to life threatening spread of infection to the brain) is relatively rare. With all cases of OM it is prudent to inspect behind the ear for inflammation, erythema, enlargement, and palpate for pain over the mastoid process. If any are noted, refer promptly to hospital for X-ray to rule out this condition

Perforation

Resolution without incident is the norm for OM (even when left untreated). Sometimes however the Increased pressure from fluid in the middle ear can create a rupture and hole in the tympanic membrane. These ruptures manifest in patient reports as spontaneous cessation of pain and draining of liquid form the ear. With cessation of infection, the perforation will heal spontaneously within 2 weeks. Refer the child for a tympanostomy consult if they experience more than 8 OM episodes per year (for fear of permanent conductive hearing loss due to scarring)

Management Plan

- Prudent approach is to implement naturopathic treatment with frequent monitoring of all pediatric presentations for any sign of exacerbation.
- In cases of recurrent OM, consider tympanostomy or prophylaxis to avoid permanent neural damage.

Guidelines for Naturopathic Treatment of OM

NPLEX

Approach: The naturopathic approach is patient-centered and aims to address the underlying nutritional, dietary, and immunologic balances, while simultaneously providing for symptomatic relief.

Shapiro,
2002
Pizzorno,
2006

1. Dietary measures

- Diet high in bioflavonoids helps decrease allergic and inflammatory responses (like mucous buildup and subsequent plugging of normal anatomic drainage).
- Allergy rotation or elimination diets are important in managing chronic OM presentations. The most common food allergies include wheat, cow's milk, soy, corn, and strawberries.
- Recommended diet: high in fresh fruits, vegetables, whole grains, beans, lean meats, and fish. Avoid mucous forming sources, such as wheat, dairy, and orange juice.
- Probiotics modulate immune function and decrease allergic response. Probiotics given within the first year of life are preventive and can significantly decrease the number of ear infections during childhood.

2. Lifestyle changes

- Parental or caregiver smoking is strongly associated with increased risk of upper respiratory conditions and OM in children.
- Pacifier use is associated with increased risk of upper respiratory tract infections and OM.

3. *Botanical medicine* (with infants, safety is as desired as efficacy)
- *Matricaria chamomila* (or *recutita*): a safe and effective antiviral, anti-inflammatory, and vulnerary that is used extensively in the treatment of OM. Strong infusions are considered excellent first-line approaches for acute or chronic OM. Chamomile is contraindicated for patients who are allergic to asters and chrysanthemums.
- *Echinacea angustifolia* and *purpurea*: well-studied botanical remedies for the prevention and treatment of colds and flu. Also safe and effective in the treatment of both acute and serous OM. Glycerinates are available for infants. Echinacea is contraindicated for patients with autoimmune disease (e.g., SLE)
- *Althea officinalis*, *Ulmus fulva*, and *Verbascum thapsus:* used to loosen and moisten any thick mucous that is blocking the eustachian tube. Mucilages are generally given as teas or lozenges, but tinctures and glycerinate are also effective.
- *Sambucus nigra* or *canadensis:* a potent immune stimulator that appears to be very promising in the treatment of OM, when mucous, allergies, sinusitis, or upper respiratory tract infections are present. Elder flower is taken as a tea, tincture, or even syrup.
- *Zingiber officinalis:* also indicated in OM accompanying a cold with clear + watery mucous. Ginger is best combined with other botanicals in tea or syrup.
- *Astragalus membranaceus:* relatively safe inducer of natural killer cytotoxicity (similar to alpha interferon), interleukin-2 production, and macrophage activity. Astragalus is usually given as a tincture or decoction.

4. *Homeopathy*
The following homeopathic remedies are most commonly chosen for acute otitis media:
- *Ferrum Phosphoricum:* the most commonly used remedy for early OM. Indications include gradual onset of symptoms, flushed face, dislike of noise or stimulation, and desire to lie still.
- *Belladonna:* recommended in right ear OM, flushed face, fever, restlessness, scant thirst, and sensitivity to noise or light.
- *Chamomilia:* indicated for OM in irritable and cranky children who cannot be appeased for a long time; one cheek is red while other is pale; and aggravation by heat.
- *Kali muriaticum:* recommended when patients experience fullness and congestion in the ear, impaired hearing, and popping or crackling sounds on swallowing. This remedy is commonly used to clear the eustachian tubes when serous fluid persists after acute OM.
- *Pulsatilla:* usually used for earaches that are accompanied with white nasal discharge, thirstlessness, and throbbing pain in the ear that is aggravated by heat. Also indicated in the treatment of OM when the child exhibits changing moods (clingy, weepy, fidgety) with a need to be consoled.

5. *Acupuncture*
The World Health Organization (WHO) approves acupuncture for the treatment of acute OM. In China, acupuncture is considered a component of first-line treatment for all presentations of OM. Assessment and point prescription should follow traditional Chinese medicine doctrine (at least until experimental studies suggest significant variation). Acupressure (by hand or seeds) and laser acupuncture may be more appropriate for younger children who may be particularly concerned about needles.

Source

Shapiro, 2002
Pizzorno, 2006

Freise, 1996

Source

6. Pain Relief

Ear oil is a traditional and effective method of providing comfort for the pediatric OM patient (and thier parents) and in many cases will be enough of an intervention to alleviate the condition altogether. Seek traditional or proprietary ear oil brands containing Olive oil with Mullein (Verbascum thapsus), St. John's Wort (Hypericum perforatum), Calendula (Calendula officinalis), Garlic (Allium sativa) extracts. Hyperosmotic glycerol "glycerine USP" ear drops, will draw fluid through the semi permeable TM and provide almost instant pain relief. Finally there are a variety of topical anesthetics that can be applied directly to the external auditory meatus to alleviate the pain while the OM takes its natural course.

7. Clinical Nutrition

- Fish oil, vitamin A, selenium containing multivitamin (trial evidence - reduce need for antimicrobials)
- N-acetylcysteine (trial evidence - reduce frequency and recurrence of OM, reduces number of indicated tympanostomies)

Breast-feeding and the Risk of Acute OM

Breast-feeding: Breast-feeding for more than 4 months significantly decreases the risk of acute OM (even in day-care settings or in later years).
- The reasons for these findings are proposed to be the ingestion of lactoferrin and IgA (immune enhancers/modulators in breast milk) and the absence of the more allergenic cow's milk (which is the basis of most infant formulae).
- Infants in day-care settings who are formula-fed are twice as likely to develop acute OM.

STREP THROAT

NPLEX
MCCQE
USMLE

Presentation

Inflammation of nasopharynx, oropharynx, and tonsils. The classic strepthroat is a subcategory of pharyngitis, which in pediatric patients may lead to rheumatic fever.

Signs and Symptoms:
- Acute onset
- Red swollen tonsils
- Purulent exudates on tonsils
- High fever
- Lymphadenopathy

Six Major Manifestations of Rheumatic Fever (Jones Criteria):
1. Fever
2. Myocarditis
3. Arthritis

Source

4. Chorea (uncontrolled dance-like movements occur 2-3 weeks after throat infection)
5. Subcutaneous nodules (rubbery nodules)
6. Erythema marginatum rash

Management Plan

NPLEX
MCCQE
USMLE

1. Determine the patient's McIsaac Score (AKA the modified Centor Criteria) by assigning a point for each of the following: Temperature > 38°C (or history thereof), absence of cough, Tender cervical adenopathy, Tonsillar exudates, or age is 3-14 years. If score < 2 points, no antibiotic or Rapid Streptococcal Antigen Test (RSAT) necessary. This is most likely a case of viral pharyngitis. Treat supportively. Risk of strep. infection <10%.
2. If score is ≥ 2 points perform in-office RSAT, if positive then recommend antimicrobial - Penicillin or Erythromycin (if penicillin allergic) + supportive treatment (Risk of strep. infection 15% if 2 criteria, 32% if 3 criteria, 56% if 4 criteria).
3. While waiting for C&S results (which take at least 3 days), initiate naturopathic treatment for pharyngitis (see below). If treatment is successful in 1 week, then antimicrobials are not indicated.
4. Be prepared to refer or prescribe penicillin if pharyngitis is refractory to 1 week of naturopathic treatment if indicated. Therapy must be initiated within 9 days of onset of symptoms to circumvent progressive rheumatic fever and sequelae.
5. Rule out rheumatic fever. The prevalence of rheumatic fever has plummeted since the introduction of penicillin. However, in underdeveloped countries, the threat of rheumatic fever remains unchanged. When it occurs, rheumatic fever affects children 5 to 15 years of age after untreated and complicated strep throat (Group A beta-hemolytic *Streptococcus pyogenes*) infections. Rheumatic fever is antibody mediated due to antibody cross reactivity between *strep* antigens and cardiac antigens. This autoimmune attack causes myocarditis and leads to valvular heart disease in susceptible patients. The extent of permanent and irreversible valve damage depends on how many times this autoimmune reaction occurs (frequency of strep throats). Unfortunately, once a patient has developed an episode of rheumatic fever, they are susceptible to recurrent bouts.

NPLEX

Guidelines for First-line Naturopathic Treatment of Pediatric Pharyngitis

Naturopathic Treatment for Pediatric Pharyngitis

Approach
- Treat presenting infection promptly.
- Provide symptom relief and supportive remedies.
- Prevent potential progression of GABS into rheumatic fever.

1. General recommendations
- Avoid most common food allergens for 2 to 3 weeks. Oligoantigenic diet (also refered to as elimination or hypoallergenic diet) may be tried.
- Increase fluid consumption (e.g., chicken soup, ginger tea with honey and lemon). Hot showers and baths are practical hydrating methods.
- Topical: gargle with salt water (1 tbsp salt/240ml of warm water) b.i.d.
- Hydrotherapy: cold water towel over the throat covered with a dry towel for 20 minutes b.i.d.

2. Clinical nutrition
- Make sure the dose is safe for your pediatric patient 'by weight'.
- Vitamin C: 500 mg q.i.d. (or to bowel tolerance if not contraindicated)
- Vitamin A: 25,000 IU b.i.d. for 1 week; or beta-carotene 200,000 IU q.d. (Caution: vitamin A at this dose is contraindicated in women of reproductive potential.)
- Bioflavonoids: 1000 mg q.d.
- Zinc picolinate lozenges: 30 mg b.i.d.
- Thymus extract: 120 mg pure polypeptide equivalent q.d.

3. Botanical medicine
- *Echinacea spp.*: 2-4 ml 1:1 fluid extract t.i.d.
- *Hydrastis canadensis:* 2-4 ml 1:1 fluid extract, or 500 mg (4:1) powdered extract standardized to 8% to 12% alkaloid content t.i.d.
- *Althea officinalis* and *Ulmus fulva* (throat-coat tea) may be used to soothe the throat and moisten any presenting thick mucous. Mucilages are generally given as teas or lozenges, but tinctures and glycerinate are also effective.

URINARY CONDITIONS

Enuresis and Encopresis

From a behavioral and neurological perspective, enuresis is considered normal up to 5 years of age, while encopresis is normal up to 4 year of age. From a naturopathic perspective, a prudent approach is to reassure the mother and child while ruling out organic etiologies (such as UTIs). Bedwetting is common in children, but concern about it should be postponed until children are 5 years or older. Approximately 25% of children at age 4 wet the bed, and this decreases to 5% to 10% of children at age 7. Other conditions that predispose to enuresis are diabetes mellitus, constipation, cystitis, obstruction, hyperthyroid, diabetes insipidus, and psychological stress. Treatment for enuresis can be difficult, and most children are embarrassed by wetting the bed. It is normally worse in social situations because the child tries to avoid leaking, and this stress usually makes them leak.

Assessment:

- Medical history: include discussion of fluid intake (especially caffeine and soda) after dinner, urination pattern, and record of bedwetting history. Medications, recent stressors, and behavioral/emotional status are also important to note.
- Physical exam: Note any abdominal masses, bladder or kidney, genital inflammation or trauma, rectal sphincter tone, and reflexes.
- Laboratory work may include urinalysis, ADH, thyroid labs, glucose, hemoglobin A1C. X-ray and ultrasound may also be beneficial for ruling out congenital abnormalities.

Source

NPLEX

Guidelines for First-line Naturopathic Treatment of Bed-wetting

- Age appropriate stress reduction and coping skills (less stress = less enuresis). Assess psychosocial stress levels in the household or peer groups manage accordingly.
- Low-Calcium Diet (effective in ADH dependant enuresis)
- Oligoantigenic (hypoallergenic) Diet (a trial therapy may be beneficial in cases of unexplained enuresis)
- Assess for food sensitivities and avoid offending foods for at least a few months followed by gradual introduction
- Refer to urologist if case is refractive to conservative treatment

SKIN CONDITIONS

NPLEX
MCCQE
USMLE

Childhood Eczema

Eczema is a chronic, pruritic skin eruption, difficult to cure due to the multitude of physiological changes that are part of the inflammatory process. Chronic eczema can present with diffuse scaling, thickening, and erythema for many years. A key risk factor is a family history of eczema, allergies, or asthma.

Evaluation:
- History, physical, diet diaries.
- For breastfeeding mothers, consider an IgE/IgG food analysis to screen for potentially sensitizing foods
- Enquire about early introduction of dairy (<6months of age)

NPLEX

Skowron, 2009
Kalliomaki, 2007

Guidelines for First-line Naturopathic Treatments for Eczema

Dietary Measures
Hypoallergenic diet (AKA oligoantigenic diet) trial for baby or breastfeeding mother is necessary to see if case is attributable to food sensitivities. If the breastfeeding mother is allergic or sensitive to foods and has an IgE or IgG response, inflammatory cytokines will be created and secreted into the breast milk. These can create symptoms in the child, including eczema. The breastfeeding mother can have IgE/IgG food analysis performed and avoid the positive foods, or go on a hypoallergenic diet trial consisting of vegetables, fruits, whole grains, and lean meats. If the child is bottle-feeding, consider the possibility that the child is reacting to the dairy or soy in the formula, especially if the eczema presented within a month of initiating the formula. Solid foods should be introduced at a slow pace with children because eczema commonly develops as a reaction to certain foods.

Probiotics
Specific probiotic strain therapy, can reduce eczema significantly during the first 7 years of life. Lactobacillus rhamnosus GG and Lactobacillus reuteri have been most thoroughly studied for their effect in improving eczema, and should be used until other forms have been researched as beneficial.

Wickens, 2008

Source

Sausen-
thaler,
2007
Kienast,
2007

> *Clinical Nutrition*
> When food elimination and probiotics have not been helpful, other nutrients have been found beneficial, especially
> - Fish oil
> - Black currant oil
> - Vitamin D
> - Zinc
> - Digestive enzymes
> - As with other nutrient therapies, they are most effective in patients who are deficient in those nutrients

PUBERTY

NPLEX
MCCQE
USMLE

Pap Smears and Screening for Chlamydia and Gonorrhea

All sexually active females, regardless of age or reason for seeking care, should be offered and educated about the benefits of the Pap smear. Chlamydia and gonorrhea screening is recommended for screening of young sexually active females.

NPLEX
MCCQE
USMLE

Tanner Stages

Tanner staging is a universal way of expressing the stage of puberty on a 1 to 5 scale. In males, advancing stages are assigned for testicular and penis growth, as well as pubic hair development. In females, advancing stages are assigned for breast, and pubic hair development. Puberty is defined as moving beyond the preadolescent tanner stage 1 (i.e, stage 2 or higher). The global average of onset of tanner stage 2 (age of puberty) is 10.5 yr for females and 11.5 yr in males.

NPLEX
MCCQE
USMLE

Delayed Puberty

Onset of Tanner stage 2 beyond 13 yr for females and 14 years for males is considered a delayed puberty. The most common cause is constitutional delay or "late bloomer," which is a normal variant that usually runs in families. The growth curve of "late bloomers" lags behind peers but will run consistently parallel to the normal growth curve. Treatment in these cases is always education and reassurance for child and parents.

Assessment:
Approach a presentation of delayed puberty as follows:
- Test serum LH +FSH
  - If LH and FSH levels are high, suspect hypothalamic/pituitary defect, gonadal dysgenesis, Turner's Syndrome (girls), Klinefelter's Syndrome (boys) or even polycystic ovarian syndrome. Request Karyotype and refer to endocrinologist for confirmation.

Ferri, 2009

  - If LH and FSH levels are normal, test serum prolactin
    * If prolactin level is high, conclude that patient has idiopathic hyperprolactinemia, or prolactin secreting pituitary adenoma. Refer to endocrinologist for confirmation.

Source

Moore, 1996

- ☀ If prolactin levels are normal, test serum GnRH, T4 and TSH
  - ◦ If T4 is low and TSH is high, patient has hypothyroidism, treat accordingly
  - ◦ If GnRH is in normal pubertal level, conclude that patient has constitutional delay and is a "late bloomer". Reassure patient and parents about the normal nature of this condition.
  - ◦ If GnRH is absent or in prepubertal levels, suspect that patient has hypogonadism or gonadotropin deficiency. Request an endocrinology consult as patient will likely need lifelong sex steroid replacement.

Precocious Puberty

NPLEX
MCCQE
USMLE

Ferri, 2009
Root, 2000

Onset of Tanner stage 2 or above (i.e., development of secondary sexual characteristics) before 8 yr in females and 9 yr in males is considered precocious puberty (PP or Pubertas precox). Incidence is between 1:5000 and 1:10,000 (Ferris 2010). Precocious puberty is diagnosed as true or idiopathic PP or when it is not secondary to other disease process or simply when the cause is not identified.

In practice, approach a presentation of PP as follows:
- Test serum LH + FSH
  - If LH and FSH levels are elevated (in the pubertal range), the patient has a GnRH dependant PP. Suspect idiopathic or true PP, GNRH producing neoplasm, CNS tumor, hypothalamic hamartoma, neurofibromatosis, tuberous sclerosis, hydrocephalus, ventricular cysts, post acute head injury, or post CNS infection.
    - ☀ Because the considerations include life threatening ones, perform a thorough physical examination + neurological exam, test serum and urine hCG, request a brain CT or MR and refer for endocrinology consult before concluding that this is a case of idiopathic or true PP.

  - If LH and FSH levels are normal for age (prepubertal or equivocal), the patient has a GnRH independent PP. Test serum DHEAS, testosterone, adostenedione
    - ☀ If adrenal hormones are elevated request a dexamethasone suppression test.
      - ◦ If adrenal hormone secretion is suppressed by 50% after 3 days. Test serum 17OH progesterone and 11-deoxycortisol
        - • If elevated, conclude that the patient has adrenal hyperplasia and refer patient to endocrinologist.
        - • If normal, suspect that the patient has normal precocious adrenarche.
      - ◦ If the adrenal hormone secretion is inadequately suppressed by dexamethasone, suspect an adrenocortical or testicular neoplasm. Request imaging and refer patient to endocrinologist.
    - ☀ If adrenal hormones are normal, test serum sex hormones (testosterone, or estrogen), T4 and TSH to confirm etiology.
      - ◦ If T4 is low and TSH is high, patient has hypothyroidism, treat accordingly
      - ◦ If sex hormones are high, suspect exogenous sex hormone exposure or testicular or ovarian neoplasm, and refer patient to endocrinologist

Pharmacologic Treatment

NPLEX
USMLE

Root, 200
Ferri, 200

When a 6 year old (or younger) child proceeds with puberty, there are social sequelae (self image, peer acceptance, bullying, etc) as well as concerns about permanently stunted growth (premature epiphyseal ossification). For true or idiopathic precocious puberty (i.e, when the cause of precocity is not an identifiable condition) the recommended treatment is temporary pharmacologic management by GnRH antagonist leuprolide 0.2-0.3 mg/kg IM every 4 weeks, until the child reaches an appropriate age for pubertal development.

Source

CHILD ABUSE

NPLEX
MCCQE
USMLE

Reporting Guidelines

In all jurisdictions, healthcare providers are required by law to report on "suspicion" of child abuse. By legal definition, as a primary healthcare provider, you are not expected to delay reporting till you acquire proof (risk of inaction) and cannot be sued for reporting your suspicion. You should share your suspicion openly with the parents of the child and inform them of your action.

- Multiple injuries in various stages of healing (burns, bruises) without logical explanation.
- Whenever the parental story does not fit the extent of a child's trauma.
- Failure to thrive (FTT) can be seen as a marker of child neglect and abuse
- Shaken Baby Syndrome (SBS) – suspect SBS in scenarios where imaging indicates subdural hematomas but there are no external signs of trauma. On physical examination you may be able to see micro retinal hemorrhages, again without external signs of trauma
- Pervasive behavioral or emotional issues in the child without logical explanation.
- Sexually transmitted diseases in a non-sexually active pediatric patient.
- Multiple personality disorder (MPD) also known as Dissociative Identity Disorder (DID). This rare personality disorder is almost exclusively caused by pediatric sexual abuse. The primary feature of MPD, is a person who displays multiple distinct identities or personalities (known as alter egos or alters), each with their own pattern of perceiving and interacting with the environment (multiple characters with dissimilar beliefs, different mannerisms, ages, genders, etc).

NPLEX
MCCQE
USMLE

Obesity

Similar to adult patient obesity pediatric obesity is usually due to overfeeding and little physical activity (>95% of child obesity). <5% is caused by organic disease (e.g., hypothyroidism, cushing's, prader-Willi syndrome).

HEMATOLOGICAL CONDITIONS

Common Pediatric Hematological Disorders

Disorder	Presentation	Key to DDx	Labs	Notes
IgA nephropathy	Children and young adults after URI	No systemic effects	Hematuria and proteinuria without systemic effects	Poorly understood, unknown etiology. Does not respond well to treatment.
Henoch-Shonlein Purpura (HSP)	Children after URI	Rash, abdominal pain, arthritis, and melena	Urine: hematuria CBC: normal	Treatment is supportive, but may need dialysis and/or transfusion in severe cases.
Hemolytic Uremic Syndrome (HUS)	Children after diarrhea (*E. coli*)	Hemolytic anemia and renal failure *without* neurologic symptoms	Acute renal failure Urine: hematuria CBC: low RBC count, low platelet count, peripheral smear shows hemolysis	Treatment is supportive.
Thrombotic Thrombocytopenic Purpura (TTP)	Young adult women	Hemolytic anemia and renal failure *with* neurologic symptoms	Acute renal failure Urine: proteinuria CBC: low RBC count, Low platelet count, peripheral smear shows hemolysis.	Recommended treatment is plasmapheresis, NSAIDs. If these patients need transfusion, platelets should be excluded (due to clot formation).

PULMONARY CONDITIONS

NPLEX
MCCQE
USMLE

Common Causes of Epistaxis in Children

Causes:

- Nose-picking
- Trauma
- Platelet problems, like leukemia or idiopathic thrombocytopenic purpura (idiopathic because no one knows why it often occurs after URIs)
- Clotting factor deficiency, like hemophilia

NPLEX
MCCQE
USMLE

Infant Respiratory Distress Syndrome (IRDS)

A feature of premature infants and those of diabetic mothers.

Signs and Symptoms:

- Breathing fast, hard, and labored
- Substernal retractions
- Cyanotic
- Grunting
- Nasal flaring

Treatment: This infant requires intubation, oxygen, and surfactant as soon as possible.

NPLEX
MCCQE
USMLE

Diaphragmatic Hernia

A defect in the diaphragm allows for bowel herniation into chest. It sounds much worse than it really is. This herniation commonly leads to respiratory problems by restricting lung inflation (atelectasis) and development (lung hypoplasia).

Diagnosis:

- Bowel sound heard in chest
- Scaphoid (concave) abdomen
- CXR

NPLEX
MCCQE
USMLE

Common Causes of Wheezing in Children Under the Age of 2

Respiratory Syncytial Virus: usually occurs in winter and causes an acute febrile condition with marked wheezing.

Asthma: the second common cause of wheezing, but a chronic history is the key to diagnosis. Classic presentation is 'chronic wheezing in allergic children' with a family history of asthma or allergies.

PSYCHIATRIC CONDITIONS

Common Causes of Mental Retardation

- Usually the cause is idiopathic.
- Pathologic causes include fetal alcohol syndrome, cerebral palsy, Down syndrome, and fragile-X syndrome.
- Approximately 85% of diagnosed cases with mental retardation are mild, with a considerable level of independence (assistance may be required during periods of stress).
- Screen affected patients annually for sleep, appetite disturbance, weight loss and general agitation to assess for depression. Begin screening for cardiovascular disease earlier and more regularly than general population.

Autism in Children

Signs and Symptoms:
- First sign is usually impaired social interaction (i.e., isolated as if temporarily deaf, blind, and mute) in a child who is less than 3 years of age.
- Also impaired verbal (babbling, strange words, repetition) or nonverbal (eye contact, head-banging, strange movements) communication.

Conduct Disorder

The pediatric form of antisocial personality disorder. The affected child manifests aggressive and cruel behavior, such as setting fires, animal abuse, cheating, stealing, and fighting.

Diagnosis: The prudent approach to assessment in such presentations is to consider the child's motive, if any. This manifestation is often associated with child abuse or dysfunctional family units (but don't make any assumptions, since conduct disorder can occur without motives).

Oppositional Defiant Disorder

- Child is hostile (but never cruel) toward authority figures.
- Behaves normally with other children.

Diagnostic Criteria for Anorexia

A serious and potentially fatal condition that can lead to starvation, electrolyte imbalance, infections, and arrhythmias. Statistics show that 10% to 15% of anorexics die from sequelae of starvation or suicide; 50% of patients exhibit bulimia.

Diagnostic Criteria:
- Body weight > 15% below normal
- Intense fear of gaining weight or 'feeling fat' despite emaciation
- Amenorrhea

Source

Considerations:
- Assess for suicide and self-mutilation.
- Consider hospitalization in cases of severe viral illness, renal or cardiac involvement, rapid weight loss, weight loss ≥ 25% body weight, suicidal tendencies.
- Consider patients' low body weight when dosing supplements/tinctures.

DSM iv

Bulimia

Common in females who want to lose weight but cannot control their desire for food.

Signs and Symptoms:
- Bulimic patients often lose control, gorge themselves, and then engage in purging behavior (vomiting, laxatives, exercise, fasting).
- The typical patient is adolescent with normal or above average weight.
- Classic findings include tooth enamel erosion and eroded skin over knuckles from purging.

Examination Board References

NPLEX (II): North American Board of Naturopathic Examiners
Naturopathic Physician Licensing Examination Part II (NPLEx II) Blueprint. Portland, OR: North American Board of Naturopathic Examiners (NABNE), 2010.

USMLE: National Board of Medical Examiners
Brochert A. Crush Step 3. The Ultimate USMLE Step 3 Review. 3rd ed. New York, NY: Saunders, Elsevier, 2008.

MCCQE: Medical Council of Canada
Dugani S, Lam D, eds. 2009. MCCQE Review Notes & Lecture Series. Medical Counsel of Canada Qualification Examination Review Notes. Toronto, ON: McGraw Hill Professional, Canadian edition, 2009.

Related References

Ali-Eissa YA. Physician's perceptions of fever in children. Facts & Myths. Saudi J Med. 2001;22:124-28.

Bandyopadhyay S, Bergholte J, Blackwell CD, Friedlander JR, Hennes H. Risk of serious bacterial infection in children with fever without a source in the post-Haemophilus influenzae era when antibiotics are reserved for culture-proven bacteremia. Arch Pediatr Adolesc Med. 2002;156:512-7,749.

Baraff LJ. Management of fever without source in infants and children. Ann Emerg Med. 2000;36:602-14.

Canadian Pediatric Society 1998. Acetaminophen and ibuprophen in the management of fever and mild to moderate pain in children. Ottawa (ON). http//www.cps.ca/english/statements/DT/dt98-01.htm

Behrman RE, Kleigman RM, Jenson HB, Stanton B. Nelson Textbook of Pediatrics. 18th ed. Philadelphia, PA: Saunders Elsevier, 2007.

Centor RM, Witherspoon JM, Dalton HP, Brody CE & Link K (1981). The diagnosis of strep throat in adults in the emergency room. Medical Decision Making. 1981;(3): 239-46.

Centers for Disease Control and Prevention. Ann Intern Med. 2001;134:509.

Dains J, Baumann L, Scheibel P. Advanced Health Assessment & Clinical Diagnosis in Primary Care. 4th ed. St Louis, MO: Mosby C.V. Co. Ltd., 2011.

Division of Birth Defects, National Center on Birth Defects and Developmental Disabilities, Centers for Disease Control and Prevention. http://www.cdc.gov/ncbddd/actearly/milestones/index.html

El-Radhi AS, Barry W. 2003. Do antipyretics prevent febrile convulsions? Arch Dis Child. 2003;88(7):641-42.

Erlewyn-Lajeunesse MD, Coppens K, Hunt LP. Randomized controlled trial of combined paracetamol and ibuprophen for fever. Arch Dis Child. 2006:91(5):414-16.

Ferri FF. Ferri's Clinical Advisor. Philadelphia, PA: Mosby Elsevier, 2009.

Friese KH, Kruse S, Moeller H. Acute otitis media in children. Comparison between conventional and homeopathic therapy. 1996;Aug;44(8):462-66.

Gerhi M. When fever, paracetamol? Theory and practice in a paediatric outpatient clinic. Pharm World Sci. 2005;27:254-57.

Gonzales, R., Kutner, J. Current Practice Guidelines in Primary Care 2009. Toronto, ON: McGraw Hill, 2009.

Harris JS. Managing fever without a source in young children: the debate continues. Am Fam Physician. 2007;75:1775-76.

Hatakka K, Blomgren K, Pohjavuori S, et al. Treatment of acute otitis media with probiotics in otitis-prone children - a double-blind, placebo-controlled randomised study. Clin Nutr. 2007 Jun;26(3):314-21.

Juntti H, Tikkanen S, Kokkonen J, et al. Cow's milk allergy is associated with recurrent otitis media during childhood. Acta Otolaryngol. 1999;119(8):867-73.

Kadish HA, Loveridge B, Tobey J, Bolte RG, Corneli HM. Applying outpatient protocols in febrile infants 1-28 days of age: can the threshold be lowered? Clin Pediatr (Phila). 2000;39:81-88.

Kalliomäki M, Salminen S, Poussa T, et al. Probiotics during the first 7 years of life: a cumulative risk reduction of eczema in a randomized, placebo-controlled trial. J Allergy Clin Immunol. 2007 Apr;119(4):1019-21.

Kienast A, Roth B, Bossier C, et al. Zinc-deficiency der- matitis in breast-fed infants. Eur J Pediatr. 2007 Mar;166(3):189-94.

Klein JO. Management of the febrile child without a focus of infection in the era of universal pneumococcal immunization. Pediatr Infect Dis J 2002;21:584-88.

Laitinen K, Kalliomäki M, Poussa T, et al. Evaluation of diet and growth in children with and without atopic eczema: follow-up study from birth to 4 years. Br J Nutr. 2005 Oct;94(4):565-74.

Koch C, Dölle S, Metzger M, et al. Docosahexaenoic acid (DHA) supplementation in atopic eczema: a randomized, double-blind, controlled trial. Br J Dermatol. 2008 Apr;158(4):786-92

Langley JM. Fever in Children. In: Therapeutic Choices. 5th ed. Toronto, ON: Canadian Pharmacists Association, 2007.

Linday LA, Dolitsky JN, Shindledecker RD, et al. Lemon- flavored cod liver oil and a multivitamin-mineral supplement for the secondary prevention of otitis media in young children: pilot research. Ann Otol Rhinol Laryngol. 2002 Jul;111(7 Pt 1):642-52.

Mayoral CE. Alternating antipyretics: in this an alternative? Pediatrics. 2000;105:1009-12.

McIsaac WJ, Kellner JD, Aufricht P, Vanjaka A & Low DE (2004). Empirical validation of guidelines for the management of pharyngitis in children and adults. Journal of the American Medical Association. 2004; 291(13):1587-95.

Moore WT, Eastman RC. Diagnostic Endocrinology. 2nd ed. St Louis, MO: Moseby, 1996.

National Center for Biotechnology Information. http://www.ncbi.nlm.nih.gov/sites/GeneTests/?db=GeneTests

Ngamphaiboon J, Chatchatee P, Thongkaew T. Cow's milk allergy in Thai children. Asian Pac J Allergy Immunol. 2008 Dec;26(4):199-204.

Ontario Government, MHLTC Newborn Screening, Disorder Fact Sheets. http://www.health.gov.on.ca/english/providers/program/child/screening/fact_sheets.html

Ovesen T, Felding JU, Tommerup B, et al. Effect of N- acetylcysteine on the incidence of recurrence of otitis media with effusion and re-insertion of ventilation tubes. Acta Otolaryngol Suppl. 2000;543:79-81.

Root AW. Precocious puberty. Pediatr Rev. 2000;21(1):10.

Sausenthaler S, Koletzko S, Schaaf B, et al. Maternal diet during pregnancy in relation to eczema and allergic sensitization in the offspring at 2 y of age. Am J Clin Nutr. 2007 Feb;85(2):530-37.

Schriger DL. Management of the young febrile child. Clinical guidelines in the setting of incomplete evidence. Pediatrics. 1997;100:136.

Skowron J. Fundamentals of Naturopathic Pediatrics. CCNM Press; Toronto, ON:CCNM Press, 2009.

Sur DK, Bukont EL. Evaluating fever of unidentifiable source in young children. Am Fam Physician. 2007;75:1805-10.

Wickens K, Black PN, Stanley TV, et al. A differential effect of 2 probiotics in the prevention of eczema and atopy: a double-blind, randomized, placebo-controlled trial. J Allergy Clin Immunol. 2008 Oct;122(4):788-94.

PSYCHIATRY

SCHIZOPHRENIA

DEPRESSION

MANIA

ANXIETY

PERSONALITY DISORDERS

SCHIZOPHRENIA

Presentation

Schizophrenia Symptoms:

Positive	*Negative*
Delusions	Flat affect (no good days or bad days)
Hallucinations	Anhedonia (loss of pleasure in previously pleasurable activities)
Bizarre Behavior	Avolition (apathy)
Thought disorder (e.g., tangentiality and clanging)	Poor attention
	Alogia (loss of speech)

Prevalence

The World Health Organization estimates that 1% of the population of almost every country has schizophrenia. It is also estimated that 10% of this population (diagnosed or not) eventually commit suicide.

- It is perhaps more worrisome that an even greater percentage exhibit functional disability (i.e., they can't do what they aspire to do), and constitute a significant burden on their social support group (partners, friends, or family, if any).
- Whether you are concerned with quantity or quality of life, and regardless of your modality of interest, these staggering statistics compel us as primary healthcare providers to screen, treat, educate as well as cooperate with other healthcare providers.

Diagnostic Criteria

These are the same five criteria that describe psychotic behavior, according to the *Diagnostic and Statistical Manual* (DSM).

1. Delusions: These are non-bizarre observations that could potentially happen, but generally don't. For example: "*The guy on* Days of Our Lives *is talking trash about me all the time*" or "*My husband has been adding rat poison to my morning coffee.*"
2. Hallucinations: These are bizarre observations that 'to the best of your knowledge' could not potentially happen. For example: "*I avoid air travel because customs officers steal body parts when you pass through their scanners.*"
3. Disorganized speech: Using words out of their intended context (be cautious with people whose mother tongue is not the same as yours), mixing words, creating new ones, or simply not making sense.

4. Grossly disorganized or catatonic behavior: Movements such as swatting at the air or repetitive movements that are clearly out of context.
5. Negative symptoms: Negative behavior, such as flat affect and poor attention.

Clinical Reasoning: The same clinical reasoning that you employ in establishing non-psychiatric diagnoses holds true for psychiatric disease. That is, a clinical reasoning that is based on preponderance of evidence rather than isolated features of any presentation. For example, while any person may experience any of the five manifestations of schizophrenia (under stressful conditions beyond the person's tolerance threshold), that person would definitely not be diagnosable with schizophrenia.

Duration of Psychotic Behavior

According to the DSM, a patient with the same psychotic symptoms is given one of three different diagnoses based only on the duration of symptoms. The following is the differential list for psychotic disorders:
1. Acute Psychotic Disorder: lasts at least 1 day but < 1 month
2. Schizophreniform Disorder: lasts 1 to 6 months
3. Schizophrenia: lasts > 6 months

Age of Onset

The typical age of onset is 15 to 25 years of age for males (the cue is behavioral and academic deterioration in high school or college), but 25 to 35 years of age for females.

Etiology of Schizophrenia

The manifestations of psychotic disorders, including schizophrenia, are multifactorial:
- Genetic predisposition
- Environmental factors
- Sustained excessive stressors

Hypotheses: Several hypotheses have been posited to account for the causes and course of schizophrenia:
- Adrenaline Hypothesis: Dr Abram Hoffer argues that psychotic behavior is, in part, a biochemical result of sustained increased secretion of adrenaline (due to severe and prolonged stress). It follows that catecholamine derivatives, such as adrenochrome and adrenolutin, are implicated in the toxic psychosis known as schizophrenia. These derivatives are metabolized first by phenolases, then by secondary pathways, such as monoamine oxidase, catechol-O-methyl transferase, and phenol sulfotransferase. The result is a net increase in circulating indolic catechols (toxic free radicals) and orthoquinones. Accordingly, the two main components of the biochemical treatment of schizophrenia must be to decrease the biochemical effects of stress and to use ample amounts of antioxidants.
- Other Hypotheses: Researchers have implicated abnormal circulating histamine levels (histapenia and histadilia), depletion of zinc + vitamin B-6, and altered membrane phospholipid metabolism in the pathogenesis of schizophrenia.

Source

MCCQE
USMLE

Conventional Treatment

Conventional approaches to managing schizophrenia revolve around the use of antipsychotic drugs (prototypes include haloperidol, chlorpromazine, and clozapine) with secondary utilization of psychosocial treatment.

Characteristics	High Potency	Low Potency	Atypical
Prototype drug	Haloperidol	Chloropromazine	Clozapine
Incidence of extra pyramidal system side effects – dystonia, akathisia, Parkinsonism, and tardive dyskinesia	High	Low	Low
Incidence of autonomic side effects – dry mouth, urinary retention, orthostatic hypotension, and sedation	Low	High	Medium
Therapeutic efficacy for positive symptoms	Effective	Effective	Effective
Therapeutic efficacy for negative symptoms	Poor	Poor	Effective

Guidelines for First-line Naturopathic Treatment of Schizophrenia

NPLEX

Approach: Naturopathic approaches range from complementary to alternative. However, following the well-documented Hoffer model, the following generalizations can be made:

Pizzorno, 2006

1. Reduce biochemical stress
- Prescribe anxiolytics or botanical alternatives.
- Avoid hallucinogenic and recreational drugs.
- Avoid exposure to allergens.
- Address food sensitivities if present.
- Avoid infections.
- Employ psychosocial or cognitive behavioral treatments.

2. Antioxidants: Antioxidants (ascorbic acid, vitamin E, and vitamin B-3) are valuable in protecting against the toxic effects of the chrome indoles on the brain.

Hoffer, 1998

3 Clinical nutrition (Hoffer's recommended treatment plan)
- Niacinamide: 1-12 g q.d. The dose is increased gradually and over a long period of time to allow the patient to adjust to the peculiar effects of vitamin B-3 at this dose. Due to possible

Hoffer, 1998

Source

but rare liver toxicity, monitoring of liver function markers (ALP, AST, ALT & Bilirubin) is recommended at 1, 3, and 6 months of treatment.

- Vitamin C: 3 g q.d. (or to bowel tolerance)
- Vitamin B-6: 250-1000 mg q.d.
- Zinc: 25-100 mg q.d.
- Calcium and magnesium supplementation: 1:1 or 2:1 ratio

DEPRESSION

Presentation

NPLEX
MCCQE
USMLE
DSM IV

The terms major depressive episode, major depression, and clinical depression refer to the same condition. The lay term 'depression' usually refers to depressed mood, one of many criteria for diagnosing a depressive episode, according to the *Diagnostic and Statistical Manual* (DSM).

- A major depressive episode is a period of > 2 weeks that exhibits at least five of the following nine signs/symptoms:
  1. Depressed mood
  2. Diminished interest in previously pleasurable activities
  3. Weight loss or gain
  4. Psychomotor agitation or retardation
  5. Insomnia or hypersomnia
  6. Fatigue
  7. Feelings of worthlessness or guilt
  8. Cognitive difficulty
  9. Suicidal ideation

Screening

Gonzales, 2009

Screening of high-risk adults and adolescents is recommended when accurate diagnosis can be made and adequate treatment can be provided. Screening can be done via PHQ, direct questioning, MDQ, or Hamilton Depression Scale

Gray, 2007

Diagnosis: To be diagnosed with major depressive disorder, patients must exhibit two or more major depressive episodes. These episodes must be at least 2 months apart. Ask about past symptoms of mania or hypomania because some depressive treatments are contraindicated in bipolar disorder. Assess for co-morbid disorders, such as anxiety, substance abuse, and endocrine/metabolic disorders.

Adjustment Disorder

Occurs when something 'bad' happens in our life (relationship break-up, failing at school, or loosing a job, for example) and we don't take it so well.

- Although we may feel 'down' and 'good for nothing', we would not fulfill the criteria (quantitative or periodic) of major depression.

Normal Grief and Pathologic Grief

Normal Grief: follows the passing of a loved one.
- Often manifests like major depression and lasts up to 1 year.
- Experiencing hallucinations about the deceased – and even searching for the deceased years after their death – is considered part of normal grief.

Pathological Grief: exhibits other features of major depression.
- Feelings of worthlessness
- Psychomotor retardation
- Suicidal ideation

Dysthymia

Simply refers to depressed mood (on most days) for more than 2 years *without* episodes of major depression, mania, hypomania, or psychosis.

Major Risk Factors for Suicide

- Age > 45 years
- Recent loss or separation
- Single, widowed, or divorced status
- Alcohol or substance abuse
- Loss of health (recent disability)
- Unemployed or retired
- History of rage or violence
- History of psychiatric disease
- History of suicide attempts
- Being male (three time more successful suicides than women; but women attempt suicide four times more than men)
- Although suicide rates are on the rise in 15 to 24 year olds, the highest rate still belongs to people over the age of 65.

Conventional Treatment Limitations

Current epidemiological studies indicate that inadequately treated mood disorders account for 60% to 75% of suicide cases.
- A recent National Institute of Mental Health survey suggests that approximately 70% of depressed people go without conventional pharmacological treatment.
- Another recent study showed that over 50% of patients receiving treatment with selective serotonin reuptake inhibitors (SSRIs) or tri-cyclic antidepressants (TCAs) discontinue treatment after 6 weeks.
- The reason for under treatment is suspected to be fear of social stigma (the implication of a mental disease label), as well as worry regarding the side effects of conventional treatment (for example, the sexual side effects of SSRIs).

Source

NPLEX

Guidelines of First-line Naturopathic Treatment of Depression

Approach: Naturopathic approach to depression is patient-centered and focuses on modulating factors that contribute to the individual patient's condition; optimizing overall nutrition; utilizing safe and effective botanicals; and counseling patients to develop positive mental attitudes.

Pizzorno, 2006

1. Dietary modifications
- Encourage eating of vegetables, grains, legumes, cold-water fish, raw nuts, and seeds.
- Avoid caffeine, nicotine, alcohol, and sugar.
- Identify and control food sensitivities.

Schnider, 2002

2. Lifestyle changes
- Counsel patient (e.g., cognitive behavioral counseling) with the goals of:
  - Developing an unconditionally positive mental attitude
  - Helping the patient set realistic goals
  - Avoiding negative behavioral patterns
  - Finding ways to include laughter and humor into the patient's life
- Since regular exercise has been shown to be as effective as antidepressants and psychotherapy, attention should be dedicated to motivating the patient to include exercise as part of daily health regime.

3. Clinical nutrition
- Enteric-coated S-adenosylmethionine (SAM-e): 200 mg q.d. to be gradually increased over 1-2 weeks to 800 mg b.i.d. Has been shown to be an effective and well-tolerated antidepressant in a number of randomized controlled trials; most patients respond within 1 week of treatment; useful in major depression; contraindicated in bipolar disorders.
- Folic acid and vitamin B-12: 800 mcg q.d. and 1000 mcg, respectively.

Coppen, 2005

- Omega-3 fatty acids: Evidence of efficacy exists for depression and bipolar disorders; recommend food sources, as well as flaxseed or fish oil supplements.
- Vitamin D: 1000-4000IU q.d. May be beneficial in cases of seasonal affect disorder.

4. Botanical medicine
- *Hypericum perforatum:* 300 mg or equivalent t.i.d. Recommended and proven to be effective for mild to moderately severe depression; well tolerated. Possible mild form of serotonin syndrome when combined with SSRI, or MOAI.
- *Griffonia simplifica:* 100-200 mg t.i.d. A natural source of 5-HTP; indicated in combination with *Hypericum* for severe depression.
- *Ginkgo biloba:* 80 mg t.i.d. Indicated for older patients, who also exhibit signs of cerebrovascular insufficiency.

Schnider, 2002

5. Acupuncture: Numerous controlled and uncontrolled trials indicate that acupuncture is promising in the treatment of depression. Two randomized trials indicate that electro-acupuncture is as effective as amitriptyline (a TCA) in the treatment of major depression; the same observation holds true for preventing recurrence. Diagnose and treat based on the patient's overall TCM presentation.

MANIA

Source

NPLEX
MCCQE
USMLE

Manic Episode

A distinct period (>1 week) of abnormally and persistently elevated or irritable mood, which exhibits the following symptoms:
- Decreased need for sleep
- Pressured speech; talkative with flight of ideas
- Exaggerated self-importance or delusions of grandeur
- Seeking high-risk pleasurable activity (sexual promiscuity, driving against traffic, etc.)

Hypomania: essentially mania, but not to the level that impedes social or occupational function.

NPLEX
USMLE

Bipolar Disorder I and Bipolar II Disorder

Bipolar Disorder: bipolar (used to be called manic-depressive) patients exhibit at least one manic episode and at least one major depressive episode.

Bipolar II Disorder: somewhat milder than Bipolar I Disorder. The patient exhibits at least one period of hypomania and major depression.

Cyclothymia (Cyclothymic Disorder)

At least 2 years of hypomania alternating with depressed mood. These patients do not experience mania or major depression.

ANXIETY

Presentation

NPLEX
MCCQE
USMLE

A number of conditions marked by irrational and involuntary thoughts and behavior. Again, the etiology seems to be a network of genetic, environmental, biochemical, and experiential factors. The defining characteristic of anxiety disorders is disruption of personal, social, and/or occupational activities by overt distress.

Screening

Gray, 2007

Because anxiety and depression often occur simultaneously, screening for depression is indicated. CBC, LV fxn tests, sTSH, and ECG to rule out secondary anxiety.

Source

Prevelance

The 13.3% prevalence of anxiety disorders in North America ranks them as the most common mental disorder (ever). To complicate matters, this condition is clearly under-diagnosed in primary care practices. (Comparing prevalence and frequency of diagnosis is how you determine whether primary care facilities are doing their mandated job or not.)

Anxiety Disorders Classifications

Class	Criteria of Diagnosis	Other Characteristics
Generalized Anxiety Disorder (GAD)	Intense worrying (about everything – career, family, future, money, relationship); occurs on most days for > 6 continuous months + three of the following symptoms: easy fatigability, difficulty in concentrating, irritability, muscle tension, restlessness, and sleep disturbance.	Patients usually complain of physical symptoms, with no awareness that their condition may be related to a mental disorder.
Panic Disorder	Discrete, unprovoked episodes of intense fear + four of the following symptoms: chest pains, chills, hot flushes, derealization, diaphoresis, dizziness, trembling, unsteadiness, fear of losing control, fear of dying, nausea, palpitation, paresthesia, and sensation of choking.	Patients are so worried about having another episode or the implications of panic that they start avoid seemingly tolerable situations.
Phobias	Irrational fears of a specific entity or situation. The most common phobias are agoraphobia, social phobia, snakes, spiders, heights, and flying.	Social phobia is the fear of being humiliated in public. This fear usually leads to avoidance of ordinary events, such as birthdays or professional gatherings.
Post-Traumatic Stress (PTSD)	This is a typical set of symptoms that develop after a person sees, gets involved in, or hears an extreme stressor.	The person persistently starts to relive the event, either in its entirety (visions/illusions/fear) or partially (fear and helplessness).

Lee, 2002

Source

NPLEX

Lee, 2002

Guidelines for First-line Naturopathic Treatment of Anxiety

1. Botanical medicine

- *Piper mythesticum* (kava): perhaps the most effective botanical for these conditions. It has been proven in seven clinical trials to be safe and effective in the treatment of mild to moderate anxiety disorders. However, case reports from Germany/Switzerland raised suspicion of hepatotoxicity. Because of these reports, the marketing of kava is under evaluation in Germany. In the United States, the FDA has decided to monitor the situation closely. *In Canada, a health advisory notice has been issued advising against the public use of kava.* It is important to note that the American Botanical Council continues to recommend kava for anxiety disorders (except in alcoholics or patients with liver disease).
- *Valeriana officinalis, Melissa officinalis, Nepeta cataria, Passiflora officinalis, Scutellaria lateriflora, Cypripedium pubescens, Datura stramonium, Vinca major, Viscum album* and *Luctica virosa* should be prescribed based on specific presenting symptoms.

Sherma, 1993

2. Mind-Body techniques

- Meditation results in remarkable improvement in people with anxiety. The challenge is to motivate the patient to start a formal or informal meditation (both equally effective) program.
- Biofeedback has also been shown to be effective (for children, too).
- Guided imagery
- Hypnosis
- Progressive muscle relaxation is also gaining acceptance.

www.nimh .ni.gov

\

3. Counseling

- Cognitive behavioral therapy has been shown to alleviate anxiety in a number of clinical studies.
- Also consider other successful techniques, such as flooding and systematic desensitization in the treatment of phobias.

www.nimh .ni.gov
Lee, 2002

4. Exercise

- Similar to its effect on depression, regular exercise (aerobic or anaerobic) is particularly effective in reducing anxiety.

5. Diet

- Avoidance of stimulants (coffee, tobacco, tea, colas, soft drinks), alcohol, and refined sugars constitutes a crucial cornerstone in the effective management of anxiety disorders.

6. Clinical nutrition

- Niacinamide: 1-12 g q.d. The dose is increased gradually and over a long period of time to allow the patient to adjust to the peculiar effects of vitamin B-3 at this dose. Due to possible but rare liver toxicity, monitoring of liver function markers (ALP, AST, ALT & Bilirubin) is recommended at 1, 3, and 6 months of treatment.
- Vitamin C: 3 g q.d. (gradual increase, not to exceed bowel tolerance)
- Vitamin B-6: 250-1000 mg q.d.
- Vitamin B-12: 1000-5000mg q.d.
- Omega-3 PUFA: 3:1 ratio of EPA to DHA 1-2 g omega-3 q.d.
- Magnesium: 50 - 200 mg t.i.d.

Hoffer, 1998
Ross, 2009
Jacka, 2009

PERSONALITY DISORDERS

Source

Presentation

NPLEX
MCCQE
USMLE
DSM IV

According to DSM-IV criteria, personality disorders are defined as "enduring subjective experiences and behavior that deviates from cultural standards, are rigidly pervasive, have onset in adolescence or early childhood, are stable through time, and lead to unhappiness and impairment." The classification of subtypes depends upon the predominant symptoms and their severity. Personality disorders can be considered a matrix for some of the more severe psychiatric problems – for example, schizotypal, relating to schizophrenia, and avoidance types, relating to some anxiety disorders.

NPLEX
MCCQE
USMLE

Diagnosis:
- Long history dating back to childhood or adolescence
- Recurrent maladaptive behavior
- Low self-esteem and lack of confidence
- Minimal introspective ability with a tendency to blame others for all problems
- Major difficulties with interpersonal relationships or society
- Depression with anxiety when maladaptive behavior fails

NPLEX
MCCQE
USMLE

Personality Disorder Classifications

Paranoid Believe that everyone is out to get them; they tend to pursue legal proceedings against accountancies.

Schizoid Loners who have no friends and no interest in having any.

Schizotypal Bizarre beliefs (e.g., cults, superstition, illusion) without psychosis.

Avoidant Social inhibition, feelings of inadequacy, hypersensitive to negative criticism. Have no friends, but have interest in forming friendships. Avoid others out of fear of rejection or criticism.

Histrionic Over dramatic, attention seekers (often seductive) who must be the center of attention.

Narcissistic Egocentric, need excessive admiration, lack empathy, and use others for their own gain.

Antisocial Long criminal record, liar, aggressive, torture animals. History of pediatric conduct disorder. Do not uphold their responsibilities. Severe presentations usually make the news because of their lack of remorse.

Borderline Lack of own identity, with rapid changes in mood, intense unstable interpersonal relationships, marked impulsivity, instablility of affect, and instability in self image. features include: suicide attempts, micropsychotic episodes, and in constant crisis.

Source

Dependent   Pervasive and excessive need to be taken care of. Cannot be or do anything alone. Difficulty making everyday decisions.

Obsessive Compulsive   Rules are more important than objectives; inflexible, stubborn; excessively orderly; perfectionist (leads to difficulty in completing tasks); and overly controlling. Exclusion of leisure activities due to work preoccupation is a main feature.

Obsessive Compulsive Disorder (OCD)

Characterized by anxiety surrounding recurrent thoughts, behaviors, or impulses that lead to marked dysfunction in inter-personal or occupational realms.

Signs and Symptoms: Patients may present with washing (hands, objects) or checking (doors, locks) rituals that occur > 30 times per day. These repetitive behaviors or mental acts are aimed at reducing distress.

ASSOCIATED CONDITIONS

Somatoform Disorder, Factitious Disorder, and Malingering

NPLEX
MCCQE
USMLE

Somatoform Disorder: somatoform disorder (or somatization) refers to psychiatric stress that manifests itself in the form of physical symptoms. This is an unconscious process where the patient does not intend for the manifestations to occur.

Factitous Disorder: in factitious disorder (or Münchausen syndrome), a patient intentionally feigns symptoms to assume the sick role.

Malingering: a patient intentionally feigns symptoms for economic gain or to avoid responsibilities (legal or vocational).

Tourette's Syndrome

NPLEX
MCCQE
USMLE

Motor tic disorder (e.g., repetitive blinking, throat-clearing, grimacing, swearing)
- Tends to be a life-long problem.
- Remits during periods of low stress.
- Males are affected more than females.

Cocaine Dependency and Amphetamine Intoxication

NPLEX
MCCQE
USMLE

Cocaine Dependency: cocaine is a sympathetic stimulant that causes hyper-alertness, tachycardia, insomnia, hypertension, aggression, paranoia, psychosis, and formications.
- Overdose often causes arrhythmia, MI, seizure, or stroke.
- Withdrawal invariably leads to sleepiness, hunger, depression, and irritability.
- Cocaine use by pregnant females causes congenital vascular disruption in the fetus.

Source

- While cocaine withdrawal is not considered dangerous, the cravings are so severe that some form of support is required for long-term compliance.

Amphetamine Intoxication: effects are similar to those of cocaine, but more psychotic manifestations prevail.

NPLEX
USMLE

Opioid Toxicity

Recreational use of heroin (and other opioids) leads to euphoria, drowsiness, analgesia, constipation, and CNS depression.
- Overdose causes respiratory depression and secondary apnea.
- Since the delivery method is often intravenous with shared needles, think HIV, endocarditis, and cellulitis.
- Although heroin withdrawal is not considered life threatening, the patient almost always perceives it to be so.

NPLEX
MCCQE
USMLE

Lysergic Acid Diethylamide (LSD) Intoxication

'Mushroom' or LSD intoxication: Features include visual hallucinations, tachycardia, and mood disturbances.
- Although overdose is not considered dangerous, there are rare reports of dangerous behavior that occurs secondary to visual hallucinations.
- Users may experience 'bad trips' while intoxicated and 'flashbacks' months or years later.

NPLEX
MCCQE
USMLE

Benzodiazepine (Tranquilizer) and Barbiturate (Sleeping Pill) Dependency

Both are sedatives that cause drowsiness and disinhibition.
- Can be particularly dangerous when combined with alcohol because of CNS and respiratory depression.
- Abrupt withdrawal from either (after a long periods of dependency) is considered to be life threatening because patients often experience seizures and cardiovascular collapse.
- Gradual withdrawal over several days is recommended (at inpatient withdrawal facilities).

Examination Board References

NPLEX (II): North American Board of Naturopathic Examiners
Naturopathic Physician Licensing Examination Part II (NPLEx II) Blueprint. Portland, OR: North American Board of Naturopathic Examiners (NABNE), 2010.

USMLE: National Board of Medical Examiners
Brochert A. Crush Step 3. The Ultimate USMLE Step 3 Review. 3rd ed. New York, NY: Saunders, Elsevier, 2008.

MCCQE: Medical Council of Canada
Dugani S, Lam D, eds. 2009. MCCQE Review Notes & Lecture Series. Medical Counsel of Canada Qualification Examination Review Notes. Toronto, ON: McGraw Hill Professional, Canadian edition, 2009.

Related References

American Psychiatric Association. Diagnostic and Statistical Manual of Mental Disorders. 4th ed. Primary Care

Version. Washington, DC: American Psychiatric Association, 1995.

Coppen A, Bolander-Gouaille C. Treatment of depression: time to consider folic acid and vitamin B12. Journal of Psychopharmacology. 2005;19(1): 59-65.

Dains J, Baumann L, Scheibel P. Advanced Health Assessment & Clinical Diagnosis in Primary Care. 2nd ed. St. Louis, MI: Mosby C.V. Co. Ltd., 2003.

Diagnostic and Statistical Manual of Mental Disorders. 4th ed. Primary Care Version. Washington, DC, American Psychiatric Association, 1995.

Gray J. Therapeutic Choices. 5th ed. Ottawa, ON: Canadian Pharmacists Association, 2007.

Gonzales R, Kutner J. Current Practice Guidelines in Primary Care 2009. Toronto, ON: McGraw Hill, 2009.

Hoffer A. Vitamin B-3 & Schizophrenia: Discovery, Recovery, Controversy. Kingston, ON: Quarry Press, 1998.

Horrobin D. Schizophrenia as a membrane lipid disorder which is expressed throughout the body. *Psychiatry Res.* 1996;63(2-3):133-42.

Jacka FN, Overland S, Stewart R, et al. Association between magnesium intake and depression and anxiety in community-dwelling adults: the Hordaland Health Study. Aust N Z J Psychiatry. 2009;43(1): 45-52.

Lee R. Anxiety. Complementary and Alternative Medicine Secrets. Philadelphia, PA: Hanley & Belfus Inc, 2002.

Massachusetts Department of Mental Retardation, University of Massachusetts Medical School's Center for Developmental Disabilities Evaluation and Research. (2007). Preventive health recommendations for adults with mental retardation. Boston (MA): Massachusetts Department of Mental Retardation, University of Massachusetts Medical School's Center for Developmental Disabilities Evaluation and Research, 2007.

National Institutes of Health. www.nimh.nih.gov

Pfeiffer C. The schizophrenias: At least three types. Mental and Elemental Nutrients. New Canaan, CT: Keats Publishing, 1975:396-421.

Pizzorno JE, Murray MT. Textbook of Natural Medicine. Vol. 1 and 2. 2nd ed. New York, NY: Churchill Livingstone, 1999.

Pizzorno JE, Murray MT. Textbook of Natural Medicine. 3rd ed. New York, NY:Churchill Livingstone, Elsevier, 2006. Schnider C. Depression. Complementary and Alternative Medicine Secrets. Philadelphia, PA: Hanley & Belfus Inc, 2002.

Ross, BM. Omega-3 polyunsaturated fatty acids and anxiety disorders. Prostaglandins Leukot Essential Fatty Acids, 2009;81(5-6): 309-12.

Sherman J. The Complete Botanical Prescriber. 3rd ed. Corvallis, OR: The National College of Naturopathic Medicine, 1979.

Sudak DM, Scherger JE Anorexia nervosa. First Consult Elsevier Inc., 2007. Online at www.mdconsult.com

PULMONOLOGY

LUNG SOUNDS

Lung Sounds

The art of documenting and interpreting lung sounds is like riding a bike – once achieved it requires minimal refresher training. It is good practice to be systematic, comparative, and unhurried while auscultating lung fields. This skill is fundamental in diagnosing pulmonary conditions. It is also tested on naturopathic medical board examinations.

INTERPRETING LUNG SOUNDS:

Auscultation	Lung Sound	Context
Late inspiratory crackles (rales) in the dependent portions of both lungs. Normal vesicular lung sound over lung fields.	*Crackles or rales:* Discontinuous 'taps' heard on inspiration.	**Left-sided heart failure**: leads to pulmonary congestion and alveolar edema.
Localized late inspiratory crackles. Localized abnormal bronchial lung sounds over affected area.	*Bronchial sounds:* Indicate consolidation = high pitch expiration note lasts longer than inspiration note (compare to vesicular below)	**Consolidation:** leads to increased conductance of sound – bronchophony, egophony, and whispered pectoriloquy.
Low pitch inspiration tone lasts 3X longer than expiration tone. Occasional transient inspiratory crackles at the bases of the lungs.	*Vesicular sounds:* The normally predominant lung sound	**Normal:** transient crackles disappear after asking the patient to cough (compare to persistent crackles above).
Normal vesicular sounds + scattered persistent crackles + rhonchi or wheeze.	*Rhonchi*: The most musical of lung sounds (low pitched continuous, like a snore); cough may clear	**Chronic Bronchitis:** absent bronchophony, egophony, and whispered pectoriloquy.
Markedly decreased breath sounds, but normal vesicular sounds predominate.	*Clear:* COPD lung fields are 'clear' except when the etiology is chronic bronchitis	**COPD:** decreased tactile fremitus and transmitted lung sounds.
Obscured lung sound due to predominance of wheeze.	*Wheeze:* High pitched, continuous, musical, squeaking sounds	**Asthma:** also exhibits resonant or hyperresonant percussion note.

Obstructive and Restrictive Pulmonary Disease

Obstructive Lung Disease (e.g., chronic obstructive pulmonary disease 'COPD' = chronic bronchitis + emphysema, asthma). Patients can inhale normally, but can't expire adequately; thus, total lung capacity (FVC) will be normal, while forced expiratory volume in one second (FEV_1) divided by the total forced expiratory volume (FEV) will be decreased (i.e., FEV_1/FEV).

Restrictive Lung Disease (e.g., muscular dystrophy, parenchymal disease, pneumothorax). Patients can't inhale normally, but expire quite well; thus, total lung capacity (FVC) will be reduced, while FEV_1/FEV will be normal. FEV_1 may be equal in both conditions, but the ratio will always tell you what is going on.

BRONCHITIS

Presentation

Acute Bronchitis: inflammation of the trachea and large bronchi. It is usually caused by bacterial or viral infection, but it can be triggered by allergic reactions. Progression: runny nose + fever + dry cough → productive cough with clear sputum → productive cough with yellow sputum. Acute bronchitis is usually self limiting and responds to conservative treatment, but in some cases it may progress to pneumonia (see below).

Signs and Symptoms:
- Cough
- Coryza
- Fatigue
- Myalgia
- Pyrexia
- Pharyngitis
- Chest pain
- Dyspnea

Auscultation:
- Scattered rhonchi
- Wheezing
- Rare crackles (rales)
- Forced expiration > 4 seconds

Etiology:
- Bacterial, viral, or allergic
- Most common in the winter after upper respiratory tract Infection (URI)
- Air pollution
- Cold climate
- Malnutrition
- Chronic sinusitis

Source

NPLEX

Pizzorno,
2006

Guidelines for First-line Naturopathic Treatment of Acute Bronchitis

1. Dietary measures
- Avoid food allergens for 2 to 3 weeks (first eliminate milk products, then try grains, especially wheat).
- Try hypoallergenic diet for 2 to 3 weeks.
- Increase fluid consumption (e.g., chicken soup, ginger tea with honey and lemon).
- Hot showers and baths are practical bronchial soothing methods.

2. Clinical nutrition
- Vitamin C: 500 mg q.i.d. (or to bowel tolerance if not contraindicated)
- Vitamin A: 25,000 IU b.i.d.
- Zinc picolinate: 30 mg b.i.d.
- NAC (N-acetyl cysteine) 500 mg t.i.d. (mucolytic + antioxidant)

3. Botanical medicine
- Formulation depends on patient's TCM presentation; drying herbs for wind cold invasion or cooling and drying herbs in wind heat invasion.
- Bot Φ of *Lobelia, Echinacea, Zingiber* and *Glycyrrhiza* in equal parts: 35 gtts in hot water 4-5 times per day
- Specific herbs, such as *Inula helenium & Marrubium vulgare*, are also indicated.

Sinusitis

NPLEX
MCCQE
USMLE

Signs and Symptoms:
- Purulent 'yellow/green' nasal discharge
- Tender sinus palpation
- Localized headache that is worse when patient leans over
- Toothache in maxillary sinusitis
- Negative transillumination

Treatment: Same approach as acute bronchitis (above), substituting antimicrobial botanicals instead of cough formula.

CHRONIC OBSTRUCTIVE PULMONARY DISEASE

Source

NPLEX
MCCQE
USMLE

Ferri, 2004

Presentation

Characterized by the presence of recurrent airflow obstruction that is irreversible or minimally reversible. COPD is a descriptive term that denotes:
1. Chronic cough >3 months
2. Dyspnea
3. Progressive reduction in expiratory air flow (i.e., diminishing FEV_1 on spirometry)

Subtypes: Based on additional predominant symptoms, signs, and sequelae, COPD is further classified into:
1. Chronic bronchitis
2. Emphysema
3. Mixed

Prevalence

- In the Unites States, approximately 16 million people are affected, with >80,000 deaths per year; 500,000 hospitalizations; and > $18 billion in direct healthcare costs.
- In Canada, approximately 2 million people are affected, with 12,000 deaths per year; 70,000 hospitalizations; $4 billion in estimated healthcare costs.

NPLEX
MCCQE
USMLE

Prognosis

- 5-year survival:
  - FEV_1 < 1.0 L = 50%
  - FEV_1 < 0.75 L = 33%
- Average decline in FEV_1: 75 mL/year for COPD (versus 25 mL/year for healthy individuals)
- Cause of death: usually related to hypoxemia and cor pulmonale (right ventricular failure RVF).

NPLEX
MCCQE
USMLE

Risk Factors

- Cigarette smoking is the most important risk factor (10% to15% of smokers develop COPD)
- Environmental factors
  - Air pollution
  - Occupational exposure to pulmonary toxins (e.g., talcum powder, cadmium)
  - IV drug abuse
- Demographic factors
  - Age > 40
  - Family history
  - Male sex

Source

- Recurrent childhood respiratory infections
- Low socioeconomic status
- Treatable factors
  - Low BMI
  - α-1 antitrypsin deficiency (rare <1% of COPD patients)
  - Bronchial hyperactivity (asthmatic bronchitis)

Pathophysiology

NPLEX
MCCQE
USMLE

1. Inflammatory cytokines → Narrowing of bronchioles → Wheeze + decreased FEV.
2. Release of lysosomal enzymes → Proteolytic digestion of connective tissue framework of the lung → Decreased parenchymal tethering of airways.
3. Loss of alveolar surface area and capillary bed → Loss of functional respiratory membrane.
4. Loss of lung elasticity (recoil) → Lung hyperinflation.
5. Reduced pulmonary ventilation triggers corrective vasoconstriction in the remaining capillaries → Increased pulmonary vascular resistance (leading to pulmonary hypertension and RVF).

Clinical Presentation

NPLEX
MCCQE
USMLE

Type	Symptoms	Signs	Complications
Chronic Bronchitis 'Blue Bloater'	■ Mild dyspnea ■ Productive cough ■ Purulent sputum ■ Hemoptysis	■ Rhonchi 'noisy' chest and crackles that are reducible by coughing ■ Cyanotic (secondary to hypoxemia and hypercapnia) ■ Peripheral edema (due to RVF) ■ Frequently obese	■ Secondary polycythemia ■ Pulmonary HTN ■ RVF
Emphysema 'Pink Puffer'	■ Significant dyspnea (+/- exercise) ■ Minimal cough ■ Tachypnea	■ Pink skin ■ Pursed-lip breathing ■ Cachectic appearance (due to increased work of breathing + anorexia) ■ Barrel chest ■ Hyperresonant percussion ■ Decreased breath sounds ■ Decreased diaphragmatic excursion	■ Pneumothorax due to formation/ rupture of bullae ■ Weight loss due to more mechanical work exerted in breathing
Mixed	■ Although pure *blue-bloater* and *pink-puffer* presentations exist, chronic bronchitis and emphysema typically coexist within the same patients. ■ In these cases, you will be faced with a combination of the above symptoms, signs, and complications. ■ In end-stage patients, it is difficult to differentiate between the two.		

Assessment

Differential Diagnosis: Because several conditions may mimic the presentation of COPD, begin with a differential diagnosis to rule out these conditions:

- CHF
- Asthma
- Respiratory infections
- Bronchiectasis
- Cystic fibrosis
- Neoplasm
- Pulmonary embolism
- Obstructive sleep apnea
- Hypothyroidism

Evaluation Strategy: To narrow down the list of differentials or to confirm your clinical suspicion, the following evaluation strategy is recommended:

1. Chest x-ray (CXR): *Look for:*
   - Hyperinflation with flattened diaphragm
   - Tending of diaphragm at rib margin
   - Increased retrosternal space
   - Predominant chronic bronchitis
     - Thickened bronchial markings
     - Enlarged right side of the heart
   - Predominant emphysema
     - Decreased vascular markings
     - Bullae formation

2. Complete Blood Count (CBC): *Look for*
   - Leucocytosis during acute exacerbations

3. Pulmonary Function Testing (PFTs): *Look for*
   - Simple Spirometry
     - Increased total lung capacity
     - Increased residual volume
     - Reduction of FEV_1
   - Diffusion capacity for carbon monoxide (DLCO)
     - Predominant chronic bronchitis exhibits abnormal diffusion capacity
     - Predominant emphysema exhibits normal diffusion capacity

4. Arterial Blood Gases (ABGs): *Look for*
   - Normocapnia
   - Mild to moderate hypoxemia

Source

Gray, 2007

Screening

In your primary care practice, screen via spirometry in all patients who are smokers ≥ 35 yo, ≥ 20 pack years of smoking (1 pack per day X 20 years = 20 pack as a year), recurrent/chronic respiratory sx, FHx of COPD, significant exposure to respiratory irritants.

Non-pharmacologic Treatments

- Patient education: allows patient to modify progression and improves compliance.
- Smoking cessation and elimination of air pollutants: reduces annual decline of FEV_1, cough, and sputum.
- Exercise rehabilitation: improves physical endurance.
- Nutritional counseling: poor nutrition is associated with increased mortality of COPD patients.
- Intermittent mechanical ventilation: relieves dyspnea and allows respiratory muscles to rest.
- Supplemental oxygen therapy: shown to decrease COPD complications such as cor pulmonale and improve survival.

Guidelines for First-line Naturopathic Treatment of Chronic Bronchitis, COPD and Emphysema

NPLEX

Pizzorno, 2006

1. Dietary measures
- Implement hypoallergenic diet.
- Increase fluid consumption (e.g., chicken soup, ginger tea with honey and lemon).
- Hot showers and baths are also practical bronchial soothing methods.

2. Clinical nutrition
COPD:
- Vitamin C: 500 mg t.i.d.
- Zinc picolinate: 30 mg b.i.d.
- Beta- carotene: 200,000 IU q.d.
- Nebulized 2 ml of 60 mg/mL of glutathione solution 5-10 min b.i.d. (caution with sulfite-sensitivities - may cause bronchoconstriction)

Lamson, 2000
Prousky, 2008

Predominant Chronic Bronchitis: *Add*
- Magnesium citrate: 300 mg b.i.d.
- NAC (N-acetyl cysteine): 500 mg t.i.d. (mucolytic + antioxidant)
Predominant Emphysema: *Add*
- Lecithin: 1200 mg t.i.d. Improves surfactant section by pneumocytes.
- Vitamin E: 400 IU t.i.d.
- Fish oil or flax oil: 2 tbs q.d.

3. Botanical medicine
- Bot Φ of *Trigonella foenum-graecum*; *Grindellia robusta*; *Boswella serrata*, and *Tussilago farfara* in equal parts: 1 tsp t.i.d.
- General respiratory tonics, such as *Inula helenium, Thymus vulgaris, Marrubium vulgare,* and *Verbascum thapsus,* are also indicated.

Sherman, 1993

Source

MCCQE
USMLE

Conventional Drug Treatment

- Bronchodilators (mainstay of drug therapy): increase airflow and reduce dyspnea.
  - Inhaled B2-agonists (salbutamol, salmeterol): fast onset of action, but significant side effects at high doses (hypokalemia).
  - Inhaled anticholinergics (ipratropium bromide): slow onset of action, more effective, and fewer side effects than B2-agonists.
- Methylxanthines (theophylline): increase strength of respiratory muscles, collateral ventilation, and mucociliary clearance.
- Corticosteroids (beclomethasone, flunisolide): although COPD involves inflamed airways, it is usually not responsive to steroids.
- Nicotine replacement (gum or patch): may aid in smoking cessation.
- Antibiotics (azithromycin, levofloxacin): warranted with febrile bacterial exacerbations.
- Diuretics (furosemide): used in patients with RVF.
- α-1 antitrypsin replacement: for documented deficiency. Evidence of efficacy is lacking and treatment is very expensive.

MCCQE
USMLE

Surgical Approaches

- Lung volume reduction therapy (LVRS): experimental intervention. Evidence suggests a transient improvement in clinical symptoms. Unknown effect on survival.
- Lung transplantation: rarely considered due to confounding factors, but is an option for severe presentations in young patients.

Bronchiectasis

A common complication of chronic bronchitis, uncontrolled asthma, or cystic fibrosis. Chronic bronchiolar suppurative infection → abnormal and irreversible dilation of bronchioles due to changes in elastic and muscle layers.

- Patient complains of long standing cough and copious foul-smelling sputum that gets worse over the years.
- This type of cough almost always occurs in exhaustive bouts on rising or with typical regularity.

Complications: Respiratory failure and cor pulmonale are the most important complications, followed by general sepsis with subsequent abscess formation.

Treatment: Treat aggressively to avoid progression of respiratory deficit.

PNEUMONIA

Source

NPLEX
MCCQE
USMLE

Presentation

The 5th leading cause of death in the United States. Pneumonia is especially dangerous in the elderly, infants, immune compromised, and alcoholics (due to aspiration and ineffectual cough reflex).

Signs and Symptoms:
- Cough, malaise, pyrexia, tachypnea, and pleuritic pain
- CBC shows leucocytosis
- Chest x-ray (CXR) abnormal and consistent with pneumonia
- Rusty-brown purulent sputum is typical

Auscultation:
- Crackles (rales), especially in base of affected lung and friction rubs (due to pleuritis)

Etiology:
- Bacterial, viral, or fungal
- Most common in the winter after influenza URI
- Smoking
- Hospitalization
- Malnutrition
- Chronic debilitating disease

NPLEX
MCCQE
USMLE

Typical and Atypical Pneumonia

Characteristic	Typical Pneumonia	Atypical Pneumonia
URI Prodrome	< 2 days	> 3 days + headache, malaise, and body aches
Fever	High > 39 C	Low < 39 C
Age	> 40 years of age	< 40 years of
CXR	One distinct lobe is involved	Diffuse or multiple lobes involved
Causative organism	*Streptococcus pneumonia*	*Hemophilus influenza, Mycoplasma, Chlamydia*, etc.
Empiric antibiotic	Penicillin or cephalosporin	Erythromycin

Causative Organisms in Pneumonia

- College student: *Mycoplasma* (look for cold agglutinins) or *Chlamydia* (positive DNA probe)
- HIV/AIDS: *Pneumocystis carinii* or *cytomegalovirus*
- Child < 1 year: RSV
- Child > 1 year: Parainfluenza (croup)
- Cystic fibrosis: Pseudomonas or *Staphylococcus aureus*
- COPD: *Hemophilus influenza*
- Immigrant from developing country: TB
- TB with pulmonary cavitation: *Aspergillus sp.*
- Exposure to central air conditioners: *Legionella sp.*
- Exposure to bird droppings: *Chlamydia psittaci* or histoplasmosis
- Alcoholics: *Klebsiella* (i.e., 'currant jelly' sputum), M. tuberculosis or *Staph. aureus*

Conventional Drug Treatment for Pneumonia

Pneumonia is serious condition with potentially lethal sequelae. According to the American Thoracic Society (ATS 2007) outpatient settings guidelines, prompt prescription for the following is indicated:

Group I

- Patients with no significant risk factors, such as chronic heart, lung, liver, or renal dz; diabetes, alcoholism, malignancies, asplenia, immunosuppresion, past drug resistant S pneumonia or MRSA.
- A Macrolide (Azithromycin "Zithromax", Clarithromycin "Biaxin") OR Doxycycline "Apo-Dox" is indicated and will provide substantial clinical improvement within a few days. Empiric prescription is needed and may be confirmed post hoc via sputum culture and sensitivity (C&S) studies.

Group II

- Patients with significant risk factors (see above)
- Two agents are required: A Beta-Lactam (Cefotaxime, Ceftriaxone, Ampicillin-sublactam) + either a Macrolide, Doxycycline, Fluoroquinolone (Ciprofloxacin), or Amoxicillin-calvulanate (Amoxi Clav "Augmentin") are indicated and will provide substantial clinical improvement within a few days. Empiric prescription is needed and may be confirmed post hoc via sputum culture and sensitivity (C&S) studies.

Curb Scale:

Refer your patient for hospitalization if they have ≥2 on the CURB-65 Scale. Give 1 point for any of the following then add them up:
C: Confusion
U: Blood urea nitrogen >19 mg/dL,
R: Respiratory rate > 30 bpm,
B: Blood pressure <90/60 mmHg, age >65 yo

Source

Guidelines for First-line Naturopathic Treatment of Pneumonia

Approach: Naturopathic treatment is recommended as adjunctive treatment.

Pizzorno, 2006

1. Dietary measures
- Because the main concern is adequate protein and caloric intake, a protein mixture (e.g., whey or rice) or meal replacement shakes are required.
- Increase fluid consumption (e.g., chicken soup, ginger tea with honey and lemon).
- Hot showers and baths are practical hydrating methods.

2. Clinical nutrition
- Vitamin C: 500 mg q.2h. Watch for osmotic diarrhea.
- Vitamin A: 50,000 IU q.d. for 1 week. C/I in women with reproductive potential because dosage may be teratogenic.
- Vitamin E: 200 IU q.d.
- Zinc picolinate: 30 mg b.i.d.
- Thymus extract (pure polypeptide fraction): 120 mg q.d.

3. Botanical medicine
- *Lobelia inflata:* 15-30 gtts of tincture t.i.d.
- *Echinacea sp.:* 150-300 mg of 3.5% echinacoside standardized solid extract (6.5:1) t.i.d.
- *Hydrastis canadensis:* 250-500 mg of 12% alkaloid standardized solid extract (4:1) t.i.d.
- Antimicrobial botanicals (see Infectious Diseases module)

4. Physical medicine
- Diathermy to chest and back 30 minutes q.d.
- Teach partner/parent to perform lymphatic massage and aid in postural drainage t.i.d.

ASTHMA

NPLEX
MCCQE
USMLE

Presentation

Signs and Symptoms:
- Wheezing
- Chest Tightness
- Shortness of Breath
- Tachypnea
- Coughing
- Symptoms are often worse at night or in response to excercise or cold air

Source

Conventional Treatment for Asthma

- Involves B2 agonists (e.g., Ventolin, salbutamol, or albuterol) in acute settings.
- Other measures include cromolyn sodium (mast cell stabilizer used only for prophylaxis) and corticosteroids.
- Beta-blockers are contraindicated in asthma and COPD because they produce bronchoconstriction.

NPLEX
Mark,
2002

Guidelines for First-line Naturopathic Treatment of Asthma

Approach: Involves a systematic process to determine defect allowing for sensitization; to address the metabolic condition causing excessive inflammation; to avoid triggering allergens; to modulate inflammatory process; and to treat for bronchoconstriction.

1. Environment

- Minimize exposure to air-borne allergens (pollen, dander, and dust mites).
- Avoid cats, dogs, upholstery.
- Allergen proof the bedroom.
- Install air purification filters (HEPA=high efficiency particulate arresting filters) to central heating or air-conditioning systems.

2. Dietary measures

- Identify and eliminate food allergens.
- Use 4-day rotation diet, hypoallergenic diet, or vegan diet.
- Eat cold-water ocean fish.

3. Clinical nutrition (adult dosage is provided)

- Vitamin B-6: 25 mg b.i.d.
- Vitamin B-12: 1000 ug oral q.d. or weekly IM injection. Re-evaluate after 6 weeks.
- Antioxidant cocktail = vitamin C 10-30 mg/kg body weight in divided doses; vitamin E 200-400 IU q.d.; and selenium 200 ug q.d.
- Magnesium citrate: 200-400 mg t.i.d. Bronchodilator - calcium channel blocker.
- Quercetin: 400 mg t.i.d. before meals. Natural mast cell stabilizer.

Pizzorno,
2006

4. Botanical medicine: (specific botanicals need to be considered)

- *Glycyrrhiza glabra:* 250-500 mg t.i.d. Inhibits phospholipase A2 and subsequent ecosanoid synthesis + expectorant.
- *Tylophora asthmatica:* 200 mg leaves or 40 mg dry extract b.i.d. Histamine receptor blocker, antispasmodic, inhibits mast cell degranulation.
- *Coleus fosrkohlii:* 50 mg (18% forskolin) b.i.d. or t.i.d. Side effects include nausea, decreased taste for salt, and slight oral soreness.

5. Counseling: Especially important for young patients with behavioral problems, as well as adults for whom asthma attacks are precipitated by emotional crisis.

Source

LUNG CANCER

Presentation

NPLEX
MCCQE
USMLE

Signs and Symptoms:
- Cough; hemoptysis; dyspnea; chest pain; increased sputum production; hoarseness; and weight loss in advanced cases.
- On percussion, there may be atelectasis, consolidation, or abnormalities in auscultation.
- Prudent management plan of such a patient would involve imaging, ruling out other causes for chronic cough (see above), then referral for bronchoscopy/biopsy.

Screening

Gonzales,
2009

There is insufficient evidence to recommend screening of asymptomatic patients, though screening of individuals at increased risk should be considered. While screening increases the rate lung cancer diagnosis, it doe s not seem to reduce incidence of death from lung cancer.

ADULT RESPIRATORY DISTRESS SYNDROME

Presentation

NPLEX
MCCQE
USMLE

ARDS Signs and Symptoms:
- Rapid onset respiratory insufficiency = severe dyspnea + cyanosis + intercostals retractions + hypoxia that is refractory to oxygen therapy.
- Results from noncardiogenic pulmonary edema secondary to alveolar injury (sepsis, inhalation of irritants, pancreatitis, shock, near drowning, and drug overdose). It usually occurs 24-48 hours after the initial insult.

Treatment: This patient needs positive end expiratory pressure (PEEP) ventilation. Call an ambulance while trying high concentration oxygen ventilation in your office.

CYSTIC FIBROSIS

Presentation

The most lethal genetic disease in Caucasians, this autosomal recessive disorder affects 1 in 2,500 newborn white babies.

- Viscous secretions accumulate (and block the flow) in the glandular lumen of the pancreas, bronchi, and gastrointestinal system.
- Subsequently, there is pancreatic fibrosis, deficiency in digestive enzymes, malabsorption, multiple nutritional deficiencies, and bronchiectasis with recurrent bouts of pneumonia.

Signs and Symptoms: The classical board examination example is a mother who claims that her baby is 'salty-tasting'. Clinically, however, suspect CF in pediatric patients with these symptoms:

- Rectal prolapse
- Meconium ileus
- Esophageal varices
- Recurrent pulmonary infections
- Failure to thrive

Treatment: Any pulmonary infection in these patients requires aggressive treatment to avoid additional irreversible damage.

- Chest physical therapy (i.e., postural drainage, lymphatic pump)
- Fat-soluble vitamins (vitamin A,D,E,K)
- Pancreatic enzyme supplementation

Solitary Pulmonary Nodule

A systematic process is required to identify the cause before secondary care can be initiated.

Presentation	*Probable Cause*
Immigrant; recent residence in developing country; tree-planting; malnourished.	Suspect tuberculosis. Request a PPD skin test and culture sputum if positive.
Recent travel to Southwest United States (Arizona, New Mexico, and Southern California) and northern Mexico.	Suspect *Coccidioides immitis* fungal infection. Request coccidioidin skin test.
Cave explorers; exposure to bird droppings; recent travel to Midwest United States (Ohio and Mississippi River valleys)	Suspect *Histoplasmosis* fungal infection. Request a histoplasmin skin test.
Smoker over the age of 50	Consider lung cancer. Request bronchoscopy and biopsy.
Person under age 40	Consider hamartoma (normal cells are arranged abnormally – i.e., a nevi is an abnormally arranged cluster of normal melanocytes)

Examination Board References

NPLEX (II): North American Board of Naturopathic Examiners
Naturopathic Physician Licensing Examination Part II (NPLEx II) Blueprint. Portland, OR: North American Board of Naturopathic Examiners (NABNE), 2010.

USMLE: National Board of Medical Examiners
Brochert A. Crush Step 3. The Ultimate USMLE Step 3 Review. 3rd ed. New York, NY: Saunders, Elsevier, 2008.

MCCQE: Medical Council of Canada
Dugani S, Lam D, eds. 2009. MCCQE Review Notes & Lecture Series. Medical Counsel of Canada Qualification Examination Review Notes. Toronto, ON: McGraw Hill Professional, Canadian edition, 2009.

Related References

Bach PB, Jett JR, Pastorino U, Tockman MS, Swensen SJ, Begg CB. Computed Tomography Screening and Lung Cancer Outcomes. JAMA 2007;297:995.

Dains J, Baumann L, Scheibel P. Advanced Health Assessment & Clinical Diagnosis in Primary Care. 2nd ed. St. Louis, MO: Mosby C.V. Co. Ltd, 2003.

Dains J, Baumann L, Scheibel P. Advanced Health Assessment & Clinical Diagnosis in Primary Care. 4th ed. St Louis, MO: Mosby C.V. Co. Ltd., 2011.

Damjanov I, Conran PB, Goldblatt PJ. Pathology: Rypins' Intensive Reviews. Philadelphia, PA: Lippincott-Raven, 1998.

Ferri F. Ferri's Clinical Advisor: Instant Diagnosis and Treatment. St. Louis, MO: Mosby Inc, 2004.

Gray J. Therapeutic Choices. 5th ed. Ottawa: ON: Canadian Pharmacists Association, 2007.

Gonzales R, Kutner J. Current Practice Guidelines in Primary Care 2009. Toronto, ON: McGraw Hill, 2009.

Lamson DW, Brignall MS. The use of nebulized glutathione in the treatment of emphysema: a case report. Alternative Medicine Review, 2000;5(5): 429-31.

Mark JD. Asthma. Complementary and Alternative Medicine Secrets. Philadelphia, PA: Hanley & Belfus Inc, 2002.

Marz RB. 1999. Medical Nutrition from Marz. 2nd ed. Portland, OR: Omni-Press, 1999.

Mills S, Bone K. Principles and Practice of Phytotherapy: Modern Herbal Medicine. New York, NY: Churchill Livingstone, 2000.

Moore R. Hematology Laboratory Diagnosis. Guelph, ON: McMaster University Press, 2001.

Pizzorno JE, Murray MT. Textbook of Natural Medicine. Vol. 1 and 2. 2nd ed. New York, NY: Churchill Livingstone, 1999.

Pizzorno JE, Murray MT. Textbook of Natural Medicine,. 3rd ed. Churchill Livingstone, Elsevier, 2006.

Prousky J. The treatment of pulmonary diseases and respiratory-related conditions with inhaled (nebulized or aerosolized) glutathione. Evidence Based Complementary Alternative Medicine. 2008;5(1) 27-35.

Saunders, PR. 2000. Herbal Remedies for Canadians. Toronto, ON: Prentice Hall-Pearson, 2000.

Sherman J. The Complete Botanical Prescriber. 3rd ed. Corvallis, OR: National College of Naturopathic Medicine, 1979.

Skidmore, LR. Mosby's Handbook of Herbs & Natural Supplements. St. Louis, MO: Mosby, 2004.

RHEUMATOLOGY

OSTEOARTHRITIS

GOUT

RHEUMATOID ARTHRITIS

RHEUMATIC FEVER

ASSOCIATED CONDITIONS

OSTEOARTHRITIS

Presentation

Osteoarthritis (OA) accounts for more than 75% of arthritis cases. OA is a degenerative joint disease, also called 'old age' or 'wear-and-tear' arthritis. OA first appears asymptomatically at age 20, then by age 40 almost all people will exhibit some characteristic pathologic changes in weight-bearing joints.

Signs and Symptoms:
- Mild early morning stiffness
- Stiffness following periods of rest
- Pain that worsens on joint use
- Loss of joint function
- Physical examination: OA exhibits few signs of inflammation without the hot, red, tender joints seen in rheumatoid, gout, pseudogout, and septic arthritis. Look for Heberden's nodes at the DIPs and Bouchard nodes at the PIPs.
- X-ray findings: While not essential in clear presentations, radiographs will show narrowed joint space, osteophytes, increased density of subchondral bone, subchondral sclerosis, bony cysts, and periarticular swelling.

Guidelines for First-line Naturopathic Treatment of OA

Approach:
- Reduce weight because this is a weight-bearing manifestation.
- Reduce joint stress.
- Promote collagen repair and eliminate foods and other factors that inhibit collagen repair.
- Control predisposing factors (obstacles to healing).
- Minimize or eliminate need for NSAIDs (while valuable in relieving pain and inflammation, they often inhibit collagen matrix synthesis and accelerate cartilage destruction).

1. Dietary measures
- Avoid simple, processed, and refined carbohydrates.
- Emphasize complex-carbohydrates and high-fiber foods.
- Minimize fats.
- Encourage flavonoid-rich berries or extracts (e.g., blue berries).
- Determine sensitivity to night shades (e.g., tomatoes, potatoes, eggplant, peppers) via a trial elimination diet because this group of plants contain an alkaloid that may aggravate symptoms of OA.

Source

2. Clinical nutrition
- Glucosamine sulfate: 500 mg t.i.d.
- Niacinamide: 800 mg t.i.d. Establish a baseline liver enzyme profile and then monitor appropriately.
- Ensure adequate intake of vitamins A, C, B-5, and B-6.
- Ensure adequate intake of boron, zinc, and copper.
- S-Adenosyl-Methionine (SAMe): 400 mg. Significantly better alternative to NSAIDs: increases cartilage formation in 91% of cases; tolerance is very good in 87% of cases; and is a mild analgesic anti-inflammatory agent.
- PUFA omega 3

3. Botanical medicine
- *Medicago sativa* (alfalfa tonic): equivalent to 5-10 g crude herb q.d.
- *Harpagophytum procumbens:* 5 ml tincture or 400 mg solid extract t.i.d
- *Boswella serrata:* 400 mg boswellic acids t.i.d.

4. Physical medicine
- Monitored daily non-impact exercise is highly recommended (e.g., swimming and isometric exercise).
- Short wave diathermy and hydrotherapy are important because they improve joint perfusion.
- TENS and acupuncture may offer symptomatic pain relief.

Medhi, 2009

5. Other
- Castor oil topically reduces inflammation.

GOUT

NPLEX MCCQE USMLE

Gout

Hyperuricimia is the underlying cause of gout. Traditionally, gout was viewed as an inherited disorder of purine metabolism with 95% of cases occuring in male patients. Joint affected is usually either a big toe, MTP of foot, or knee. Alcohol- and protein-rich foods may precipitate an attack.

Signs and Symptoms:
- Acute onset
- Frequently nocturnal
- Typically monoarticular joint pain with asymptomatic periods between attacks
- Joint is red, hot and swollen
- Elevated serum uric acid

ray, 2007

Medical: Atherosclerosis, diabetes, drugs (alcohol, cyclosporine, diuretics, salicylates, theophylline, levodopa, nicotinic acid), hyperlipidemia, hypertension, renal dz, ischemic heart dz, obesity

Source

Risk Factors:
- Dietary causes account for 12% of gout cases
- Consumption of alcohol, fructose-sweetened drinks, meat, seafood

Conventional Treatment:
- NSAIDs
- Colchicine
- Steroids

NPLEX

Guidelines for First-line Naturopathic Treatment of Gout

Pizzorno, 2006

Approach:
- Reduce intake of pruine forming foods.
- Increase elimination of purine metabolic by products.
- Reduce predisposing factors (Alcohol, red meat, seafood).
- Minimize or eliminate need for NSAIDs (see OA).

1. Dietary measures
- Eliminate alcohol especially beer and liquor.
- Implement low-purine diet.
- Increase complex-carbohydrates.
- Minimize fats.
- Limit protein intake (0.8g/kg body weight), especially red meat and seafood.
- Increase pure water consumption.
- Encourage consumption of 0.25 kg flavonoid-rich berries per day or equivalent supplementation (e.g., blue berries, cherries).
- Monitor compliance with 24-hour urine uric acid on a monthly basis.

2. Clinical nutrition
- Eicosapentanoic acid (EPA): 1.8 g q.d. Anti-inflammatory, inhibits synthesis of leukotrienes.
- Vitamin E: 400-800 IU q.d. Antioxidant, lowers leukotriene levels.
- Folic acid: 10-40 mg q.d. Inhibits xanthine oxidase, thus uric acid production.
- Bromelain: 125-250 mg t.i.d. Anecdotal evidence of effective anti-inflammatory activity.
- Quercetin: 125-250 mg t.i.d. Alternative to allopurinol, inhibits xanthine oxidase, leukotriene release, and neutrophil aggregation.

3. Botanical medicine
- *Harpagophytum procumbens:* 5 ml tincture or 400 mg solid extract t.i.d.
- *Vaccinium myrtillus:* equivalent to 80 mg anthocyanoside q.d.

RHEUMATOID ARTHRITIS

Presentation

Signs and Symptoms:
- Prolonged morning stiffness
- Vague joint pain preceding visible swelling
- Joint stiffness that is ameliorated by motion (compare to OA)
- Progressive joint involvement

Assessment

Diagnosis:
- Key to diagnosis is systemic symptoms (fever, malaise, subcutaneous nodules, uveitis, pericarditis, or pleural effusion).
- Look for ulnar deviation, swan neck, and Boutonnière deformities during your physical examination.

X-ray Findings:
- Bilaterally symmetrical soft tissue swelling, pannus formation, erosion of cartilage margin, and joint space narrowing.

Lab Tests:
- Rheumatoid factor (RF) is present in most adult patients, but absent in children.
- Antinuclear antibodies (ANA) are elevated in 20% to 60% of patients.

Psoriasis

Can cause arthritis in the hands and feet that resembles RA. However, RF is almost always negative in psoriatic arthritis.

Diagnosis: Key to diagnosis is observing psoriatic skin lesions on physical examination.

Ankylosing Spondylitis (AS)

Signs and Symptoms:
- Typically, a 20- to 40-year-old man with positive family history complaining of back pain and morning stiffness.
- The SI joints are primarily affected.
- Since this is an autoimmune disorder, you would expect a low-grade fever as well as microcytic anemia.

X-ray findings:
- 'Bamboo spine'
- Syndesmophytes

Source

Lab Tests:
- Positive human leukocyte antigen B27 (HLA-B27)
- Elevated ESR
- High C-reactive protein

Reiter's Syndrome

NPLEX
MCCQE
USMLE

Linked to the mnemonic "can't see, can't pee, can't dance with me" by generations of healthcare providers.

Signs and Symptoms:
- Conjunctivitis
- Urethritis (due to chlamydial infection)
- Arthritis
- Superficial oral and penile ulcers (possible)

Lab Tests:
- Reiter's syndrome is HLA-B27 positive (which is not required for diagnosis).

Treatment:
- This condition follows bacterial infections (STDs or, rarely, enteric pathogens). Therefore, the target of treatment is the causative organism.
- Also treat the patient's sexual partner where applicable.

Hemophilia

NPLEX
MCCQE
USMLE

This condition can cause arthritis, but the patient would know about the condition long before hemarthrosis causes debilitating arthritis – an easy diagnosis.

Lyme Disease

NPLEX
MCCQE
USMLE

The tick-borne *Borrelia burgdorferi* causes erythema chronicum migrans 'bull's-eye lesion' and late onset migratory arthritis. Lyme disease can cause myriad manifestations (similar to meningitis or cranial nerve palsies), but the bull's-eye is the tell-tale sign.

Diagnosis: ELISA or western blot test.

Ischemic Arthralgia

NPLEX
MCCQE
USMLE

Due to sickle cell crisis, which is usually a manifestation of avascular necrosis of the femoral head. Refer to the Hematology module for diagnosis of sickle-cell anemia.

Source

NPLEX
MCCQE
USMLE

RHEUMATIC FEVER

Presentation

Prevalence has plummeted after the introduction of penicillin; however, in underdeveloped countries, the threat of rheumatic fever remains. When it occurs, rheumatic fever affects children 5 to 15 years of age after untreated and complicated strep throat (Group A beta-hemolytic *Streptococcus pyogenes*, or GABS) infections. Rheumatic fever is antibody mediated due to antibody cross reactivity between *strep* antigens and cardiac antigens.

Complications: This autoimmune attack causes myocarditis and leads to valvular heart disease in susceptible patients. The extent of permanent and irreversible valve damage depends on how many times this autoimmune reaction occurred (frequency of strep throats). Unfortunately, once patients have developed an episode of rheumatic fever, they are susceptible to recurrent bouts.

Strep Throat Manifestations:
- Acute onset
- Red swollen tonsils
- Purulent exudates on tonsils
- High fever
- Lymphadenopathy

Major Manifestations of Rheumatic Fever (Jones criteria):
- Fever
- Myocarditis
- Arthritis
- Chorea (uncontrolled dance-like movements occurs 2-3 weeks after throat infection)
- Subcutaneous nodules (rubbery nodules)
- Erythema marginatum rash

Managing Pharyngitis in Children:
1. Perform a rapid strep screen on suspected cases.
2. If positive, then antimicrobials are required.
3. If negative, do culture and sensitivity (C&S) on a throat swab. If C&S indicates *Streptococcus pyogenes* infection, then antimicrobials are required.
4. While waiting for C&S results (which takes at least 3 days), initiate naturopathic treatment for pharyngitis. If treatment is successful in 1 week, then antimicrobials are not indicated.
5. Be prepared to refer or prescribe penicillin if pharyngitis is refractory to 1 week of naturopathic treatment. There is published evidence that shows a decline of in incidence of GABS induced rheumatic complications if therapy is successful in the first 9 days of being infected.

ASSOCIATED CONDITIONS

Charcot Joints (Neuropathic Peripheral Joints)

Lack of sensation causes abuse of joints, which, in turn, leads to joint deformity and pain.
- Seen in diabetics; patients with neuropathy, pernicous anemia; tertiary syphilis.
- The best treatment is prevention and treatment of the cause of neuropathy.

Autoimmune Disorders

Signs and Symptoms:
- Elevated ESR and C-reactive protein
- Fever
- Anemia of chronic disease (microcytic)
- Fatigue
- Weight loss
- Incidence of autoimmune disease is significantly higher in women of reproductive age.

Systemic Lupus Erythematosus (SLE)

Signs and Symptoms:
- Well demarcated rash (malar or discoid)
- Photosensitivity
- Kidney damage
- Poly-arthritis (more than one joint is involved)
- Possible pericarditis/pleuritis
- Oral ulcers
- Neurological disturbances (depression, psychosis, and seizures)

Diagnosis: It is a difficult diagnosis in early stages before the classical clinical presentation is recognized.
- Use Anti-Nuclear Antibody (ANA) titer as a screening test.
- Confirm with Anti-Smith antibody test.
- CBC disorders (thrombocytopenia, leukopenia, anemia, or pancytopenia).

In practice, it is important to differentiate between SLE flare ups and infections. Remember also that the common causes of mortality SLE patients is nephritis and infection (makes the case for screening urinalysis and CBC).

Hallmarks of Scleroderma

Signs and Symptoms:
- Classically presents with CREST symptoms:
  - **C**alcinosis
  - **R**aynaud's phenomenon
  - **E**sophageal dysmotility with dysphagia
  - **S**clerodactyly
  - **T**elangectasia + heartburn and mask-like leathery face

Source

Lab Tests:

1. Use ANA titer as a screening test.
2. If positive, perform anticentromere antibody test (this is positive in CREST patients).
3. If positive, perform antitopoisomerase antibody test (a positive result here indicates full blown scleroderma).

NPLEX
MCCQE
USMLE

Sjogren Syndrome

Signs and Symptoms:

- Causes keratoconjunctivitis sicca (dry eyes) and xerostomia (dry mouth).
- Often a feature of autoimmune diseases.

Fibromyalgia, Polymyositis, and Polymyalgia Rheumatica

Differential Feature	Fibromyalgia	Polymyositis	Polymyalgia Rheumatica
Class age/sex	Young adult women	Female 40-60 years of age	Female >50 years of age
Location	Various	Weakness and stiffness of proximal muscles	Severe pain and stiffness in pectoral and pelvic girdles; neck is usually involved.
ESR	Normal	Elevated	Markedly elevated
Electromyography and/or biopsy	Normal	Abnormal	Normal
Classic findings	Anxiety, stress, point tenderness over affected muscles	Elevated creatine phosphokinase (CPK)	Temporal arteritis, gelling phenomenon (stiffness after inactivity), malaise, fever, depression, and weight loss).

NPLEX
MCCQE
USMLE

Chronic Fatigue Syndrome (CFS)

Suspected when there is profound fatigue that disrupts daily activities in absence of identifiable pathology. CFS is a diagnosis of exclusion.

Signs and Symptoms:

- Hypotension
- Mild fever
- Recurrent sore throat
- Painful lymphadenopathy
- Muscle weakness, muscle pain
- Prolonged fatigue after exercise

Blackwell,
2002

- Recurrent headaches
- Migratory joint pain
- Depression
- Hypersomnia or insomnia

Guidelines for First-line Naturopathic Treatment of CFS

Source

NPLEX

Approach: The first-line naturopathic approach is aimed at identifying underlying factors (e.g., food sensitivities), restoring hepatic detoxification, and supporting proper GI and immune functions.

1. Dietary measures
- Identify and control food allergies, increase water consumption, and eliminate caffeine and alcohol.
- Encourage consumption of whole organic foods and regular healthy small meals.
- Control hypoglycemia (if suspected) by eliminating sugar and refined foods.
- Support detoxification through the use of oligoantigenic diets.

Pizzorno, 2006

2. Lifestyle modification
- Encourage regular low intensity aerobic exercise (>3X per week).
- Involve patient in meditation and/or progressive relaxation activities.
- Counsel to support mental-emotional well-being.

Clinical trials indicate that exercise, antidepressants (fluoxetine) and cognitive behavioural therapy reduce fatigue, depression and improve physical functioning in the short term. Long term benefits are uncertain as most trial exhibit significant drop rate.

3. Clinical nutrition
- Vitamin C: 500-1000 mg t.i.d.
- Vitamin E: 200-400 IU q.d.
- Pantothenic acid: 250 mg q.d. Valuable in treating associated depression.
- Magnesium citrate and/or malate: 200-300 g t.i.d. Deficiency in Mg causes symptoms similar to CFS.
- L-carnitine: 500 mg b.i.d.
- Vitamin B12: 1000 mcg q.d.
- Vitamin D: 1000 - 4000 IU

Rossini, 2006

4. Botanical medicine
- *Eleutherococcus senticosus:* 200 mg solid extract t.i.d. Supports adrenals, adaptogen, increases T-helper cells and NK activity, published evidence of efficacy in treatment of CFS.
- *Glycyrrhiza glabra:* 250-500 mg t.i.d. Antiviral and glucocorticoid potentiating properties. Monitor blood pressure on monthly basis since prolonged use may produce hypertension.
- *Hypericum perfoliatum* 300 mg eq. t.i.d. May also be indicated in cases presenting with moderate depression. Immune support; suspected SSRI activity; published evidence of efficacy in mild-moderate depression; C/I with SSRIs, MAOI, and tricyclic antidepressants.

Bercovitz, 2009

Juvenile Rheumatoid Arthritis

Signs and Symptoms:
- Uvetis
- Arthritis
- Negative rheumatoid factor

Paget's Disease

Usually occurs in men >40 years of age. Patients often complain of bone pain, arthritis, nerve deafness, and paraplegia. Classic cases involve the pelvis and the skull. These patients may tell you that they had to buy larger hats to accommodate their growing head. The risk of osteosarcoma is increased in affected bones.

Lab Tests: Markedly elevated Alkaline Phosphatase (ALP) indicating increased bone remodeling.

X-ray Findings: Cortex thickening, blade of grass sign, frontal bossing, and coarse bizarre trabeculae (once you have seen a Pagetoid skull you will not confuse it with anything else).

Examination Board References

NPLEX (II): North American Board of Naturopathic Examiners
Naturopathic Physician Licensing Examination Part II (NPLEx II) Blueprint. Portland, OR: North American Board of Naturopathic Examiners (NABNE), 2010.

USMLE: National Board of Medical Examiners
Brochert A. Crush Step 3. The Ultimate USMLE Step 3 Review. 3rd ed. New York, NY: Saunders, Elsevier, 2008.

MCCQE: Medical Council of Canada
Dugani S, Lam D, eds. 2009. MCCQE Review Notes & Lecture Series. Medical Counsel of Canada Qualification Examination Review Notes. Toronto, ON: McGraw Hill Professional, Canadian edition, 2009.

Related References

Berkovitz S, Ambler G, Jenkins M, Thurgood S. Serum 25-hydroxy vitamin D levels in chronic fatigue syndrome: a retrospective survey. In Journal of Vitamin Nutritional Research, 2009;79(4) 250-54.

Blackwelder R. Chronic Pain Syndrome. Complementary and Alternative Medicine Secrets. Philadelphia, PA: Hanley & Belfus Inc, 2002.

Dains J, Baumann L, Scheibel P. Advanced Health Assessment & Clinical Diagnosis in Primary Care. 4th ed. St Louis, MO: Mosby C.V. Co. Ltd., 2011.

Damjanov I, Conran PB, Goldblatt PJ. Pathology: Rypins' Intensive Reviews. Philadelphia, PA: Lippincott-Raven, 1998.

Edmonds M, McGuire H, Pric, J. (2004). Exercise therapy for chronic fatigue syndrome. Cochrane Database Systematic Review: CD003200

Hsia EC, Sisson, SD. (2007). Systemic lupus erythematosis. First Consult Elsevier Inc, 2007. Online at. www.mdconsult.com

Medhi B, Kishore K, Singh, U., Seth, SD. (2009). Comparative clinical trial of castor oil and diclofenac sodium in patients with osteoarthritis. Phytotherapy Research. 2009; 23(10):1469-73.

Mills S, Bone K. Principles and Practice of Phytotherapy: Modern Herbal Medicine. New York, NY: Churchill Livingstone, 2000.

Moore R. Hematology Laboratory Diagnosis. Guelph, ON: McMaster University Press, 2001.

Pizzorno JE, Murray MT. Textbook of Natural Medicine. 3rd ed. New York, NY: Churchill Livingstone, Elsevier, 2006.

Price JR, Mitchell E, Tidy E, Hunot V. Cognitive behaviour therapy for chronic fatigue syndrome in adults. Cochrane Databse Systematic Review. 2008;(3):CD001027.

Rossini M, Di Munno O, Valentini G, et al. Double-blind, multicenter trial comparing acetyl l-carnitine with placebo in the treatment of fibromyalgia patients. Clinical Exp Rheumatology, 2007;25(2):182-88.

Saunders, P. Herbal Remedies for Canadians. Toronto, ON: Prentice Hall-Pearson Canada Inc., 2000.

Shaver SL. Osteoarthritis. Complementary and Alternative Medicine Secrets. Philadelphia, PA: Hanley & Belfus Inc, 2002.

UROLOGY

MALE CONDITIONS

URINARY TRACT INFECTIONS

Source

MALE CONDITIONS

Presentation

NPLEX
MCCQE
USMLE

Urogenital Examination: Always conduct an examination if the following signs and symptoms are present:
- Penile discharge
- Dysuria
- Lesions reported by patient
- Pain (abdominal or pelvic)
- Hernias
- Dermatological disease (e.g., redness and excoriation)

Prepuce Retraction: Retract the prepuce during routine male genital to detect chancres and carcinomas.

Penile Discharge: If a patient presents with penile discharge, the most prudent approach is to conduct a male genital examination, followed by Gram stain and culture of any urethral discharge.

Testicular Torsion and Epididymitis

NPLEX
MCCQE
USMLE

Characteristics	*Testicular Torsion*	*Epididymitis*
Age of onset	< 30 years of age	> 30 years of age
Appearance	There is notable testicular swelling. Testes may be elevated into the inguinal canal.	Swollen testes; scrotal erythema; urethral discharge; urethritis; and possible prostatitis.
Prehn's sign	Pain is not alleviated by testicular elevation	Pain decreases upon testicular elevation.
Treatment	This is an emergency condition because immediate surgical intervention is required to prevent irreversible damage to the testes.	Naturopathic supportive treatments, as well as antimicrobial botanicals, are recommended.

Testicular Cancer

NPLEX
MCCQE
USMLE

Gonzales,
2009

Usually presents as a painless (often firm) mass in young men (20 to 40 years of age). The main risk factor is cryptorchidism (undescended testes).

Diagnosis:
- Confirmed via testicular ultrasound, biopsy, and tumor marker assay – for example, Alfa-fetoprotien (AFP) and human chorionic gonadotropin (HCG).

Source

ACS, 2004
AAFP, 2008
USPSTF,
2004

Screening:

While the American Cancer Society (ACS 2004) recommends routine screening during physical exams, the American Academy of Family Physicians (AAFP 2008) and the United States Preventive Services Task Force (USPSTF 2004) recommend against screening, arguing that treatments are effective at all stages of the cancer, while the false positive findings would cause harm from undue investigative procedures.

Treatment:

- Because testicular cancer is one of the most aggressive cancers (this is true for all germ-cell tumors), the recommended treatment is radiation and orchiectomy (for refractive tumors).
- For metastatic presentations, antineoplastic chemotherapy is the mainstay of treatment.

Orchitis

Presents as a painful and swollen testis. Mumps is touted for its propensity to cause orchitis (especially in post-pubertal males). Orchitis will rarely cause infertility.

Benign Prostatic Hypertrophy (BPH)

As men age, BPH is extremely common, affecting 5% to10% of men at age 30 and more than 90% of men over age 85.

Symptoms and Sequelae:

- Increased progressive urinary frequency, especially at night (nocturia)
- Weak urine stream
- Straining and dribbling on urination
- Feeling that the bladder cannot be completely emptied
- Urine of abnormal color
- Erectile dysfunction
- Burning on urination

Pizzorno,
2006

Risk Factors:

1. Aging
2. Inadequate zinc intake. Zinc inhibits the activity of 5-alpha reductase enzyme (the enzyme that converts testosterone to dihydrotestosterone 'DHT') and prolactin secretion by the pituitary gland.
3. Regular beer consumption. Hops increases circulating prolactin levels (prolactin increases the prostatic uptake of testosterone).
4. Stress. Considerable and excessive stress physiologically induces both thyroid hormones, as well as prolactin.
5. Low protein diet (70% carbohydrate; 10% protein; 20% fat) has been shown to stimulate 5-alpha reductase.
6. Alcohol consumption of >740ml per month (especially wine and sake) is associated with increased incidence of BPH.
7. Smoking (even second-hand) is major source of cadmium, which is an antagonist of zinc.

Assessment

- The most effective work-up is accomplished by screening symptomatic patients via a digital rectal examination (DRE) and/or transrectal prostatic ultrasound, along with a serum prostate specific antigen (PSA) assay to rule out prostatic carcinoma. Because symptoms of BPH and prostate cancer can be similar, the PSA test is added to this work-up.
- In men over 50 years of age with an immediate relative diagnosed with prostate cancer, a yearly DRE, as well as a PSA test, are highly recommended (combined will identify 90% of prostate cancers).
- Normal value for PSA is < 4ng/ml; a level >10ng/ml is highly suggestive of prostatic carcinoma.

Screening:

According to ACS 2004, all men >50 yo should be screened regardless of FHx, but the AAFP 2008 and USPSTF 2004 argue against screenings as they would lead to interventions (and side effects) in cases where the undetected cancer would not have caused significant morbidity.

Conventional Treatments for BPH

Conventional approaches are recommended for severe cases (significant urinary retention of > 150ml residual urine volume after voiding):
- Alpha-1 blockers: e.g., prazosin (Cardura) and terazosin (Hytrin).
- Gonadotropin releasing hormone analogs: e.g., flutamide and finasteride (Proscar).

Transurethral resection of the prostate (TURP) is reserved for even more advanced cases, especially with recurrent urinary tract infections.

Guidelines for First-line Naturopathic Treatment of BPH

Approach:
- Reduce progressive growth of prostate gland.
- Provide sympton relief (improve urine flow; reduce burning on urination).
- Induce regression of the size of the prostate gland.
- Circumvent associated congestion and tissue inflammation.

1. Prevention
- Limit alcohol consumption.
- Avoid smoking (first-hand and second-hand smoke).
- Increase consumption of soy foods (genistein and daidzein in soy compete for estrogen receptors).
- Avoid pesticides (inducers of 5-alpha reductase) in the environment, as well as in foods.
- Increase consumption of omega-3 EFA-containing foods, such as cold-water fish, nuts, and seeds (e.g., flaxseed and walnuts).
- Maintain healthy cholesterol levels.

2. Dietary measures
- Encourage a high-protein diet (40% protein) of nuts, seeds, fresh vegetables, whole grains, legumes, and liberal amounts of soy products.

Source

3. Clinical nutrition
- Zinc: 45-60 mg q.d.
- Flaxseed oil or fish oil: 1 tbsp q.d.
- Glycine, glutamic acid, and alanine: 200 mg q.d. In controlled studies, this combination of amino acids provided significant symptomatic relief for men with BPH.

Ferri, 2004

4. Botanical medicine
- *Serenoa repens:* 160 mg of standardized (85% to 95% fatty acids and sterols) extract b.i.d. Clinical studies indicate that saw palmetto is 90% effective in diminishing all major symptoms of BPH. The effect is similar (and demonstrably faster in action) to the drug finasteride (e.g., Proscar, an anti-androgenic drug).
- *Pygeum africanum:* 100 mg of standardized (14% triterpenes) extract b.i.d. When combined with saw palmetto, the net synergistic effect is marked reduction of the presenting symptoms, as well as the clinical signs of BPH.
- Other complementary phytotherapeutics, include Cernilton (flower pollen) and *Urtica dioica.*

NPLEX
MCCQE
USMLE

Erectile Dysfunction (ED)

History often indicates the etiology in cases of psychogenic-erectile-dysfunction, which is a common presentation in general practice.

Signs and Symptoms:
- Patients will present with a normal pattern of nocturnal erections.
- In addition, they will exhibit some level of selective dysfunction – for example, where the patient has normal erections on masturbation, but not with his sexual partner.
- Other cues include stress, anxiety, and fear.

O'Hanlo,
2007

Organic Causes:
- Vascular insufficiency secondary to atherosclerosis and diabetes.
- Uncontrolled diabetes can also cause ED through diabetic autonomic neuropathy (see Diabetes module).
- Some prescription medications (antihypertensives and antidepressants) are known to cause ED as a side effect.
- Alcohol, smoking, and elicit drugs can contribute to the problem.

Thorough history is necessary to establish cause. Fasting blood glucose and HbA1C should be ordered in all cases. Testosterone, prolactin and TSH may follow depending on presenting case. Inquire about ED in male patients with multiple vague complaints, evasive answers and frequent visits.

NPLEX
MCCQE
USMLE

Hydroceles and Varicoceles

Hydroceles: will transilluminate, generally cause no symptoms, and do not require treatment.

Varicoceles: will not transilluminate; on palpation feel like a 'bag of worms' (more common over the left testis); disappear in the supine position; and may cause pain and/or infertility.

Cryptorchidism

Arrested descent of the testes from their embryological place of origin (renal area) to the scrotum. It is common in premature infants. Most cases of cryptorchidism eventually resolve within the first year of life (warm sitz baths may encourage descent). After 1 year of age, if the testis is showing no sign of descent, surgical orchiopexy is considered to preserve fertility.

Risk Factor: Cryptorchidism is a major risk factor for testicular cancer; it increases the incidence of this cancer up to 40 times the normal rate. Note that while surgical reduction of cryptorchidism improves fertility, it does not reduce testicular cancer risk significantly.

Epispadias and Hypospadias

Both conditions are congenital penile defects. As the name implies, epispadias refers to a urethra that opens on the top-side of the penis, while hypospadias refers to a urethra that opens on the bottom-side of the penis (the non-anatomical terms 'top' and 'bottom' are chosen so as to avoid any spatial confusion).

Treatment: Surgical intervention is recommended to improve both functions (i.e., urination and ejaculation) and to circumvent the resulting susceptibility to UTIs.

URINARY TRACT INFECTIONS

Presentation

Signs and Symptoms:
- Urgency
- Dysuria
- Distorted stream (in females)
- Incontinence
- Suprapubic pain (both genders) and/or low back pain (more common in males when prostate is inflamed)

Causes: In > 75% of cases, UTIs are caused by *Escherichia coli*. Other causes include *Staphylococcus saprophyticus*, *Proteus*, *Pseudomonas*, *Klebsiella*, *Enterobacter*, and *Enterococcus*.

Urethral Discharge

Absence of urethral discharge is generally considered the norm for males as well as females. In fact, scanty white or clear urethral discharge is a common sign of non-gonococcal urethritis and requires gram stain and culture to rule out infectious etiology.

Source

NPLEX
MCCQE
USMLE

Urinary Tract Infections (UTIs) Classifications

Upper Urinary Tract Infection: The convention is to call the renal nephron, pelvis, and ureter the upper urinary tract.

Lower Urinary Tract: Anything below the ureter is termed the lower urinary tract (i.e, bladder, prostate, and urethra).

NPLEX
MCCQE
USMLE

Risk Factors

Predisposing Factors for UTI:

- Females are more susceptible because of their short urethra: 90% of cases occur in women; 10% to 20% of all women have UTIs at least once a year.
- Any condition that promotes urinary stasis (BPH, pregnancy, stones, neurogenic bladder, vesicourethral reflux) or bacterial colonization (indwelling catheters without proper maintenance, fecal incontinence, urethral trauma).
- Diabetes predisposes to infections, including UTIs (rule it out if recurrent).
- Ureteric valve incompetence causes urine reflux into ureter and is a leading cause of recurrent UTIs (but you will most likely catch it in children).
- Some females acquire recurrent lower UTIs from sexual intercourse (treat prophylactically and encourage urination after intercourse).
- Recurrent kidney infection secondary to UTIs is associated with progressive damage of renal tissue, leading to scarring and, rarely, kidney failure.

NPLEX
MCCQE
USMLE

Assessment

UTI Diagnosis:

1. Definitive diagnosis constitutes clean-catch urinalysis showing WBCs, positive leukocyte esterase, and/or positive nitrite; with urine microscopy exhibiting > 100,000 colony-forming units (CFU) of a specific kind of bacteria per ml of urine.
2. If urine culture exhibits >100,000 Colony-forming Units (CFU)/ml of 'mixed flora', then sample was contaminated with vaginal flora or otherwise and should not be used to diagnose or treat the condition.
3. If the signs and symptoms are typical of uncomplicated UTI, a urine dipstick test showing positive leukocyte esterase and/or positive nitrite will suffice.
4. However, if urine dipstick test is negative for leukocyte esterase, urine microscopy and culture should still be performed.
5. Approximately 40% of women with classic symptoms of UTI do not exhibit a significant level of bacteruria. Some references recommend treatment of classic presentations even without definitive laboratory evidence.

NPLEX
MCCQE
USMLE

UTIs in Infants and Children

Infants can't verbalize symptoms of UTIs the way children and adults can. To complicate matters, the presentation of UTIs in infants is atypical and elusive, accounting for most cases of fever without source (FWS = febrile condition without identifiable origin).

Source

Diagnostic Procedure:
1. For any FWS in an infant, the first action should be to obtain a urine sample for urinalysis.
2. If positive for infection, treat.
3. If urinalysis is negative and you still suspect UTI, the gold standard is a clean-catch urine culture.

UTI in Children: In children less than 5 year of age, a UTI may be the presenting symptom of genitourinary malformations (such as vesicourethral reflux or posterior urethral valves). The alarm should sound when UTI occurs recurrently in a patient < 6 years of age.

Treatment: Refer or consult with urologist because you will require a voiding cystourethrogram to ascertain your hypothesis.

Asymptomatic Bacteruria

NPLEX
MCCQE
USMLE

Hoffman,
1996

In general, do not treat. Bacteria may exist in urine without causing malice (remember that urine is not a sterile medium). However, you should treat asymptomatic bacteruria in pregnant females because of lowered immunity and high risk of progression to pyelonephritis.

Treatment:
- Use only botanical and nutritional agents that are safe in pregnancy, such as *Arctostaphylos uva-ursi* (Bearberry), *Agropyron repens* (Couchgrass), *Agathosma betulina* (Buchu), *Hydrangea arborescense* (Hydrangea), and *Zea mays* (Cornsilk).
- There are also a select few antibiotics considered safe for use during pregnancy (e.g., penicillin, amoxicillin, and erythromycin).

Saunders,
2000

Guidelines for First-line Naturopathic Treatment of UTIs

NPLEX

Approach:
- Reduce predisposing factors.
- Provide symptom relief.
- Treat infection.
- Circumvent information.

1. Adjust urinary pH: A significant amount of controversy continues regarding the role of urinary pH in the treatment of UTIs. On the one hand, low urinary pH is considered protective against *Proteus* & *Klebsiella* (both are urease producers that like alkaline environments). On the other, alkalinization has long been the cornerstone for successful naturopathic treatment and prophylaxis of UTIs. In addition, many of the herbs used to treat UTIs work better in an alkaline environment.

Bhat-
tachara,
2002

2. Dietary and lifestyle measures
- Consider food sensitivities.
- Avoid consumption of simple sugars, refined carbohydrates, and concentrated fruit juices.
- Encourage ingestion of watermelon (natural diuretic) and liberal amounts of garlic and onion.
- Advise patient to drink plenty of filtered water and cranberry or blueberry juice, which prevents *E. coli* adhesion to the endothelial cells of the bladder.

Pizzorno,
2006

Source

3. Clinical nutrition

- Vitamin C: 500 mg q.2h. for the first day of infection (or until bowel tolerance), then reduce dose.
- Bioflavonoids: 1000 mg q.d.
- Vitamin A: 25,000 IU q.d. May not be safe during pregnancy.
- Zinc: 30 mg q.d.
- Choline: 1000 mg q.d.
- D-mannose: 1 tsp q.i.d.

4. Botanical medicine

- *Hydrastis canadensis*: Berberine works better in alkaline environment; specific antimicrobial spectrum against *E. coli, Staphylococcus, Proteus, Pseudomonas, Klebsiella,* and *Enterobacter.* May not be safe during pregnancy.
- *Arctostaphylos uva ursi*: Arbutin is hydrolyzed into hydroquinone, which alkalinizes the urine; crude plant is more effective than isolated arbutin; recent clinical trials established efficacy in treatment of recurrent cystitis; narrow therapeutic window; toxic signs include tinnitus, N/V, and shortness of breath.

Hoffman, 1996

- Traditional herbalists recommend a mixture of *Arctostaphylos uva-ursi* (bearberry), *Agropyron repens* (couchgrass), & *Achillea millefolium* (yarrow) in equal parts as a tea: 1 cup q.2h. until condition improves, then t.i.d. for a week or two for total cure.

Saunders, 2000

- Other beneficial herbs in the treatment of UTIs include *Juniperus communis* (juniper berries), *Agathosma betulina* (buchu), *Hydrangea arborescense* (hydrangea), and *Zea mays* (cornsilk).
- Note that of the above mentioned herbs, the following are not considered safe for use during pregnancy: *Hydrastis canadensis* (goldenseal), *Achillea millefolium* (yarrow), and *Juniperus communis* (juniper berries).

Morrison, 1998

5. Acute Homeopathic Remedies: Most homeopaths recommend giving the constitutional remedy in a 12C or 30C strength, especially if the remedy covers urinary tract disorders.

- *Cantharis*: indicated for intense dysuria when every drop feels like scalding acid as it passes + feeling that emptying bladder would bring relief + pain is the primary symptom.
- *Nux Vomica*: indicated for constant urging and full sensation, but only small, unsatisfying amounts are passed + frequent urging is the main symptom.
- *Petroselinum*: indicated for intense itching or tingling deep in urethra or neck of bladder + itch or irritation is the main symptom.
- *Pulsatilla*: indicated for pain that increases every moment the urge is postponed + pain is irregular, paroxysmal or with spurting.
- *Sarsaparilla*: indicated for copious urination with marked burning pain at the end of urination.
- *Staphysagria*: indicated for post-coital and honeymoon cystitis + burning and tenesmus + unsatisfied after urination.

Ferri, 2004

Conventional Treatment: Antimicrobial treatment should be considered for any patient with persistently positive urine cultures or recurrent infections despite naturopathic treatment.

Interstitial Cystitis (IC)

A peculiar presentation of a severe bladder disorder of at least 12 months duration that causes chronic suprapubic pain, urinary frequency, and nocturia. Routine urine cultures are negative, and symptoms do not respond to antimicrobials.

Causes: Possible causes include:

- Autoimmune reaction toward bladder antigens
- Deficiency of glycosaminoglycan (GAG) mucosal layer
- Mast cell infiltration of bladder interstitium
- Food sensitivities

Diagnosis:

- Common differentials of cystitis must first be ruled out before diagnosing this condition.
- Consider bladder tumors, bladder calculi, and side effects of medications in chronic presentations.
- Cystoscopy may identify ulcers in 10% cases, though lack of ulceration does not rule out IC (90% of cases).
- 24h voiding log may help establish baseline and assess pattern (average void frequency is 16 times per day for IC patients)

Treatment:

- Conventional therapies include antihistamines, tricyclic antidepressants (amitriptyline) to reduce nociception, bladder wall coating agents (pentosan polysulfate), temporary hydrodistention and surgery.
- Although clinical studies are pending, conservative naturopathic treatments, including a trial oligoantigenic (elimination) diet and acupuncture, quercetin, as well as the herb *Centella asiatica* or gotu kola (contraindicated during pregnancy), have been shown to be effective in the treatment of IC.
- Hyperbaric oxygen therapy may be an effective option according to some current publications

Pizzorno,
2006

Bat-
tacharya,
2002

Tanaka,
2011
Van
Ophoven,
2006

Examination Board References

NPLEX (II): North American Board of Naturopathic Examiners
Naturopathic Physician Licensing Examination Part II (NPLEx II) Blueprint. Portland, OR: North American Board of Naturopathic Examiners (NABNE), 2010.

USMLE: National Board of Medical Examiners
Brochert A. Crush Step 3. The Ultimate USMLE Step 3 Review. 3rd ed. New York, NY: Saunders, Elsevier, 2008.

MCCQE: Medical Council of Canada
Dugani S, Lam D, eds. 2009. MCCQE Review Notes & Lecture Series. Medical Counsel of Canada Qualification Examination Review Notes. Toronto, ON: McGraw Hill Professional, Canadian edition, 2009.

Related References

Bhattacharya B. Urinary Tract Infection. Complementary and Alternative Medicine Secrets. Philadelphia, PA: Hanley & Belfus Inc, 2002.

Cutler P. Problem Solving in Clinical Medicine: From Data to Diagnosis. 3rd ed. Baltimore, MD: Lippincott, Williams & Wilkins Press, 1998.

Dains J, Baumann L, Scheibel P. Advanced Health Assessment & Clinical Diagnosis in Primary Care. 4th edition. St Louis, MO: Mosby C.V. Co. Ltd., 2011.

Damjanov I, Conran PB, Goldblatt PJ. Pathology: Rypins' Intensive Reviews. Philadelphia, PA: Lippincott-Raven, 1998.

Ferri F. Ferri's Clinical Advisor: Instant Diagnosis and Treatment. St. Louis, MI: Mosby Inc, 2004.

Gonzales R, Kutner J. Current Practice Guidelines in Primary Care 2009. Toronto, ON: McGraw Hill, 2009.

Hoffmann D. The Complete Illustrated Holistic Herbal. Boston, MA: Element Books Ltd, 1996.

Metts JF. (2001). Interstitial cystitis: urgency and frequency syndrome. American Family Physician. 2001;64:1199-1206.

Moore R. Hematology Laboratory Diagnosis. Guelph, ON: McMaster University Press, 2001.

Morrison R. Desktop Companion to Physical Pathology. Nevada City, CA: Hahnemann Clinic Publishing, 1998.

O'Hanlon KM, Pearson RL, Baustian GH, Kabongo ML, Aliotta PJ, Chopra AK. (2007). Erectile dysfunction. First Consult Elsevier Inc., 2007. Online at www.mdconsult.com

Pizzorno JE, Murray MT, Textbook of Natural Medicine. 3rd ed. New York, NY: Churchill Livingstone, 2006.

Saunders, P. Herbal Remedies for Canadians. Toronto, ON: Prentice Hall-Pearson Canada Inc., 2000.

Tanaka T, Nitta Y, Morimoto K, et al. Hyperbaric oxygen therapy for painful bladder syndrome/interstitial cystitis resistant to conventional treatments: long-term results of a case series in Japan. BMC Urology. 2011;11(1):11.

Van Ophoven A, Rossbach G, Paionk F, Hertle L. Safety and efficacy of hyperbaric oxygen therapy for the treatment of interstitial cystitis: a randomized, sham controlled, double-blind trial. Journal of Urology. 2006;176(4 Pt 1): 1442-46.

REVIEW QUESTIONS

PROBLEM-BASED QUESTIONS

KNOWLEDGE COMPETENCIES

Answering the following questions is the first step in acquiring the knowledge to succeed in family medicine and primary care courses before proceeding into your practical clinical rotations. Use them to guide your knowledge and skill development. These questions may be posed in grand-rounds style during class or assigned to your team to work-up for delivery in seminars.

These questions correspond to the current standards and guidelines presented in this textbook. Be sure to keep abreast of new standards and guidelines as they are published by medical associations and authoritative journals. Use the margin column to cite the source of new information.

To practice primary care successfully, you should be able to answer the following questions:

PART 1
Standards and Guidelines

Evidence-Based Medicine
1. What is the definition of evidence-based medicine (EBM)?
2. What are the weaknesses in the EBM approach?
3. Can complementary and alternative medicine (CAM) be evidence based?
4. Why is evidence-based medicine relevant to naturopathic primary care?
5. How is EBM generally practiced?
6. What are the differences in the quality of medical evidence?
7. What is an experimental study?
8. What are prospective studies?
9. What is a retrospective study?
10. What are case series studies?
11. What are prevalence surveys good for?
12. How is the sensitivity of a test defined? What are highly sensitive tests used for clinically?

13. How is the specificity of a test defined? What are highly specific tests used for?
14. What is the definition of positive predictive value?
15. How do the concepts of sensitivity, specificity, and predictive value affect your interpretation of any diagnostic test result?
16. What would an abnormal test result mean?
17. Is there any single test that can rule in or out a particular disease?
18. What subtypes of bias that can exist in a clinical study?
19. What is the NNT? How should it be interpreted?

Part 2
Case Management Guidelines

Cardiology
1. What is an ECG?
2. How do you read an ECG?
3. How is chest pain managed?
4. What findings on ECG should make you suspect an MI?
5. What is the character of pain in MI?
6. What are other clinical findings that would suggest an MI?
7. What characteristics of the patient history indicate a diagnosis of MI?
8. What are the common noncardiac causes of chest pain?
9. What is stable angina and how is it managed?
10. What is unstable angina?
11. What is variant or Prinzmetal's angina?
12. What is the first-line naturopathic treatment of stable angina?
13. What are functional heart murmurs?
14. Which adventitious sounds are considered normal?
15. What are common abnormal heart sounds?
16. What is the general guideline for endocarditis prophylaxis?
17. What are the risk factors for deep venous thrombosis (DVT)?
18. What is the clinical presentation of DVT?
19. Can superficial thrombophlebitis cause pulmonary embolism (PE)?
20. What is the prognosis of DVTs?
21. Can DVT lead to a stroke?
22. What are the symptoms and causes of PE?
23. What are the hallmarks of congestive heart failure (CHF)?
24. How are right and left CHF distinguished?
25. How is CHF classified and treated?
26. What is the first-line naturopathic treatment for chronic CHF?
27. What is the definition and presentation of Cor Pulmonale?

28. What is a cardiomyopathy? How is it classified?
29. What are the causes of restrictive and constrictive pericarditis?
30. Which cardiomyopathy is likely in a young athlete who passes out while exercising?
31. What ECG abnormalities indicate cardiac arrhythmias?
32. What endocrine disease is suggested in sinus tachycardia or atrial fibrillation?
33. How does Wolf-Parkinson-White (WPW) syndrome present?
34. What is hypertension? Why should it be treated?
35. Are there any exceptions to the two-measurement rule?
36. What is hypertensive urgency versus hypertensive emergency?
37. What causes hypertension?
38. What are the most common secondary causes of hypertension?
39. What are less common secondary causes of hypertension?
40. How often should you screen for hypertension?
41. What laboratory evaluations should be always be ordered with a diagnosis of hypertension?
42. What is the first-line treatment for non-urgent hypertension?
43. What are the first-line medications for the treatment of hypertension?
44. Can patients with hypertension successfully stop their medication by changing their diet?
45. What is the first-line botanical treatment for hypertension?
46. What is the first-line clinical nutrition treatment for hypertension?
47. What are the suggested management plans for hypertension in out-patient clinics?
48. From a Traditional Chinese Medicine perspective, what are the differential Zang-Fu syndromes for hypertensive presentations?
49. Why are lipid levels important clinically?
50. What are the risk factors for atherosclerosis and coronary artery disease (CAD)?
51. What are lipoproteins?
52. What is reported on a complete lipid panel?
53. Is LDL-C a predictor of disease risk?
54. How is LDL cholesterol calculated?
55. Should patients fast before lipid profile testing?
56. What are the most recent guidelines of the ATP III for lipid lowering interventions?
57. What clinical physical findings would possibly indicate hyperlipidemia?
58. How often should you screen for dyslipidemia?
59. What is the portfolio diet for lowering LDL-C? How does it compare to the NCEP diet and drug intervention?

60. What dietary recommendations can further increase the efficacy of the portfolio diet?
61. Will these interventions address the more significant concern of TC:HDL-C ratio?
62. What medications are used in the treatment of hyperlipidemia?
63. What is the first-line naturopathic clinical nutrition treatment for dyslipidemia?
64. What is the first-line naturopathic botanical treatment for dyslipidemia?

Ear, Nose & Throat

1. What is presbyacusis? When would you suspect other causes of hearing loss?
2. What is the most common cause of acute onset deafness?
3. What is the definition of otosclerosis?
4. What is the Weber test used to evaluate?
5. What is the Rinne test used to evaluate?
6. What are the most common causes of vertigo?
7. How does myringitis present?
8. How does sinusitis present?
9. What are the causes and risk factors for sinusitis?
10. How is sinusitis diagnosed?
11. What is the first-line naturopathic approach to sinusitis?
12. What causes parotid gland swelling?
13. What is the most common cause of lower motor neuron (LMN) facial nerve paralysis?
14. What are the other causes of LMN facial nerve paralysis?

Endocrine Disorders (Diabetes Mellitus)

1. What are the chief presentations of diabetes?
2. What are the current recommendations for diabetes mellitus screening?
3. What are the differences between type 1 and type 2 DM?
4. What is syndrome X? How is it diagnosed?
5. What are the goals of management of diabetes in terms of glucose levels?
6. What is a good measure of long-term diabetes control or compliance with treatment?
7. What is diabetic ketoacidosis (DKA)?
8. What is hyperosmolar non-ketotic state (HONK)?
9. What is lactic acidotic coma (LA)?
10. What are the common long-term complications of diabetes mellitus?
11. How bad can peripheral neuropathy be?

12. What is the first-line naturopathic treatment for diabetes mellitus?
13. What is the recommended evaluation strategy for every patient with a diagnosis of diabetes?
14. What are the oral hypoglycemic medications used in the treatment of DM II?
15. What is the treatment for proliferative diabetic retinopathy?
16. How does hypoglycemia present?
17. What are the indications for insulin?
18. What are some of the adverse effects of insulin therapy?
19. What are the different types of insulin preparations?
20. How do the Somogyi effect and the Dawn phenomenon present?
21. What is the concern with beta-blockers and diabetes?
22. What is the best single treatment for DM type II?
23. How would you manage a case of diabetes?
24. When would you refer to a family physician?
25. When would you refer to the ER?

Gastroenterology

1. What does the term gastroesophageal reflux disease (GERD) mean?
2. What is the role of stomach acid levels in GERD? Is it too much or too little?
3. How can you tell if stomach acid is excessive or deficient?
4. How do you diagnose GERD?
5. What are the first-line naturopathic treatments for GERD?
6. Is HCl supplementation effective?
7. What is a useful GERD management plan?
8. What are the sequelae of GERD?
9. What is a hiatal hernia? How is it different from paraesophageal hernia?
10. When do you know you are dealing with peptic ulcer disease (PUD)?
11. What are the differences between duodenal and gastric ulcers?
12. How can you confirm your suspected diagnosis of PUD? Do you have to confirm the diagnosis?
13. What is the most worrisome complication of PUD?
14. What is the first-line naturopathic treatment of PUD?
15. List the surgical options for ulcer treatment.
16. What causes achlorhydria?
17. What are the diagnostic differences between upper and lower gastrointestinal (GI) bleeding?
18. How is a gastric bleeding treated?
19. What radiological imaging studies can be done to localize a GI bleed?
20. When is surgery indicated?

21. What are the complications of diverticulosis.
22. How is diarrhea categorized according to etiology?
23. How would you explain systemic diarrhea?
24. How can a diagnosis of osmotic diarrhea be made?
25. What is secretory diarrhea?
26. What are common causes of malabsorption diarrhea?
27. What are the common clues to infectious diarrhea? What are the common causes?
28. What causes exudative diarrhea?
29. How do you manage a case of diarrhea?
30. How is constipation defined?
31. What are the common causes of constipation?
32. What are first-line naturopathic treatments of constipation?
33. How do you recognize irritable bowel syndrome?
34. What is the first-line naturopathic treatment for patients with IBS?
35. What are the classic differences between Crohn's disease and ulcerative colitis?
36. What are the extra-gastrointestinal manifestations of inflammatory bowel disease (IBD)?
37. How is IBD treated conventionally and naturopathically?
38. What is a toxic megacolon?
38. How do you know that you are dealing with acute liver disease?
39. What are the common causes of acute liver disease?
40. What presentations suggest hepatitis A?
41. What is the classic abnormality on LFTs in patients with alcoholic hepatitis?
42. How is hepatitis B contracted?
43. What is the serology of hepatitis B infection?
44. What are possible sequelae of chronic hepatitis B or C?
45. What should be administered to persons acutely exposed to Hepatitis B?
46. What are the causes of hepatitis C?
47. When does hepatitis D present?
48. How is hepatitis E transmitted?
49. What drugs may induce drug-induced hepatitis?
51. What is the first-line treatment of acute viral hepatitis?
52. When should you suspect idiopathic autoimmune hepatitis?
53. What are the usual causes of chronic liver disease?
54. How do you recognize hemochromatosis?
55. What is the recommended treatment for Wilson's disease?
56. What are the clues to diagnosing alpha-1 antitrypsin deficiency?

57. What metabolic disorders result from liver failure?
58. What signs and symptoms indicate biliary tract obstruction as a cause of jaundice?
59. What are the common types of biliary tract obstruction?
60. What are the two major causes of common bile duct obstruction?
61. What is first-line naturopathic treatment of gallstones?
62. What are the most common causes of cholestasis?
63. What presentations suggest primary biliary cirrhosis?
64. What are the indications for primary sclerosing cholangitis?
65. What are the signs of esophageal disease?
66. How is achalasia diagnosed and treated?
67. What are the symptoms and signs of esophageal spasm?
68. What clues suggest that scleroderma is causing esophageal complaints?
69. What is the role of naturopathic medicine in managing esophageal cancer?
70. What causes acute pancreatitis?
71. How do you recognize acute pancreatitis?
72. What are the complications of acute pancreatitis?
73. What causes chronic pancreatitis?

Geriatrics
1. What is the percentage of the population above 65 years of age?
2. What age group constitutes the most rapidly growing segment of the population?
3. What percentage of the people over the age of 65 live in nursing homes?
4. Does an 80-year-old need fewer calories than a 30 year old? Why?
5. Does an 80-year-old need fewer vitamins and minerals than a 30 year old? Why?
6. What are the most common challenges that a primary care provider faces when dealing with geriatric patients?
7. Are hearing and vision changes a normal part of aging? When are they not?
8. Is brain atrophy is a normal part of aging?
9. How does undifferentiated dementia present to the primary care provider?
10. What are the guiding principles of managing undifferentiated dementia?
11. What percentage of patients over the age of 65 exhibit some type of dementia?
12. When do suspect that your patient has alzheimer disease (AD) or senile dementia of the alzheimer type (SDAT)?

13. How is AD diagnosed?
14. What is vascular dementia?
15. What are fronto-temporal dementia (FTD) and Pick's disease?
16. What are common organic diseases that present with dementia in the elderly?
17. How does pseudodementia present in practice?
18. Why is it important to assess cognitive function in the elderly preventively?
19. How do you assess cognitive function in daily practice?
20. What tools does the PCP need to have on hand?
21. What is hepatic encephalopathy?
22. What is renal encephalopathy?
23. What is the appropriate approach to evaluation of first incident of syncope?
24. What are the common causes and first-line management options for syncope?
25. What are the first-line approaches to management of vertigo in the elderly?
26. When do you suspect that your patient has BPV (benign paroxysmal positional vertigo)?
27. How do you manage BPV?
28. When dealing with osteopenea or osteoprosis, what are the best practices in avoidance of hip fractures?
29. How is aggression or psychosis managed in the elderly?
30. How is hypertension and CHF managed in the elderly?
31. What are the best approaches to managing diabetes in the elderly patient?
32. What is the first-line approach to heartburn in the elderly?
33. Should mammography screening be discontinued in elderly female patients?
34. Is impotence and lack of sexual desire normal in elderly people?
35. What are the best practices to avoid pressure ulcers in immobilized patients?
36. How do the normal changes in sleep habits in elderly people affect your standard lifestyle modification approaches?

Gynecology

1. What is the most common cause of preventable infertility?
2. What is the most likely cause of infertility in normally menstruating women under the age of 30?
3. How do you recognize PID in practice?

4. What are the symptoms and signs of endometriosis?
5. How is endometriosis diagnosed and treated?
6. What is the most likely cause of infertility in menstruating women over the age of 30 without a history of PID?
7. For which of these vaginal infections should you seek out and treat the patient's sexual partner: Candida albicans, T. vaginalis, G. vaginalis, HPV, Herpes virus, syphilis (stage I), syphilis (stage II), C. trachomatis, Neisseria gonorrhea, Moluscum, pediculosis.
8. What is the typical clinical presentation of common sexual transmitted infections? When do you suspect? How do you manage?
9. Should you recommend treating patients with gonorrhea for presumed chlamydia infection?
10. What are the indications, contraindications, and side effects of contraceptive methods?
11. How do you educate your female mpatients seeking contraception?
12. What is adenomyosis and how does it typically present?
13. What are fibroids?
14. How commonly do fibroids become malignant?
15. What is the relationship between uterine leomyomas and hormones?
16. What is the first-line treatment?
17. What is the first test to order in any woman of reproductive age with abnormal uterine bleeding?
18. What is dysfunctional uterine bleeding [DUB].
19. When is it physiologic?
18. Why is dilation and curettage recommended in women over 35 with DUB?
19. What causes DUB other than PCOS?
20. How do you recognize PCOS in practice?
21. What is the most likely cause for infertility in women under 30 with abnormal menstruation?
22. What is the first-line treatment of PCOS?
24. Is infertility usually a male or a female issue?
25. Assuming that the history and physical exam offer no clues, what is the first step in evaluating a couple for infertility?
26. What are the relevant characteristics of normal semen?
27. What is the next step after semen evaluation?
28. What radiologic test is commonly used to examine the fallopian tubes and uterus?
29. What points in the history may lead you to suspect a uterine or tube defect?
30. What test is the last resort in the work-up for infertility?

31. What medications can be used to try to restore female fertility?
32. What is the main risk associated with medical induction of ovulation?
33. What distinguishes primary from secondary amenorrhea?
34. Until proven otherwise, what is the cause of secondary amenorrhea?
35. Can excessive exercise cause amenorrhea?
36. What are the common causes of secondary amenorrhea?
37. When is primary amenorrhea diagnosed?
38. When in doubt, what is the best way to evaluate any type of amenorrhea?
39. What are the signs and symptoms and natural course of menopause?
40. What are the likely causes of a breast mass in a woman under 35 years old?
41. Should mammography be done for any suspicious breast lesion in a woman under 35?
42. What are the likely causes of a breast mass in a woman over 35 years old?
43. Should you proceed directly to biopsy for a new breast mass in a post menopausal woman over the age of 50?
44. Is mammography an effective tool to evaluate a palpable breast mass?
45. What is thermography?
46. What causes pelvic relaxation and vaginal prolapse?

Hematology

1. What are the diagnostic criteria, signs, and symptoms of anemia?
2. What causes anemia?
3. What should you inquire about when faced with a case of anemia?
4. What medications can cause anemia?
5. What tests should be ordered first to work-up the cause of anemia?
6. What test is automatically performed by the laboratory if the CBC indicates abnormalities?
7. What are the causes of microcytic, normocytic, and microcytic anemia?
8. What is the most common cause of anemia in North America?
9. What are the typical laboratory abnormalities in iron deficiency anemia?
10. What cravings are sometimes associated with iron deficiency anemia?
11. What is Plummer-Vinson syndrome?
12. How is iron deficiency treated?
13. What causes folate deficiency?
14. What causes vitamin B-12 deficiency?
15. How is thalassemia differentiated from iron deficiency anemia?

16. What is sickle cell disease and how is it diagnosed?
17. What lab test is positive in patients with autoimmune anemia?
18. What clues point to lead toxicity as a cause of anemia?
19. How do you recognize anemia of chronic disease?
20. How do you recognize G6PD in your clinical practice?
21. What are the most common causes of disseminated intravascular coagulation (DIC)?
22. How do you recognize DIC in clinical settings?
23. What conditions lead to eosinophilia?
24. What do you typically see on laboratory studies of a patient with infectious mononucleosis?
25. What do clotting tests measure?
26. What conditions prolong coagulation tests?
27. What causes thrombocytopenia?
28. What clinical manifestations are associated with it?
29. What causes petechiae in the absence of thrombocytopenia?

Immunology and Genetics

1. What are the four types of hypersensitivity reactions?
2. What is type I hypersensitivity?
3. What type of testing can identify an allergen if it is not obvious?
4. What type of hypersensitivity explains food sensitivities?
5. What causes type II hypersensitivity?
6. What type of testing can identify type II hypersensitivity if it is not obvious?
7. What causes type III hypersensitivity?
8. What causes type IV hypersensitivity?
9. What sexually transmitted disease should you consider when a patient presents with sore throat and mononucleosis-like syndrome?
10. How is HIV diagnosed?
11. How long after exposure does the HIV test become positive?
12. What is the most common primary immunodeficiency?
13. What usually causes hereditary angioedema?
14. Complement deficiencies of C5 through C9 cause recurrent infections due to what?
15. What is chronic mucocutaneous candidiasis?
16. If both parents are carriers of an autosomal recessive condition, what are the odds that their child will develop the condition?
17. If a father has an X-linked recessive disorder, what are the odds that his child will be affected if the mother is not a carrier?

18. If a mother is a carrier of an X-linked recessive disorder and the father is healthy, what are the odds that their son or daughter will develop the disease?
19. How do you recognize Down syndrome?
20. What is the second most common cause of inherited mental retardation?
21. What is Patau's syndrome?
22. How do you recognize Turner's syndrome?
23. What causes Klinefelter's syndrome?
24. What causes Marfan's syndrome and how do you recognize it?
25. What is cri-du-chat syndrome?
26. When would you suspect galactosemia in an infant?

Infectious Diseases

1. What is the etiology of fever?
2. What is normal body temperature?
3. What localizing symptoms indicate the source of fever?
4. Do infectious diseases always present as a febrile condition?
5. What conditions are naturopathic physicians obligated to report to public health officials?
6. What are the signs and symptoms that indicate serious febrile diseases?
7. What is your clinical response to fever without identifiable source (FWS) in children?
8. What are the basic concepts of that guide the selection of antimicrobial drugs in clinical practice?
9. What are the antimicrobial drugs of choice that are used to treat common bacterial pathogens?
10. What is the value of enquiring on sputum characteristics in cough presentations?
11. What is the causative organism for classic presentations?
12. What is the role of probiotic therapy in managing infectious presentations?
13. What homeopathic remedies are used in infectious diseases?
14. What botanical remedies are commonly used as immune modulators or stimulants?
15. What botanical remedies are commonly used as nti-inflammatories?
16. What botanical remedies are commonly used as an antipyretic or diaphoretic?
17. What are commonly used botanical antimicrobials?

Nephrology

1. What is azotemia?
2. What is the definition of acute renal failure?
3. What are the three categories of renal failure?
4. What medications commonly cause renal insufficiency or failure?
5. What is the presentation of Goodpasture's syndrome?
6. What are the main causes of chronic renal failure?
7. What are the symptoms of chronic renal failure?
8. How is chronic renal failure treated?
9. What is pephrotic syndrome and how is it diagnosed?
10. What is nephritic syndrome and how is it treated?
11. What is the presentation of acute glomerulonephritis?
12. What is the most common glomerular disease diagnosed in clinical practice worldwide?
13. How are urinary tract infections classified?
14. What are the signs and symptoms of UTIs?
15. What factors increase the likelihood of UTI?
16. How do you diagnose UTIs?
17. Why are UTIs in infants and children a special concern?
18. How should asymptomatic bacteruria be treated?
19. What are the signs and symptoms of kidney stones?
20. What causes kidney stones?
21. How do you differentiate among the common pediatric hematological disorders that affect the kidney?

Neurology

1. What are the characteristics of motor neuron lesions?
2. How does multiple sclerosis typically present?
3. How can the history of common neurological symptoms lead you to the correct diagnosis?
4. What is the classic presentation of Gullain-Barré syndrome (GBS)?
5. What are the signs and symptoms of myasthenia gravis (MG)?
6. What vitamin deficiencies present with neurologic manifestations?
7. What are the characteristics of amyotrophic lateral sclerosis (ALS)?
8. How would you describe the muscle weakness seen in botulism?
9. How would you describe the muscle weakness seen in tick paralysis?
10. When is syncope a cause for concern?
11. How are the various types of headache diagnosed?
12. What are the causes of tension headaches?
13. What are the common types of seizure?
14. What are the presentations of dementia?

15. How can delirium and dementia be differentiated?
16. What is the first-line naturopathic treatment for dementia?
17. What are the signs and symptoms of Alzheimer disease?
18. What is the conventional treatment for Parkinson's disease?
19. What is the first-line naturopathic treatment of Parkinson's disease?
20. What are the symptoms of stroke and TIA?
21. What is the management plan and first-line naturopathic treatment post-stroke?

Ophthalmology
1. What are the most common sources of eye pain?
2. What are the most common causes for loss of vision?
3. What is the most common ocular complaint?
4. What are absolute ocular emergencies?
5. What are the common causes or uveitis?
6. What adjunct naturopathic treatments are there for uveitis?
7. What are the common causes of conjunctivitis?
8. What are the common causes of keratitis?
9. What conditions can cause sensation of a foreign body in the eye?
10. What is the difference between a sty and a chalazion?
11. What are the types of glaucoma?
12. What are the first-line medications used in treatment of glaucoma.
13. What are the preventive and first-line naturopathic treatments for glaucoma?

Orthopedics
1. What features of musculoskeletal pain help in identifying the underlying cause of the condition?
2. What is a compartment syndrome?
3. What are the main motor and sensory functions of the cardinal peripheral nerves?
4. How do you test the cruciate ligaments of the knee joint?
5. What fracture is likely after a fall on an outstretched arm?
6. What are the most important orthopedic tests?
7. What are the most common locations for intervertebral disk herniation?
8. What are charcot joints?
9. What bacteria are the most common cause of septic arthritis?
10. What are the most common types of bone tumors?
11. To what site is pain form hip inflammation or dislocation commonly referred?

12. What is the presentation of the most common pediatric hip disorders?
13. How is Osgood-Schlatter disease recognized and treated?
14. How do you assess scoliosis?

Pediatrics
1. What are common congenital heart defects?
2. What are normal heart rates for children?
3. What changes occur in the circulation as a neonate adapts to extrauterine life?
4. What are the presentations for otitis media?
5. What GI malformations are common in children?
6. What is the most common cause of diarrhea in children?
7. Is IBS seen in children?
8. What should you watch for in children after a bout of diarrhea?
9. How do you manage a case of yellow-infant?
10. What causes physiologic neonatal jaundice?
11. How do you recognize pediatric pathologic jaundice?
12. How is pathologic jaundice treated?
13. How do you manage presentations of pharyngitis in pediatric patients? When does current evidence support recommending antibioticss?
14. What are the first-line naturopathic treatment guidelines for pediatric pharyngitis?
15. What are cavernous hemangiomas? How are they treated?
16. What are Caput succedaneum and Cephalhematoma? How can you distinguish them? How are they treated?
17. When does the anterior fontanel usually close? What disorder should you suspect if fails to close?
18. Is milky-white or blood-tinged vaginal discharged normal in the first week of life?
19. Should adult vital sign parameters be used when assessing children?
20. When are commonly referenced developmental milestones achieved?
21. How should you approach a presentation of fever in a pediatric patient?
22. What are the clinically important facts about pediatric pyrexia?
23. What is the evidence based approach to pediatric fever without source (FWS)?
24. What are physical methods of pyrexia reduction? Which ones are counter-productive? When are they recommended?
25. What are first-line pharmacologic antipyretics? Which ones are safe?

Which combinations are not?

26. Which botanical remedies are commonly used as antipyretic or diaphoretic?

27. Which botanical remedies are commonly used as immune modulators or stimulants?

28. What are the commonly performed screening tests for metabolic and congenital disorders?

29. What is anticipatory guidance?

30. Are screening and preventive care important mainly during a well checkup?

31. How often should height, weight, head circumference be measured? Why? What can growth charts tell you?

32. What is ailure to thrive?

33. How are hearing and vision screened?

34. In what situations would you suspect hearing loss?

35. How do you diagnose and treat acute otitis media (AOM) in children?

36. Is it normal to have strabismus up to a certain age? When should you be concerned?

37. Should you screen your pediatric patients for anemia? Why or why not?

38. Should you give all infants prophylactic iron supplements?

39. How and when do you screen for lead exposure?

40. Are there any circumstances where fluoride supplementation is indicated?

41. Do breastfed infants need vitamin D supplementation?

42. Should children be screened for tuberculosis?

43. Is there a benefit in performing routine urinalysis in children?

44. When should you be concerned about enuresis? How do you manage?

45. Do sexually active teen-aged girls need pap smears and screening for chlamydia and gonorrhea?

46. When should you recommend that child see a dentist for the first time?

47. What are the tanner stages? Why are they important?

48. What is considered delayed puberty? What is the most common cause? What are the pathological reasons for delayed puberty?

49. What is considered precocious puberty? What is the most common causes? What are the pathological reasons for precocious puberty?

50. If the cause of precocious puberty is unknown or not correctable, should you recommend that the child receives pharmacologic treatment? Why or why not?

51. What findings should make you suspect child abuse?

52. Do you need proof before reporting child abuse?

53. What should you remember when you think of aspirin use in a child?

54. Are there any conditions where aspirin is recommended to a pediatric patient?
55. What are the main causes of obesity in children?
56. How do you manage a case of childhood eczema?

Psychiatry

1. What are the five main diagnostic criteria for schizophrenia?
2. Why is the duration of psychotic behavior a crucial factor in establishing a diagnosis?
3. What are the positive and negative symptoms of schizophrenia?
4. What is the difference in age of onset for schizophrenia in males and females?
5. What is the etiology of schizophrenia?
6. What are implications for treatment and management?
7. What is a major depressive episode?
8. What is the approach of naturopathic medicine to the treatment of depression?
9. What is mania or a manic episode?
10. What is hypomania or a hypomanic episode?
11. What is dysthymia?
12. What is bipolar disorder and bipolar II disorder?
13. What is cyclothymia or cyclothymic disorder?
14. What are the major risk factors for suicide?
15. What population exhibits the highest suicide rate?
16. What is adjustment disorder?
17. How do you distinguish between normal grief and pathologic grief?
18. What are anxiety disorders?
19. What is a somatoform disorder?
20. What are factitious disorders and malingering?
21. How is personality disorder recognized?
22. What characterizes each subtype of personality disorders?
23. What is an obsessive compulsive disorder (OCD)?
24. What are the common causes of mental retardation?
25. How do you recognize autism?
26. What are the characteristics of conduct disorder?
27. What characterizes oppositional defiant disorder?
28. What are the diagnostic criteria for anorexia?
29. How does bulimia manifest?
30. What is the prognosis of Tourette's syndrome?
31. How is bed-wetting treated?

32. What are the symptoms of cocaine dependency, amphetamine intoxication, and opioid toxicity?
33. What are the features of "magic mushroom" or lysergic acid diethylamide (LSD) intoxication?
34. What are the risks of benzodiazepine (tranquilizer) and barbiturate (sleeping pill) dependency?

Pulmonology

1. What distinguishes acute bronchitis from chronic bronchitis?
2. What are the characteristics of bronchiectasis?
3. How is emphysema recognized?
4. What are the characteristics of pneumonia?
5. What is the difference between obstructive and restrictive pulmonary disease on pulmonary function testing (spirometry)?
6. How is asthma treated?
7. What is a common cause of wheezing in children under the age of 2?
8. What is the typical presentation of lung cancer?
9. How do you recognize and treat adult respiratory distress syndrome (ARDS)?
10. What is the difference between typical and atypical pneumonia?
11. What are the classic clinical clues for the causative organisms in pneumonia?
12. What should you suspect if a child has recurrent pneumonias?
13. How do you recognize and manage sinusitis?
14. What are the most common causes of epistaxis in children?
15. What is infant respiratory distress syndrome (IRDS)?
16. In pediatric settings, when would you suspect diaphragmatic hernia?
17. What is the most-common lethal genetic disease in Caucasians?
18. How should cystic fibrosis be managed?

Rheumatology

1. What is the most common form of arthritis?
2. What presentations point to a diagnosis of osteoarthritis?
3. What are the first-line recommendations for the naturopathic management of OA?
4. What signs and symptoms lead you to suspect gout?
5. What are the first-line recommendations for the naturopathic management of gout?
6. What is the presentation of rheumatoid arthritis (RA)?
7. Can psoriasis cause arthritis similar to RA?

8. What are the hallmarks of ankylosing spondylitis (AS)?
9. How do you recognize Reiter's syndrome as a cause of arthritis?
10. Can hemophilia cause arthritis?
11. Can Lyme disease cause arthritis?
12. Sickle cell patients are susceptible to what kind of joint pain?
13. What are the hallmarks of rheumatic fever?
14. When do you see Charcot joints?
15. What generalized systemic signs of inflammation suggest autoimmune disorders?
16. How is systemic lupus erythematosus (SLE) recognized?
17. What are the hallmarks of scleroderma?
18. What is the presentation of Sjogren syndrome?
19. How do you distinguish among fibromyalgia, polymyositis, and polymyalgia rheumatica?
20. How do you recognize and treat chronic fatigue syndrome (CFS)?
21. If a pediatric patient has uveitis, arthritis, and a negative rheumatoid factor, what disease should you suspect?
22. What is Paget's disease?

Urology

1. What are the reasons for conducting a male urogenital examination?
2. What should you do if a patient presents with penile discharge?
3. What are the risk factors for sexually transmitted disease?
4. Is it essential to retract the prepuce during routine male genital examinations?
5. What are the most common non-genital manifestations of sexually transmitted disease?
6. Does scanty white or clear urethral discharge require further evaluation?
7. What are the differences in presentation between testicular torsion and epididymitis?
8. How does testicular cancer usually present?
9. What are the major risk factors for testicular cancer?
10. What is the classic cause of orchitis?
11. Does orchitis affect fertility?
12. What are the symptoms, risk factors, preventive measures, and first-line naturopathic treatment for benign prostatic hypertrophy (BPH).
13. What are the common causes of erectile dysfunction (ED)?
14. How do you distinguish between a hydrocele and a varicocele?
15. What is cryptorchidism?
16. What are epispadias and hypospadias?

17. How are urinary tract infections classified?
18. What are the signs and symptoms of UTIs?
19. What factors increase the likelihood of UTIs?
20. How do you diagnose UTIs?
21. What is the first-line naturopathic treatment of UTIs?
22. What is chronic interstitial cystitis (IC)?
23. What are the signs and symptoms of kidney stones?

The following sample questions are included to illustrate the interplay of the clinical knowledge and reasoning skills required to pass Primary Care objective-structured clinical evaluation examinations. These multiple choice questions simulate concepts and criteria tested by the North American Board of Naturopathic Examiners (NABNE). The following questions offer a realistic 'look and feel' of the physical clinical diagnosis and laboratory diagnosis component of the Naturopathic Physician Licensing Examination (NPLEx).

Directions: Circle the ONE answer that BEST fulfills the objective of each question.

1. Which of the following is a feature of secretory diarrhea?

   a) Persistent diarrhea despite fasting
   b) Malodorous, often floating stools
   c) Blood and/or pus in the stools
   d) Elevated levels of leucocytes in stool

2. A 35-year-old female patient seeks your opinion regarding four episodes of chest pain that she experienced during the last month. She is anxious because her husband died of a heart attack 3 months ago and hands you a typed list of laboratory tests that her niece (second-year naturopathic student) recommends to rule out heart attacks. She has no family history of heart disease. Your physical examination reveals no abnormalities. What is your plan?

   a) Recommend avoidance of coffee, alcohol, spicy foods, and milk
   b) Send this patient to ER
   c) Tell this patient that the cause of her episodes is psychologic
   d) Order routine electrocardiography and serum creatine kinase

3. In a 5-year-long observational study published in a peer-reviewed journal, researchers documented an inverse relationship between average
serum beta-carotene level and incidence of coronary artery disease
(CAD). What can you confidently conclude from this study?

   a) B-carotene is an appropriate marker to screen for CAD
   b) B-carotene supplementation can be used to treat CAD
   c) Low serum B-carotene causes CAD
   d) None of the above

4. A 52-year-old healthy woman comes to your office for her annual
check-up. Your usual intake is unremarkable as well as your age-specific laboratory screening tests. However, on her CBC report, hemoglobin level was slightly elevated. What do you do?

   a) Send patient to her family doctor, as this condition requires
prescription medications
   b) Treat her polycythemia vera with proven antineoplastic
botanical *Ganoderma lucidum*
   c) Nothing; monitor her CBC during her next visit
   d) Reassure patient that the test result does not indicate any
abnormality

5. Abdominal pain of psychogenic origin can be distinguished from
organic pain based on history. Which of the following reasoning criteria distinguish organic from functional pain?

   a) Psychological stress rules out organic pain
   a) Acute persistent pain rules out functional pain
   a) Abdominal pain that awakes patient strongly suggests organic
etiology
   a) Anxiety, fever, and anemia strongly suggests functional etiology

6. A mother brings her 1-year-old infant with a chief complaint of abdominal colic, insomnia, and fussiness. She describes the stool as 'mucousy'
and blood tinged. Your work-up is unremarkable, with the exception
of a 1 cm x 3 cm palpable mass in the hypogastrum. You decide to send
the patient to your local children's hospital for which of the following
diagnostic procedures?

a) A blood sample for liver enzymes
b) Lower GI computed tomography scan
c) Lower GI radiological study with barium
d) Kidney and urinary bladder ultrasound scan

7. Which of the following is not a considered first-line naturopathic treatment of gallstones?

   a) Phosphatidylcholine: 500 mg q.d.
   b) Fiber supplementation: 2 g t.id.
   c) Complete avoidance of saturated fat, animal protein, and fried foods
   d) Drinking 1/2 cup of lemon juice t.i.d.

8. What precaution should be taken when complementing oral hypoglycemic drugs with botanicals?

   a) None; oral hypoglycemic drugs and botanicals are contraindicated
   b) Gradual introduction with daily glucometer journaling
   c) Patient should take oral hypoglycemic agents before meals and botanicals afterwards
   d) Dose of oral hypoglycemics should be reduced before starting naturopathic treatment

9. B. F. is a 16-year-old type 1 diabetic male who has been seeing you for adjunct naturopathic therapy. He tells you that his glucometer test shows high levels in the morning. What is your assessment?

   a) He has been taking less insulin than required
   b) He has been taking more insulin than required
   c) His insulin dose is adequate but his diet is poor
   d) It is impossible to determine appropriateness of insulin dose from data provided

10. Acute wheezing in pediatric presentations is most common with which of the following conditions?

    a) Klebsiella pneumonia
    b) RSV infection
    c) Legionnaire's disease
    d) Bronchial asthma

11. Detection of white blood cells in the stool is a sign of which of the following conditions?

    a) Colon cancer
    b) Ulcerative colitis
    c) Malabsorption syndrome
    d) Irritable bowel syndrome

12. A 12-year-old boy complains of aching knees and elbows, a fever, and loss of appetite. Physical examination reveals painless subcutaneous nodules near his hips and shoulders. What is the most important question to ask this child?

    a) "Did you fall down in the last week?"
    b) "Has your fever been getting worse?"
    c) "Have you had a sore throat recently?"
    d) "Do you have any skin irritation?"

13. A 36-year-old Mediterranean female is assigned to you at the clinic as a new patient. She complains of chronic low back pain that is "better after hot showers." Otherwise, she has an unremarkable medical history. Physical examination reveals decreased lordosis, tenderness on palpation, and decreased range of motion of low back and hips. Your laboratory work-up indicates an elevated ESR. Which of the following statements is correct regarding this patient?

    a) Presence of ANAs would strongly suggest rheumatoid arthritis
    b) Bilateral sacroiliitis on plain film radiology would strongly suggest ankylosing spondylitis
    c) Ameliorating factors indicate functional low back pain that is best treated by massage
    d) CT is required to confirm lumbar disk herniation, which is the most likely diagnosis

14. A 45-year-old Caucasian female presents with difficulty breathing due to progressive sharp pain in the left side of her chest. She tells you that she has tried some of her father's nitroglycerin to no avail, and then she came promptly to see you. Her medical history includes cholecystectomy at age 31. Pressure on the indicated point of pain causes it to worsen and radiate into her shoulder. Given a normal ECG and cardiac enzymes, what is your diagnosis?

a) Costochondritis
b) Myocardial infarction
c) GERD
d) Cholangitis

15. A 6-year-old girl complains of abdominal pain. Which of the following would be included in your differential diagnosis?

a) Gastroenteritis, musculoskeletal origin, strangulated hernia, UTI
b) Gastroenteritis, fibroids, strangulated hernia, UTI
c) Intussusception, strangulated hernia, constipation, hypothyroidism
d) Alcohol abuse, lactose intolerance, fibroids, hyperthyroidism

16. A 41-year-old female presents with nervousness and insomnia. She reports a significant increase in her appetite without weight gain. How would you proceed with this patient?

a) Order laboratory tests, then refer to the emergency department
b) Refer to a nearby hospital outpatient clinic
c) Order laboratory tests
d) Prescribe a nervine tincture of *Humulus lupulus* and *Valeriana officinalis*

17. The 2002 edition of the *Merck Manual* lists polydipsia, polyuria, polyphagia, fatigue, and weight loss as diagnostic criteria for diabetes mellitus. Why is progressive weight loss considered a feature of this disease given that obesity is an etiological factor?

a) Because catabolic metabolism maintains fasting hyperglycemia despite progressive glycosuria
b) Because there is a net gain in body stores of glycogen, fat, and protein
c) Because there is a net loss of body water; thus, the loss of weight represents dehydration in these cases
d) The *Merck Manual* is wrong; a naturopathic physician would not consider diabetes in a patient who is losing weight

18. Which of the following options is true? A patient with acute renal failure is likely to be _____, while a patient with chronic renal failure is likely to be _____.

   a) Afebrile; Febrile
   b) Symptomatic; Asymptomatic
   c) Polyuric; Anuric
   d) Jaundiced; Pale

19. This ECG tracing of a patient presenting with bouts of palpitation exhibits which of the following conditions?

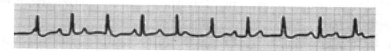

   a) Increasing PR interval until a QRS complex is dropped
   b) Multiple P waves but when beats are conducted PR intervals are unvarying
   c) Ventricular rhythm is regular while atrial rhythm is not
   d) ST segment is elevated

20. How is irritable bowel syndrome diagnosed?

   a) Air-fluid levels on abdominal plain films
   b) Through a process of exclusion
   c) History of stress
   d) Small intestinal biopsy

21. Recently, investigators working with your municipal health department collected the following cancer statistics. As of 31 December 2006: 1,000 cases of prostate cancer were counted, 200 of which were diagnosed since 01 January 2006. As of the same date, the adult population of the municipality was 100,000; 60% of whom are female. Based on the statistics provided, which of the following fractions correctly indicates the rate of incidence of prostate cancer in the municipality in the year 2006.

   a) 200/100,000
   b) 200/40,000
   c) 200/39,800
   d) 200/39,200

22. Sickle cell anemia patients are susceptible to what kind of joint pain?

    a) Ischemic arthralgia
    b) Osteoarthralgia
    c) Autoimmune arthralgia
    d) Hemarthrosis arthralgia

23. Which of the following laboratory tests reliably indicate autoimmune disorders?

    a) Decreased hematocrit
    b) Decreased erythrocyte sedimentation rate
    c) Increased C-reactive protein
    d) Increased serum alkaline phosphatase

24. CREST syndrome is described as calcinosis, Raynaud's phenomenon, esophageal dysmotility with dysphagia, and telangiectasia. This syndrome is a less severe manifestation of which of the following conditions?

    a) Systemic lupus erythematosus
    b) Scleroderma
    c) Sjogren's syndrome
    d) Reiter's syndrome

25. A 28 year-old female presents with a complaint of progressive fatigue. The following are the highlights of your chart: normal vitals; bilateral periorbital edema; no cyanosis; normal capillary refill; normal heart and lung examination; normal jugular venous pressure; negative kidney punch; bilateral ankle swelling; and grade 3 pitting edema of ankles. Your in-house urinalysis indicates marked proteinuria without hematuria. What is the most likely diagnosis?

    a) Nephrotic syndrome
    b) Nephritic syndrome
    c) Acute glomerulonephritis
    d) Chronic pyelonephritis

26. Persistent fever without identifiable etiology (FWS) in infants necessitates laboratory investigation to rule out which of the following conditions?

   a) Juvenile rheumatoid arthritis
   b) Upper urinary tract infection
   c) Upper respiratory tract infection
   d) Hemolytic uremic syndrome

27. A 60-year-old vegetarian male is referred to you for nutritional counseling. The CBC you ordered exhibits decreased Hct, low RBC count, increased MCV, and hyper-segmented neutrophils. What would you advise this patient to do?

   a) Increase his consumption of green leafy vegetables
   b) Avoid spicy and bitter foods
   c) Supplement with vitamin B-12 and folic acid
   d) Get retested during his next scheduled visit

28. A 48-year-old male has been seeing you regularly for annual checkups. As part of your work-up, you obtain a CBC and lipid profile. The CBC results are suggestive of iron deficiency anemia. Given the patient's exemplary dietary habits, you decide to perform a stool occult test, which returned a positive result. What would you do next?

   a) Retest during next annual check-up
   b) Advise patient to supplement with iron succinate 100 mg t.i.d.
   c) Refer patient for flexible colonoscopy
   d) Inquire about family history of sickle cell disease

29. With regards to microcytic hypochromic anemia, which of the following statements is incorrect?

   a) Elevated hemoglobin A2 level indicates thalassemia
   b) Basophilic stippling indicates lead poisoning
   c) Increased total iron binding capacity (TIBC) indicates anemia of chronic disease
   d) Elevated serum ferritin levels rule out iron deficiency anemia

30. A 14-year-old female patient tells you that she has been suffering from extreme tiredness for the last 3 days. You noted in your chart that the patient appears pale; temp 38.6C; BP 109/76; RR 14; generalized lymphadenopathy; pharynx is erythematous and tender w/o discharge. Which laboratory tests would you order to confirm your suspicions?

   a) CBC & Indirect Coombs test
   b) CBC & Schilling test
   c) CBC & transferrin
   d) CBC & Monospot test

31. Which of the following statements is not true with regards to penile discharge?

   a) Clear discharge is normal
   b) Yellow discharge occurs with gonococcal urethritis
   c) White discharge is common sign of non-gonococcal urethritis
   d) Scanty discharge is a common sign of chlamydial urethritis

32. Which finding in the prostate suggests prostatic cancer?

   a) Symmetrical smooth enlargement
   b) Diffuse hardness
   c) Extreme tenderness
   d) Boggy soft enlargement

33. Your attending supervisor inquires about the rationale for your decision to prescribe the antimicrobials *Hydrastis canadensis* and *Arctostaphylous uva-ursi* to a 26-year-old female who exhibits classical signs of lower urinary infection, but does not show laboratory evidence of bacterial colonization. What is your response?

   a) Mention that 15% of all women have UTIs at least once a year
   b) Accept his criticism and inform patient that she does not have a urinary tract infection
   c) State that 40% all UTIs do not exhibit a significant level of bacteruria
   d) Argue that the predictive value of urinalysis has not been established yet

34. What condition is suggested by the following presentation: headache that follows URIs; associated with pyrexia; anorexia; and neck rigidity?

    a) Subarachnoid hemorrhage
    b) Sinusitis
    c) Meningitis
    d) Intracranial hypertension

35. During an initial intake, your 22 year-old male patient appears to be detached from his surroundings; his behavior and speech are disorganized; and he tells you that your receptionist tried to "double swipe" his credit card and warns you to keep an eye on her. He is also concerned about the "racial practices" pervasive in his university program that resulted in his placement on academic probation for the last year or so. What is your most likely diagnosis?

    a) Paranoid personality disorder
    b) Acute psychotic disorder
    c) Schizophrenia
    d) Panic disorder

36. Which of the following behaviors does a manic episode not exhibit?

    a) Depressed mood
    b) Decreased need for sleep
    c) Talkative with flight of ideas
    d) Impedance of social or occupational functions

37. A 54-year-old man has become forgetful, preoccupied, withdrawn, irritable, and disheveled. His physical examination is unremarkable. This patient has been with his company for 22 years and was considered an excellent employee. Which of the following is the most likely diagnosis?

    a) Senile dementia
    b) Schizophrenia
    c) Alcoholism
    d) Major depression

38. A young mother is very focused on the health of her 8-month-old infant. She keeps her house immaculate for fear that dirt will harm her baby. She checks the locks on the door at least ten times before going to bed, and she has to get up and check that her child is still breathing at least three times a night. She knows that her fears are a bit irrational, but persists with these behaviors. Which of the following is the most likely diagnosis?

    a) Post-partum depression
    b) Obsessive compulsive disorder
    c) Generalized anxiety disorder
    d) Paranoid personality disorder

39. A 52-year-old man comes walking slowly into your office, stooped over, and holding his hand to his back. He complains of acute onset back-pain and bilateral leg pain. He is unable to void and has not had a bowel movement for 1 week. Examination reveals a lax anal sphincter and an absent cremasteric reflex. Which of the following is the most likely diagnosis?

    a) Upper motor neuron lesion
    b) Central disk herniation
    c) Benign prostatic hypertrophy with urinary obstruction
    d) Spondylolisthesis

40. You are called in to assess an acute presentation of leg pain in a 28-year-old male. The patient started getting these debilitating pains after starting an intensive running program in preparation for a marathon. Your physical examination reveals bilateral hypertonicity of lateral leg muscles; decreased posterior tibial and dorsalis pedis pulses; decreased pain, touch, and two-point discrimination over the dorsum of both feet. What is your diagnosis?

    a) Deep venous thrombosis
    b) Atherosclerosis
    c) Fibular nerve palsy
    d) Anterior compartment syndrome

41. What is the most common location for traumatic intervertebral disk herniation?

    a) L2-L3
    b) L3-L4
    c) L4-L5
    d) L5-S1

42. As you were conducting a screening physical examination on an 8-year-old female, you noted vertebral column listing suggestive of scoliosis. This finding seems to disappear when the patient bends forward. What would you do next?

    a) Recommend a vertebral column brace to address the structural scoliosis
    b) Recommend a vertebral column brace to alleviate the functional scoliosis
    c) Perform a complete musculoskeletal examination to find the cause of her scoliosis
    d) Nothing; scoliosis is a self-limiting finding in children of that age

43. A 42 year-old male presents with vertigo that occurs with particular head movements. On examination, you note that he experiences vertigo and nystagmus when his head is laterally bent and rotated toward the left side; there is no sign of conductive or sensorineural hearing loss. This condition started 2 weeks ago and has a steady course. What is the most likely diagnosis?

    a) Meniere's disease
    b) Labyrinthitis
    c) Multiple sclerosis
    d) Benign positional vertigo

44. How would you best evaluate a presentation of a firm non-tender testicular mass?

    a) Transilluminate, and request radioactive iodine uptake scan
    b) Transilluminate, and request PSA levels and local X-ray
    c) Transilluminate, and request ultrasound and biopsy
    d) Reevaluate in 3 weeks as condition will likely subside

45. A 3-year-old is brought to you with what appears to right ear pain. The girl cries incessantly and fusses with her right ear. The crying began last night. The parents report some clear discharge from the ear. Otoscopic examination reveals vesicles and erythema of the right tympanic membrane; the left ear is unaffected. What is the most likely diagnosis?

    a) Purulent otitis media
    b) Serous otitis media
    c) Infectious myringitis
    d) Acute mastoiditis

46. When should you recommend or prescribe IM penicillin for the management of pediatric streptococcal pharyngitis that is refractory to naturopathic treatment?

    a) 3 days
    b) 7 days
    c) 10 days
    d) 14 days

47. An expecting mother is a carrier of the X-linked recessive, glucose-6-phosphate-dehehydrogenase deficiency. Her family history reveals that both male siblings as well as her mother have the enzyme defect. Her husband never exhibited any symptoms suggestive of this condition. What are the odds of that their daughter will develop this condition?

    a) 75%
    b) 50%
    c) 25%
    d) 0%

48. A 53-year-old male patient presents to your office with localized weakness in his legs and feet. The condition has been getting worse over the past month or so and has begun to interfere with his ability to perform daily activities. Your neurological examination reveals: no paresis in the upper extremity in contrast to the lower; bilateral loss of ankle and knee tendon reflex; no sensory deficits in vibration, temperature, pain or two-point discrimination. How would you best confirm your diagnostic impression of this presentation?

a) CSF analysis & Evoked nerve potential testing
b) Tensilon test
c) Indirect Coomb's test & Electromyography
d) Spinal cord computed tomography (CT) scan

49. Plummer-Vinson syndrome is characterized by which of the following presentations?

a) Iron-deficiency anemia
b) Cerebellar ataxia
c) Ascending paralysis
d) Pernicious anemia

50. Senile tremors may resemble Parkinsonism, but senile tremors do not include which of the following presentations?

a) Nodding the head as if responding yes or no
b) Rigidity and weakness of voluntary movement
c) Tremor of the hands
d) Tongue protrusion

Answers

1.	a	11.	b	21.	d	31.	a	41.	d
2.	d	12.	c	22.	a	32.	b	42.	c
3.	d	13.	b	23.	c	33.	c	43.	d
4.	c	14.	a	24.	b	34.	c	44.	c
5.	c	15.	a	25.	a	35.	c	45.	c
6.	c	16.	c	26.	b	36.	a	46.	b
7.	d	17.	a	27.	c	37.	d	47.	d
8.	b	18.	b	28.	c	38.	b	48.	a
9.	d	19.	c	29.	c	39.	b	49.	a
10.	b	20.	b	30.	d	40.	d	50.	b